PROGRESS IN CLINICAL AND BIOLOGICAL RESEARCH

RECENT TITLES

See pages following the index for previous titles in this series.

THE S-POTENTIAL

THE S-POTENTIAL

Editors

Boris D. Drujan
Miguel Laufer

Venezuelan Institute of Scientific Investigations
Center of Biophysics and Biochemistry (IVIC)
Caracas, Venezuela

ALAN R. LISS, INC. • NEW YORK

Address all Inquiries to the Publisher
Alan R. Liss, Inc., 150 Fifth Avenue, New York, NY 10011

Library of Congress Cataloging in Publication Data

Main entry under title:

The S-Potential

  (Progress in clinical and biological research;
v. 113)
  Prepared in honor of Gunnar Svaetichin.
  Includes bibliographical references and index.
  1. Retina. 2. Action potentials (Electrophysiology)
I. Drujan, Boris D. II. Laufer, Miguel.
III. Svaetichin, Gunnar, 1915–1981. IV. Series.
[DNLM: 1. Evoked potentials, Visual. 2. Retina—
Physiology. 3. Retina—Cytology. W1 PR668E v. 113 /
WW 270 S111]

QP479.S17 1982   596'.01823   82–20394
ISBN 0-8451-0113-7

Contents

Contributors ✗

Alexey L. Byzov [105]
Institute for Problems of Information Transmission, Academy of Sciences, Moscow, USSR

David R. Copenhagen [77]
Departments of Physiology and Ophthalmology, University of California, San Francisco, California

Mustafa B.A. Djamgoz [235]
Departments of Zoology and Physics (Biophysics), Imperial College, London, England

Boris D. Drujan [xi,281]
Centro de Biofísica y Bioquímica, Instituto Venezolano de Investigaciones Científicas (IVIC), Caracas, Venezuela

Masaaki Fujimoto [151]
Department of Physiology, St. Marianna University School of Medicine, Kawasaki, Japan

Antonio Gallego [9]
Departamento de Fisiología, Facultad de Medicina, Universidad Complutense, Madrid, Spain

Otto-Joachim Grüsser [207]
Physiologisches Institut der Freien Universität Berlin, Berlin, West Germany

Leo M. Hurvich [307]
Department of Psychology, University of Pennsylvania, Philadelphia, Pennsylvania

Dorothea Jameson [307]
Department of Psychology, University of Pennsylvania, Philadelphia, Pennsylvania

Robert Kretz [51]
Division of Neurobiology and Behavior, College of Physicians and Surgeons, Columbia University, New York, New York

The bold face numbers in brackets following each contributor's name indicate the opening page number of that author's paper.

Toru Kujiraoka [151]
Department of Physiology, St. Marianna University School of Medicine, Kawasaki, Japan

Miguel Laufer [xi,257]
Centro de Biofísica y Bioquímica, Instituto Venezolano de Investigaciones Científicas (IVIC), Caracas, Venezuela

Harold F. Leeper [77]
Department of Physiology, University of California, San Francisco, California

David O. Lightfoot [51]
Jules Stein Eye Institute and Departments of Ophthalmology and Anatomy, School of Medicine, University of California, Los Angeles, California

Edward F. MacNichol, Jr. [1]
Laboratory of Sensory Physiology, The Marine Biological Laboratory, Woods Hole, Massachusetts

Genyo Mitarai [137]
Research Institute of Environmental Medicine, University of Nagoya, Japan

Ken-ichi Naka [193]
National Institute for Basic Biology, Okazaki, Japan

Jacques Neyton [161]
Laboratoire de Neurobiologie de l'Ecole Normale Supérieure, Paris, France

Valentin Parthe [31]
Centro de Biofísica y Bioquímica, Instituto Venezolano de Investigaciones Científicas (IVIC), Caracas, Venezuela

Marco Piccolino [161]
Istituto di Neurofisiologia del Consiglio Nazionale delle Ricerche, Pisa, Italy

Sonia H. Reynolds [235]
Departments of Zoology and Physics (Biophysics), Imperial College, London England

Keith H. Ruddock [235]
Departments of Zoology and Physics (Biophysics), Imperial College, London, England

Masanori Sakuranaga [193]
Department of Physiology, Nippon Medical School, Tokyo, Japan

Josef Skrzypek [181]
Electronics Research Laboratory, University of California, Berkeley, California

William K. Stell [51]
Department of Anatomy, Faculty of Medicine, University of Calgary, Alberta, Canada

Jun-Ichi Toyoda [151]
Department of Physiology, St. Marianna University School of Medicine, Kawasaki, Japan

Yu A. Trifonov [105]
Institute for Problems in Information Transmission, Academy of Sciences, Moscow, USSR

Kosuke Watanabe [123]
Department of Physiology, Tokyo Women's Medical College, Tokyo, Japan

Frank S. Werblin [181]
Electronics Research Laboratory, University of California, Berkeley, California

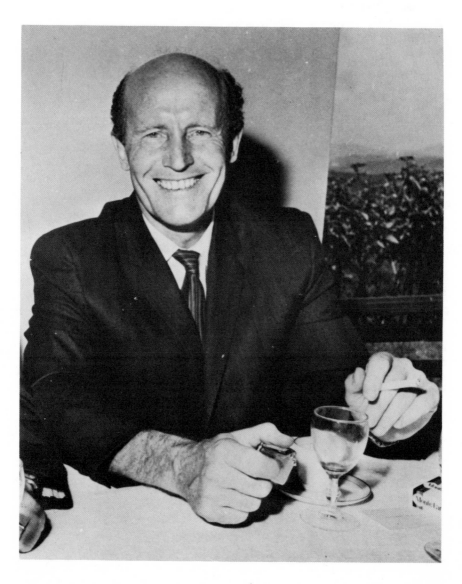

Gunnar Svaetichin
1915–1981

Foreword

This book has been conceived to honor the personality and scientific contributions of our friend and mentor Gunnar Svaetichin (1915–1981). Almost thirty years have elapsed since he first described his recordings of intracellular potentials from the fish retina. In this period, important advances in visual physiology have been made through research stemming directly from his fundamental observations. In recognition of this fact, his friends decided to gather, in a single volume, reviews of the most relevant research carried out recently on the nature and properties of the neural activity he had discovered. This was thought to be the most fitting acknowledgment of our admiration and indebtedness to him.

Practically all the colleagues who were asked to contribute to the volume answered enthusiastically, and so was Gunnar's reaction to the idea. The time elapsed since the inception of the project has resulted in the addition of more and newer data to the contents of the book, but a tragic event veiled the atmosphere. On the morning of March 24, 1981, Gunnar was found lifeless in his laboratory. Nobody was able to admit his departure, unexpected, unsuspected, unaccepted.

Gunnar Svaetichin committed himself to neurophysiology from the very days he started his scientific endeavors in his native Finland until his death. His career was extraordinarily fertile and he was able to integrate many unconventional findings into new concepts. Investigators in the field agree that his contributions to the understanding of retinal function deserve special acknowledgment. The publication was to continue despite his demise, to honor his lifelong dedication to the unraveling of the mysteries of the retina with courage, with new ideas, with a permanent will to defeat the secrecy of nature.

The S-potential, the term coined in honor of Svaetichin to identify the characteristic electrical response of the horizontal cells to illumination of the retina, is used as the title of the book. The contributors review, through their own experimental findings, the structure of horizontal cells in different vertebrate retinas, their connectivity and functional properties, as well as biochemical and pharmacological aspects in species spanning from fish to mammals. After Gunnar's death it was decided, as we believe would have been his wish, not to change anything in the original planning of the book. But one thing had to be changed to our deepest regret. This book, which was to be dedicated to a friend, is now dedicated to his memory. To the memory of a man whose smile and whose delicate and jovial personality will always live in the minds of those who knew him.

Boris D. Drujan
Miguel Laufer

The S-Potential, pages 1–8
© 1982 Alan R. Liss, Inc., 150 Fifth Avenue, New York, NY 10011

The Discovery of the S-Potential and Its Influence in the Development of Retinal Physiology: Something Was Fishy in Los Altos de Pipe

Edward F. MacNichol, Jr.

The discovery by Svaetichin in 1953 [1] of what he then considered to be the "Cone Action potentials" in the retinas of fishes marked the beginning of what has proved to be an extraordinarily productive era in understanding the neurophysiology of the retina. The technique which he pioneered is the use of intracellular micropipette electrodes in studying the responses of individual retinal cells. The remarkable result which he obtained is the discovery of cells which are maintained in a state of depolarization in the dark and which hyperpolarize during illumination, revolutionizing our concepts of how the retina operates. Indeed, due to the work of many gifted investigators that have followed up the exciting leads and provocative (even if sometimes incorrect) conclusions of Svaetichin and his co-workers, the outlines of the mechanisms of transmission of information from the receptors to the optic nerve fibers have been largely worked out, and the responses of each cell type in the retina unequivocally identified [2–10].

This is not to say that our knowledge of the mechanisms underlying retinal function is now essentially complete, far from it. The basic mechanisms of receptor excitation, synaptic transmitter release, positive identification of transmitter substances at specific synapses and their mechanism of action, and many details of the image processing functions of the retina remain to be worked out. Finally, we lack a detailed quantitative correspondence between visual theories and electrophysiological and psychophysical data. However, many of the pieces of the jigsaw puzzle that is the retina, are now understood, so that the task of fitting them into place in order to obtain a clear and complete picture of retinal structure and function no longer appears to be insuperable.

After Svaetichin's 1953 paper and a more complete series [11] describing the slow, graded intracellular potentials of the retina appeared, they were greeted with disbelief in many quarters. The brilliant work of Eccles and his colleagues in elaborating the function of motoneurons understandably had given the impression that these are the prototypes for all nerve cells. Starting from a nearly constant resting potential of about -70 mV, the graded subthreshold excitatory and inhibitory postsynaptic potentials (EPSPs and IPSPs) were clearly established. When the EPSPs depolarized the cell sufficiently, one or more regenerative action potentials would be evoked and sweep down the axon, releasing a chemical transmitter at the distant terminals. The data were consistent with those obtained from the studies of electrically and chemically stimulated axons, which had been in progress for many years, and with data on the few sensory neurons that had been studied with intracellular microelectrodes, such as the eccentric cells of the lateral eyes of Limulus [12]. Thus, the finding that what appeared to be intracellular compartments had variable resting potentials of about -20 to -40 mV and gave sustained, graded hyperpolarization which could reach -70 mV or more when the eye was illuminated, and no impulse discharge under any conditions, appeared to many to be, as one well-known neuroscientist put it in 1959, "elaborate artifacts." Poor technique involving photosensitivity of the chlorided silver electrodes, amplifier grid-current, and various other causes for the unexpected behavior were invoked by a variety of distinguished scientists. Furthermore, when Svaetichin reported in 1956 [11] that some of the cells he had studied gave hyperpolarizing responses in one region of the spectrum and depolarizing responses in another, and that at least one type of fish had cells with different wavelengths of peak hyperpolarization and depolarization (R-G and B-Y) cells, responses reminiscent of Hering's opponent color theory, the limits of credulity of many visual scientists were far surpassed. Accordingly, when Svaetichin and Fernández-Morán invited me to spend the first 6 months of 1957 in Caracas, I lept at the opportunity to observe this mystery directly. This experience turned out to be at the same time one of the most rewarding, fascinating, and frustrating periods of my life. It was a turning point in my career because I had the opportunity to learn how to study the isolated vertebrate retina, and to discover the particular advantages of fishes in retinal physiology (I had previously concentrated on invertebrate vision). It was also rewarding because we were able to extend the studies already underway and to obtain at least a rough idea of the structures from which we had been recording. It was frustrating because of the turbulent situation in the laboratory at that time, from an initial failure to get results, and because of prolonged separations from my wife and children.

Svaetichin, with the help of Jonasson, MacPherson, and Krattenmacher, had assembled a superb set-up for stimulation recording and micromanipulation, permitting precise control of position, wavelength, intensity, and duration of the stimulus, precise and stable positioning of micropipette electrodes, and stable amplification and recording of both electrophysiological data and stimulus-parameters. There was obviously nothing wrong with the equipment or the way it was being used, yet initially no responses whatever were obtained despite every precaution. After careful review of old protocols and manuscripts, Svae-tichin found that, whereas he had previously used pure oxygen bubbled through warmed water to keep the retina moist, he was now using compressed air. A change to oxygen and both the luminosity (L) and chromatic (C) potentials appeared as if by magic exactly as previously described.[1] Grid current appeared to be negligible. In fact it was not found possible to affect either the resting potential or the change upon illumination with any amount of current that could be passed through a micropipette without breaking the tip. Strong illumination of the Ag–AgCl pipette and reference electrodes produced no photoelectric effect. Clearly, the potentials were not artifacts.

Having established that everything was in working order we concentrated on two main topics during the rest of my visit: (1) The effects of background illumination upon the responses, and (2) the histological localization of the sites from which recordings were made [16,17].

We used background intensities sufficient to push the resting potentials toward saturation and, thereby, to reduce the responses to test flashes but not sufficiently to cause appreciable bleaching of photopigments. This appears to be the cause for the discrepancies between our results and those of Naka and Rushton [18], who evidently used much stronger background illumination. We found that in the case of chromatic (C-type) responses, red background light would suppress the depolarizing responses to longwave flashes and enhance the hyperpolarizing responses to shortwave flashes. Blue background light did just the reverse. However, in the case of the luminosity (L-type), responses to background light of any wavelength sufficient to produce a given amount of hyperpolarization would cause a proportional decrease in responses to flashes of all wavelengths. After the background light was turned off, the responses soon returned to their original amplitudes in all cases, indicating negligible pigment bleaching or long-term adaptation. Thus, it appeared to us that neural adaptation of the C-responses by background illumination as well as excitation was opponent in nature, whereas the receptors feeding the L-cells had synergistic effects both in respect to excitation and adaptation.

The problem of electrode localization was a very important and a very difficult one. From the difference between the depth of the electrode tip when contact was made with the retina and the depth at which recordings were made, as measured with a machinist's dial indicator mounted on the micromanipulator, it could be concluded that recordings were made from the inner segments of the cones, which are large in the species that were used. The fact that most of the

---

[1]We now know that the retinas of some teleost fishes have an unusually high requirement for oxygen [13]. Diffusion through even a thin film of solution on the surface of the retina may not be adequate. Furthermore, these fishes concentrate oxygen within the eye at a partial pressure several times that of the arterial blood by counter current flow in structures called pseudobranches and in the choroid plexus [14,15].

cones were either doubles or unequal twins, both having closely apposed inner segments, made very plausible the hypothesis that the recordings were made directly from the cones themselves; and that the L-responses came from single cones or one member of a pair having the same photopigment or mixed pigments, whereas the C-responses came from one member of a pair containing different pigments. On the other hand, the retinas were receptor-side-up in air with only a thin film of moisture covering them. When a micropipette touched a retina, wetting forces would pull the moisture film and the retina along with it up the taper of the electrode, thus making the point penetrate deeper than the dial indicator showed. This effect readily could be observed with a high-power dissecting microscope. For this and other reasons Tomita, who was attending a symposium at the Institute, expressed strong reservations about the depth measurements. Thus, we set out to try to make accurate measurements by electrophoresing dye or metallic pigment from the electrode tip and finding it in histological sections. The requirements were that the dye or pigment must not interfere with the electrical recordings, that it must not block the tip, that it have an electric charge, and that it must remain in a single cell throughout processing. Up to this point no dye having all these properties had been described. We tried everything that was at hand or available in Caracas, including some fluorescent dyes. We finally had some success filling the pipettes with crystal violet, fixing in ammonium molybdate, infiltrating with gelatin and glycerol, and cutting frozen sections with a pathologist's microtome. This avoided the use of alcohols which promptly dissolved out the dye. We obtained sufficiently good sections to show that all the recordings we marked came from the horizontal cell layer, the C-responses being proximal to the L-type. This sequence was also found as the electrode was advanced, as confirmed by others [19–21] and reviewed by Kaneko [10].

We now know that the responses of the cones, horizontal cells, and bipolar cells are very much alike, but at that time the criteria for distinguishing them by their response characteristics had not yet been worked out (this awaited the application of a really satisfactory dye-marking technique). Thus the "S-potentials," as they later were named by Japanese workers, first described by Svaetichin could have come from any or all of these three cell types. However, the comparatively low resistance of the micropipettes then used (20 to 50 Mohms filled with 2–3 M KCl), the high frequency of successful penetrations, and the results of our admittedly crude dye-marking experiments, would argue that the great majority of the units studied were the large and numerous horizontal cells. Thus, the current almost universal use of the term "S-potential" to mean specifically the horizontal cell response is probably amply justified.

Further clarification of the responses of the retinal cells had to await the development of better dyes than the ones we had available. The discovery of first Niagara Sky Blue and then the fluorescent Procion dyes in the Harvard

Neurobiology Laboratory, the very strongly fluorescent Lucifer Yellow at NIH and the use of $CoCl_2$ and horseradish peroxidase have since made precise identification of recorded cells possible. Receptor cells were unequivocally identified by Tomita et al [22], and later all cell types were identified by Kaneko [23] in the goldfish and by Werblin and Dowling [24] in the mudpuppy.

Meanwhile Svaetichin and his co-workers turned to other pursuits. One of these was an attempt to elucidate the role of the horizontal cells of fishes. Because these cells lack Nissl substance and some other light and electronmicroscopic characteristics of ordinary neurons, and because of their resemblance to astroglia in the brain, and above all because of their peculiar electrical responses, this group adopted the hypothesis that they are specialized glial elements which act as controller cells which set the sensitivity of the neuronal elements in accordance with prevailing light conditions [25]. In following this hypothesis, they did many pioneering and ingenious experiments on retinal metabolism, O_2 consumption, intraretinal pH and pO_2 changes, enzyme systems, and inhibitors [26–28]. These were invariably brilliant in conception and execution and often far ahead of their time,[2] though the interpretations are often difficult to follow.

Soon after Marks published his thesis [29] on the three types of photopigments in goldfish cones and indicated some morphological differences between cones bearing different pigments, Svaetichin et al [30] converted the photostimulator into a microspectrophotometer and studied the cones of a considerable number of species, showing the morphology of each type and its arrangement in the retinal mosaic.

The earliest and least commonly appreciated pioneering achievement of Svaetichin, probably because he made so little use of it himself, was the metal microelectrode for recording extracellular action potentials from single neurons. The use of such electrodes has been extremely valuable in studying all parts of the central nervous system. In the visual system the retinal ganglion cells, the lateral geniculate, the visual cortex, and the colliculus have been extensively studied using this technique. Although the materials and methods of electrode fabrication are many and varied, Svaetichin is probably the first to have demonstrated the principle. He evidently started working on such electrodes in 1937, but they were not described until 1939 in a paper by Granit and Svaetichin [31].

---

[2]Particularly remarkable was the excellent action spectrum obtained of retinal pO_2 as a function of wavelength of illumination in the presence of CO. This spectrum appears indistinguishable from that of a member of the cytochrome system. It indicates that absorption of light by this enzyme system reverses the depression of oxygen uptake in the presence of CO as Warburg had found in yeast suspensions. The fact that cytochrome pigments can absorb light and produce metabolic effects in the retina may be of considerable current interest because of present concern in regard to the effects of strong light on the eye. It may be no coincidence that the lowest threshold for light damage is at or near the peak absorption of the pigments of the cytochrome system at about 425 nm.

A fuller description of an improved electrode design was not written until 1951 [32].

Wilska [33] also developed a metal microelectrode and also used it to record from single retinal ganglion cells. Though each claims priority, the electrodes were constructed by such entirely different methods that I strongly suspect that the inventions were made quite independently. In any case, Svaetichin developed an effective microelectrode and he and Granit put it to good use in investigating retinal ganglion cell activity. This was certainly a great advance in the methodology of the study of the nervous system by the responses of single cells. Although even earlier, Hartline [34] had developed the technique of studying single retinal ganglion cells by dissecting single optic nerve fibers in their course across the retina to the optic nerve head, this method is very difficult and lacks the universal applicability of the microelectrode in the study of single cells in the brain.

Although most of Svaetichin's work has been on the retina, he also made recordings from single dorsal root ganglion cells of the frog and analyzed the spread of potential from the nerve fibers [35]. As with his work on the eye, this investigation is marked by a high degree of imagination and technical competence.

In summary, this brief account can only mention some of the highlights of a long and productive career. It obviously can not do justice to Svaetichin's many accomplishments. However, he and his colleagues have accumulated an impressive list of publications which clearly show the original thought, scientific leadership, and technical expertise which began a revolution in the study of the physiology of the retina. The phenomena he first described, the conclusion he reached,[3] and the controversies that ensued have stimulated others to make extraordinary advances in understanding how the vertebrate retina works. It now appears that the epoch of data gathering which he began is drawing to a close, and that the period of synthesis in which the experimental facts are fitted into a solid theoretical framework which will yield a quantitative and satisfying explanation of visual behavior, may have begun.

---

[3]Some of Svaetichin's conclusions, such as his initial assumption that he was recording from cones and later that the horizontal cells are glial elements instead of highly specialized neurons, now appear to be incorrect. However, they were based upon reasonable assumptions and evidence that appeared highly plausible at the time. His formulation and tenacious adherence to an unfashionable hypothesis until the experimental evidence for or against it became overwhelming, has led to many stimulating discussions, and has spurred others into significant experimental programs; for example, the brilliant work of Kuffler and Nicholls on glial cells, and the investigations of Naka and Rushton, Werblin and Dowling, Stell, Witkovsky and many others, on the horizontal cells. The situation was in many ways similar to the tenacious adherence by Eccles to the electrical theory of transmission at synapses which stimulated others to show conclusively that most synaptic transmission is chemically mediated.

REFERENCES

1. Svaetichin G: The cone action potential. Acta Physiol Scand 29 Suppl 106:565, 1953.
2. Fuortes MGF: "Handbook of Sensory Physiology VII 2 Physiology of Photoreceptor Organs." Berlin, Heidelberg, New York: Springer, 1972.
3. Rodieck RW: "The Vertebrate Retina. Principles of Structure and Function." San Francisco: Freeman, 1973.
4. Daw NW: Neurophysiology of color vision. Physiol Rev 53:571, 1973.
5. Werblin FS: Organization of the vertebrate retina. In Davson and Graham (eds): "The Eye, Vol. 6, Comparative Physiology." New York, London: Academic Press, 1974.
6. Zettler F, Weiler R (eds): "Neuronal Principles in Vision." Berlin, Heidelberg, New York: Springer–Verlag, 1977.
7. Cold Spring Harbor Symposia on Quantitative Biology. Vol. 15, 1975.
8. Barlow HB, Fatt P (eds): "Vertebrate Photoreception." New York, London: Academic Press, 1977.
9. Marks LE, MacNichol EF Jr (eds): "Sensory Processes 2, No. 4." 1978.
10. Kaneko A: Physiology of the retina. Ann Rev Neurosci 2:169, 1979.
11. Svaetichin G et al: Acta Physiol Scand 39, Suppl 134:1–112, 1956.
12. Hartline HK, Wagner HG, MacNichol EF Jr: The peripheral origin of nervous activity in the visual system. Cold Spring Harbor Symposium 17:125, 1952.
13. Negishi K, Svaetichin G: Effects of anoxia, CO_2 and NH_3 on S-potential producing cells and on neurons. Pflügers Arch ges Physiol 292:218, 1966.
14. Whittemberg JB, Whittemberg BA: Active secretion of oxygen into the eye of fish. Nature (London) 194:106, 1962.
15. Copeland DE: Functional vascularization of the teleost eye. In "Current Topics in Eye Research," Vol. III, New York: Academic Press, 1980.
16. MacNichol EF Jr, Svaetichin G: Electrical responses from the isolated retinas of fishes. Amer J Ophthalmology Ser 3, 46 Part II:26, September 1958.
17. Svaetichin G, MacNichol EF Jr: Retinal mechanisms for chromatic and achromatic vision. Ann NY Acad Sci 74, 2:385, 1958.
18. Naka KI, Rushton WAH: The generation and spread of S-potentials in fish (Cyprinidae). J Physiol London 192:437, 1967.
19. Laufer M, Millán E: Spectral analysis of L-type S-potentials and their relation to photopigment absorption in a fish (Eugerres plumieri) retina. Vision Res 10:237, 1970.
20. Mitarai G, Asano T, Miyake Y: Identification of five types of S-potential and their corresponding generating sites in the horizontal cells of the carp retina. Japan J Ophthalm 18:161, 1974.
21. Hashimoto Y, Kato A, Inokuchi M, Watanabe K: Re-examination of the horizontal cells of the carp retina with Procion Yellow electrode. Vision Res 16:25, 1976.
22. Tomita T, Kaneko A, Murakami M, Pautler EL: Spectral response curves of single cones in the carp. Vision Res 7:519, 1967.
23. Kaneko A: Physiological and morphological identification of horizontal, bipolar, and amacrine cells in the goldfish retina. J Physiol London 207:623, 1970.
24. Werblin FS, Dowling JE: Organization of the retina of the mudpuppy, Necturus maculosus. II. Intracellular recording. J Neurophysiol 32:339, 1969.
25. Svaetichin G, Laufer M, Mitarai G, Fatehchand R, Vallecalle E, Villegas J: Glial control of neuronal networks and receptors. In Jung R, Kornhuber H (eds): "The Visual System: Neurophysiology and Psychophysics" Berlin, Gottingen, Heidelberg: Springer–Verlag, 1961.
26. Fatehchand R, Svaetichin G, Negishi K, Drujan B: Effects of anoxia and metabolic inhibitors on the S-potential of isolated fish retinas. Vision Res 6:271, 1966.
27. Negishi K, Svaetichin G, Laufer M, Drujan B: Polarographic and electrophysiological studies

of retinal respiration. Vision Res 15:527, 1975.

28. Drujan BD, Svaetichin G, Negishi K: Retinal aerobic metabolism as reflected in S-potential behavior. Vision Res 11 Suppl 3:151, 1971.

29. Marks WB: "Difference spectra of visual pigments in goldfish cones." Baltimore: PhD. Dissertation, Dept. of Biophysics, John Hopkins University, 1963.

30. Svaetichin G, Negishi K, Fatehchand R: In Wolstenholme GEW, Knight JE (eds): "Ciba Foundation Symposium on Physiology and Experimental Psychology of Colour Vision." London: Churchill, 178 p, 1965.

31. Granit R, Svaetichin G: Principles and techniques of electrophysiological analysis of colour reception with the aid of microelectrodes. Uppsala Lakaref Forhandl 45:161, 1939.

32. Svaetichin, G: Low resistance micro-electrodes. Acta Physiol Scand 24 Suppl 86:5, 1951.

33. Wilska A: Action potential discharges of single retinal elements in the frog. Acta Soc Med (Finland) Duodecim 22 (AI):63, 1940.

34. Hartline HK: The response of single optic nerve fibers of the vertebrate eye to illumination of the retina. Amer J Physiol 121:400, 1938.

35. Svaetichin G: Analysis of action potentials from single spinal ganglion cells. Acta Physiol Scand 24 Suppl 86:23, 1951.

The S-Potential, pages 9–29
© 1982 Alan R. Liss, Inc., 150 Fifth Avenue, New York, NY 10011

Horizontal Cells of the Tetrapoda Retina

Antonio Gallego

In a comparative study of the tetrapoda retina, two basic types of horizontal cells have been described [1]: (a) The short axon horizontal cell described by Cajal [2], who classified it as "external" and "internal" in mammals and amphibians and as "brush" and "stellate" in birds and reptiles, and (b) the axonless horizontal cell found by Gallego [3, 4]. These two cell types are clearly different in their morphological features and functional connections.

The short axon horizontal cell has been found in all tetrapoda retinas. Described first by Cajal in low mammals, reptiles, birds, and amphibians, it was also studied in primates by Polyak [5]. This cell type shows morphological differences according to the class and orders of tetrapoda and even in the same retina according to its location, central or peripheral. The differences refer to the number of dendrites and retinal area covered by them, the axon length, and the structure of the axon terminal. In all the retinas studied, its dendrites form the lateral component of the cone triads and its axon terminals penetrate into the synaptic complex of rods as has been shown in mammals [6–9] and birds [10].

The axonless horizontal cell, described first by Gallego [3] in nonprimate mammals' retinas, was found afterward in the retinas of birds [11–13] and reptiles [14]. The axonless horizontal cells build plexuses which extend all over the retina, forming a well-defined single layer. These cells establish wide membrane-to-membrane contacts between themselves, suggesting electrical coupling. Their thin terminal fibers form the lateral components of cone triads, as shown up to now in mammals [8, 9] and birds [10].

According to their connections, these two types of horizontal cells seem to have different functional meanings: The short axon horizontal cell relates the cone–cone bipolar synapse with the rod–rod bipolar synapse, whereas the axonless horizontal cells are connected to only a single type of photoreceptor, the cones in tetrapoda.

In fishes the two types of horizontal cells have been also described. The short axon horizontal cell has been studied by Stell [15, 16] in the fish retina. It shows two main differences with the same cell type of the tetrapoda retina: Its axon ends by a large, elongated structure located at the vitreal side of the inner granular layer with no apparent contact with photoreceptors, and the somas establish wide membrane-to-membrane contacts between themselves as the axonless horizontal cell in tetrapoda. Two or three layers of this cell type have been described in several teleost retinas [17, 18]. In all cases the dendrites penetrate into the cone synaptic complex and the connections of the axon terminals are not known. The axonless horizontal cells form one layer in teleosts [19], and two or three layers in the selachian retina [20, 21]. Wide membrane-to-membrane contacts are established between themselves. Its cell processes penetrate into the synaptic complex of rods [20, 21].

These two basic types of horizontal cells, with few exceptions, are present in all vertebrate retinas. Nevertheless, some differences appear between classes and orders of tetrapoda which refer to the number of cells of each type and to their morphology.

MAMMALS

Retinas of the orders of primates, lagomorpha, rodentia, carnivora, artiodactyla, and perissodactyla have been studied.

Primates

Primates appear to be an exception among tetrapoda because the axonless horizontal cell has not been found in their retinas. Instead, two types of short axon horizontal cells have been described: type I, described by Polyak [5], and type II, recently found in the monkey retina [10, 11, 22].

Type I short axon horizontal cell. This cell type (Fig. 1) has been widely studied since its first description by Polyak in the monkey retina. Its morphology changes progressively from the proximity of the fovea to the periphery of the retina. Near the fovea (Fig. 1A,B,C) there is a small cell, with a cell body diameter of 8 to 10 μm, which gives out five to eight dendrites directed toward the synaptic bodies of the photoreceptors. The dendrites branch out into thinner processes which end in round clusters of endings with small enlargements at their tips. Each cluster has a diameter of 6–8 μm, which is the same size, or slightly smaller, than that of the basis of the cone synaptic body [23–25]. Golgi electron microscopic (EM) studies have shown that each ending of a cluster forms the lateral component of a triad [6, 24]. The area covered by the dendrites of this cell type, near the fovea, is round and its diameter is 25–30 μm. The cell body gives out a thick axon (1–2 μm in diameter) which runs straight, without branching for a length of 1500 to 2000 μm (Fig. 1A). The axon widens into a thicker process which branches out several times. Thin processes arise from the branches of the axon terminal directed toward the synaptic bodies of the photoreceptors. These terminals (Fig. 1D) end in knobs which form the lateral elements of the rod synaptic complex [6, 7]. The type I horizontal cell, close to the fovea, connects six to nine cones through its dendrites and with 350–500 rods, 1500–2000 μm away, through its axon terminal.

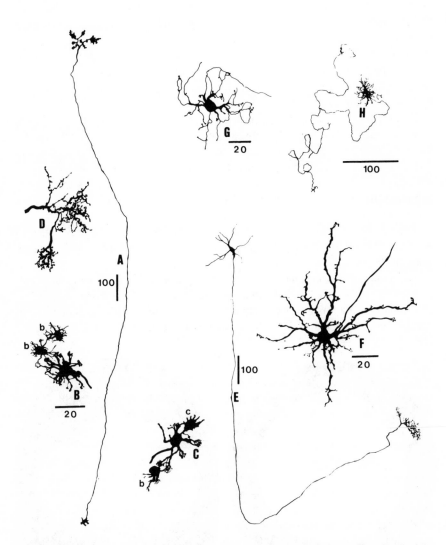

Fig. 1. Short axon horizontal cells of the primates retina, Golgi method. (A) Type I cell of the parafoveal area; (B, C) details of a type I cell dendrites of the parafoveal area (b, bipolar dendrites; c, cone synaptic body); (D) type I axon terminal; (E) type I cell of the peripheral retina; (F) detail of a peripheral type I cell dendrites; (G) detail of a type II cell dendrites; (H) type II cell of the parafoveal area. (The drawing of Figs. 1 and 3–6 have been made using microphotographs of the cells.)

The morphology of type I cells changes progressively with their distance from the fovea. This change refers mainly to the size and distribution of their dendrites and the area covered by them; the axon length and axon terminals are similar to those of the cells close to the fovea.

In the parafoveal retina, practically all the cones located in the area covered by the type I cell dendrites make contact with them. The areas covered by two neighboring type I cells do not overlap, although an occasional cluster terminal formed by dendrites from two cells can be seen.

Dendrites of cells located 5–6 mm away from the fovea and, especially the more peripheral ones (Fig. 1E), cover more irregular areas. These cells usually have one dendrite considerably longer than the others. The number of clusters formed by each cell, which determines the number of cones connected, increases with distance from the fovea (Fig. 1F). The peripheral cell shows great overlapping of the areas covered by their dendrites, but each individual cell does not contact all the cones in that area.

The number of horizontal cells in the parafoveal zone has been calculated to be of the order of 1400/mm². This number decreases progressively with distance from the fovea.

The axons of neighboring cells are randomly oriented in all directions, as can be seen in well-stained, whole, flat-mounted retinas. Considering an average axon length of 2000 μm, it means that the cones in one circular area of 500 μm diameter are connected to the rods, located in a circular band, as seen in Figure 2.

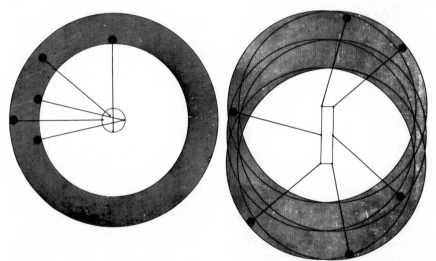

Fig. 2. The shadowed area above shows monkey retina distribution of the axon endings of type I short axon horizontal cells, enclosed in circular (500 μm in diameter) and rectangular (200 × 1000-μm) areas of the retina, for axon lengths of 2000 and 1700 μm, respectively.

A clear distinction between the short axon horizontal cell and the axonless horizontal cell is that the former does not show membrane contacts among themselves, neither at their soma nor at their axon terminals.

Type II short axon horizontal cell. This cell type has been recently described [10, 11, 22]. Its structural features and functional connections are different from those of cell type I. Its cell body, 8–10 μm in diameter, gives out several very fine dendrites in a disorderly array, which gives the cell a typical appearance (Fig. 1G). Its dendrite endings do not show terminal clusters, but only one or two small enlargements. A very thin short axon arises from the cell body and, instead of the straight course followed by the axon of type I cell, it meanders around giving some branches. The axon and its branches end by small clusters (Fig. 1H) of endings, which, in Golgi-EM studies [22], have been seen to end up as lateral or central components of the cone triads. Of the few cells studied, the dendrites of one cell located at 1 mm from the fovea made contact with 10 cones, whereas those of another cell at 4 mm from the fovea made contact with 22 cones.

The axon terminals also form the lateral components of the cone triads. Cell type II connections are similar to those of axonless horizontal cells of the non-primate mammalian retina.

The area covered by type II cell dendrites varies with their distance from the fovea, but not as much as for the type I cell dendrites.

Nonprimates

Two basic horizontal cell types found in the vertebrate retina have been described in several species of nonprimate mammals: the short axon horizontal cell [2], and the axonless horizontal cell [3].

Short axon horizontal cell. This cell type (Fig. 3) was first described by Cajal [2] in the retinas of cat, dog, rabbit, pig, sheep, and ox, having been also named in the past as "small" [25] and as horizontal "B" cell [9].

In the cat retina, where this cell type has been widely studied, it does not show the morphological differences relative to its location as described in the retina of the primate. Due to the dispersion of their dendrites, only slight differences can be seen between the central area horizontal cells and the more peripheral ones. The cat retina does not have short axon horizontal cells with the morphology of the primate retina parafoveal horizontal cells, but rather resembles the intermediate or peripheral primate cell.

In cat the horizontal cell body is about 10 μm in diameter and gives out 8–12 dendrites which branch out dichotomically two or three times. These branches show thin terminal fibers which end in small clusters of knobs. The number of knobs in each cluster is lower than in the primate retina, because of the smaller number of triads in the cone synaptic bodies of the cat than in the primate retina.

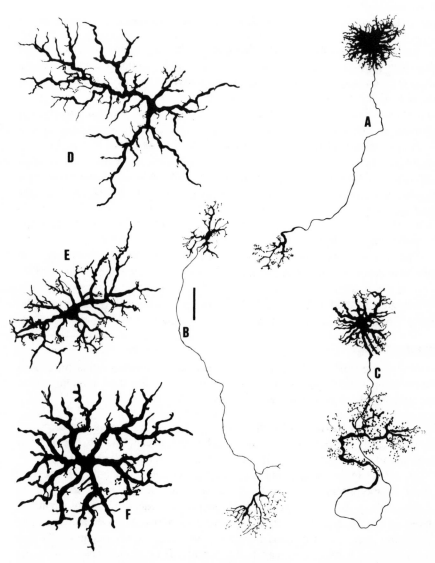

Fig. 3.   Horizontal cells of the low mammal retina, Golgi method. (A) short axon horizontal cell of a 1-month-old cat; (B) short axon horizontal cell of the adult cat; (C) short axon horizontal cell of a newborn dog; (D) axonless horizontal cell of the rabbit; (E) axonless horizontal cell of a newborn dog; (F) axonless horizontal cell of the cat. (The bar length is 50 μm.)

The cell dendrites cover a circular area of 100–150 μm in diameter and in each cell 35–45 clusters can be seen, which means that it connects to the same number of cone pedicles. Dendrite endings form the lateral component of the cone triads, as has been observed in Golgi electron microscopy [8, 9].

When one horizontal cell is completely stained (Fig. 3A,B,C) the main differences with the same cell type of primate retina can be seen in whole flat mounted preparations. These are: (a) the lesser length of the axon which usually is not longer than 400 μm; (b) the larger size of the axon terminal arborization which covers retinal areas of the order of 150 × 250 μm; and (c) the number of knobs per terminal area of the same size is larger than in the primate retina.

Golgi-EM studies of the axon terminal have shown [8, 9] that the endings penetrate into the rod synaptic complex. The number of rods, connected through one axon terminal, has been estimated to be of the order of 3000 to 4000. This number of rods is connected by one horizontal cell to 35–45 cones located 400 μm away [1].

Axonless horizontal cell.   This cell type (Fig. 3) was first described by Gallego [3, 4] with the name of "amacrine cell of the outer plexiform layer" in low mammal retinas. It was subsequently studied by electron microscopy [9, 27, 28], in Golgi-stained retina sections [26, 28], and in Golgi-stained, whole flat mounted retinas [25, 26]. This cell type was also named "large" [25] or horizontal "A" cell [9].

The technique of whole retina silver impregnation [29] shows these cells forming a single layer which extends all over the retina, including the area centralis, in cat and rabbit. The neurofibrillar staining methods, especially Balbuena and Cajal's reduced silver methods, stain this cell type very easily. On the contrary, the rapid Golgi technique used by Cajal infrequently stains it, which may explain why it was not noticed by Cajal in his study of the vertebrate retina. The number of cells varies with the retinal area [30]: In the cat it was found to be 100–140 cells/mm^2 in peripheral retina; 250–300 cells/mm^2 in yuxtapapilar zone, and 500/mm^2 in area centralis.

By using whole, flat mounted retinas stained by the Golgi method, these cells can be seen isolated. The cell body has a diameter of about 10–14 μm, and gives out four to six cell processes spreading horizontally and branching dichotomically. At their origin these processes are as thick as the cell body, making it difficult to delineate the cell body's morphological limits. These processes give out thin fibers directed toward the photoreceptor synaptic bodies. These fibers end in a very small knob cluster or in a single knob. The number of knobs in each cluster is not higher than four. The retinal area covered by the cell processes varies with their location. At the periphery, the area covered by a single cell is practically circular, 150 to 200 μm in diameter, the diameter being only 50 μm in the area centralis. Great overlapping of neighboring cell areas is always observed. This cell type size varies for different mammalian species (Fig. 3D,E,F).

This cell type contacts the cone synaptic bodies, its terminal knobs forming the lateral component of the cone triad [8]. Wide membrane-to-membrane contacts between neighboring cells can be observed, suggesting electrical coupling among them.

BIRDS

Three different types of horizontal cells have been found in the avian retina: A single type of short axon horizontal cell which corresponds to the "brush" cell described by Cajal [2], and two types of axonless horizontal cell recently described [10–13].

Short axon horizontal cell. Cajal achieved a complete staining of this cell type ([2] plate IV, Fig. 5) which he named "brush" horizontal cell. In whole flat mounts of Golgi-impregnated retinas (Fig. 4A,B,C), this cell type shows a small body (10 µm diameter), an axon from 200 to 800 µm long, depending on the avian species, and the axon terminal. The cell body gives out five to eight dendrites that run toward the synaptic bodies of the photoreceptors. These dendrites branch out a couple of times and end by small knobs clusters, similar to those found in the horizontal cell of the mammalian retina. Each cluster is formed by four to six knobs covering an area slightly smaller than the one covered by a cone's synaptic body (6 µm in diameter). The total area covered by one horizontal cell dendrite has a diameter of 30 µm. The axon, 1–2 µm thick, is 100 µm long in the newborn chick, 300–400 µm in the hen, 600–800 µm in the falconidae, and 700–900 µm in the owlet retina. In all the avian retinas, the axon ends in a wide enlargement which gives out thin terminal fibers [31]. These axon terminals, when stained independently of their axon, look like individual cells, a fact that mislead Cajal to consider them as an independent cell type: his "stellate" horizontal cell. The axon terminal ramifies into thinner branches which spread out giving rise to delicate endings that run toward the photoreceptors synaptic bodies ending in isolated knobs without forming clusters. These knobs are larger than the ones found in the dendrite clusters.

Cross-sections of the retina show the short axon cell bodies located in the outer row of nuclei of the inner granular layer. The dendrites, directed toward the photoreceptors synaptic bodies, end mainly at the outer row of synaptic bodies in the plexiform layer, but, very often, dendrites directed toward the straight and oblique cones can be seen [1].

The axon endings are located above the cell body as well as below the first row of synaptic bodies, intermingled with the synaptic bodies of the straight and oblique cones. Their thin terminal fibers end by thick knobs at the level of the external row of synaptic bodies.

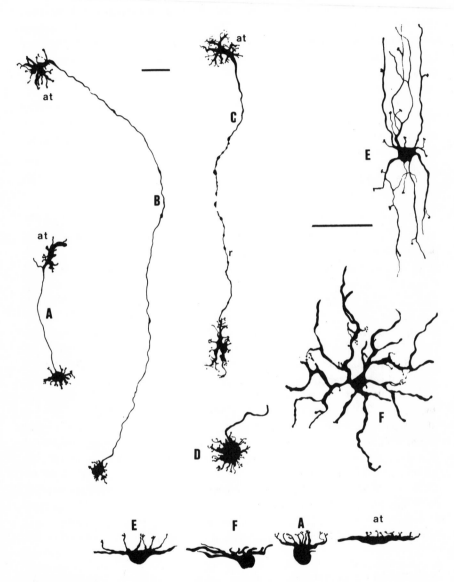

Fig. 4. Horizontal cells of the bird retina as seen in whole flat mounted preparations and in perpendicular sections, Golgi method. (A) short axon horizontal cell of the chicken; (B) short axon horizontal cell of the owlet; (C) short axon horizontal cell of the eagle; (at) axon terminal; (D) detail of the short axon horizontal cell dendrites; (E) axonless horizontal cell type I; (F) axonless horizontal cell type II. (The small bar length, for A, B and C, is 50 μm; the large bar length, for E and F, is 50 μm).

The cell body and terminals of the short axon horizontal cell have been identified by electron microscopy and studied [31, 32] both in cross and horizontal sections. The observations on the axon terminals are of great interest; they form a plexus with numerous membrane-to-membrane contacts among them. These contacts are of the gap-junction type, but they constantly show vesicles at either sides of the membranes.

Golgi EM studies have shown that the short axon horizontal cell dendrites establish contacts with the double cones of the outer row, the straight cones of the middle row, and the oblique cones. The axon terminals penetrate the rod synaptic complex [10, 32].

Axonless horizontal cells. Two types of axonless horizontal cells have been described in the avian retina [10–13].

Axonless horizontal cell type I. This cell type (Fig. 4E) is very characteristic of the avian retina [10, 11]. It has a round body, 7–9 μm in diameter, which gives out in a horizontal plane, five to seven processes, from opposite poles, giving the cell a "bitufted" aspect. These cell processes branch a few times into thinner processes. These processes are 50–60 μm long expanding through a width of 25–30 μm; this means that the area covered by the dendrites is a 120 × 25-μm rectangle. These processes give out very thin terminal fibers which, isolated and without branching, reach the outer row of the photoreceptors synaptic bodies. Each thin terminal ends in a small knob cluster. Each cluster is formed by no more than two to four knobs. Each cell shows from 16 to 24 clusters. Each cluster connects with one cone which means that each cell contacts with 16 to 24 cones in a 120 × 25 μm rectangular area. The distance between connected cones is from a minimum of 5 to a maximum of 20 μm.

The terminal knobs are located at the outer row of photoreceptor synaptic bodies [33] as can be seen in cross-sections and in whole flat mounted retinas. The endings are located at the same level of dendrite clusters and short axon horizontal cell axon terminals.

The processes of neighboring cells intermingle and because they are bitufted, they look as if they form parallel rows.

Preliminary Golgi EM studies have shown that the terminal knobs of these cells penetrate into the double cone synaptic complex [10].

Axonless horizontal cell type II. This cell type (Fig. 4F) has recently been fully described [10–13], although it was already noticed by Cajal, who drew it [34] in a cross-section of the retina and made a brief description of it under the name of "stellate" or "subepithelial." Nevertheless, Cajal [2] subsequently described, in the avian retina, the "brush" horizontal cell and its axon terminal, but thinking that this terminal was an independent cell, he also named it "stellate" horizontal cell (looking at Cajal drawings, it is clear that the "stellate" cell of the 1888 paper [34] is completely different from his "stellate" cell of the 1893 study [2]).

The cell body of 8–10 μm diameter gives out three to four thick processes which branch out several times covering a circular area of 100 μm in diameter. These cell processes give out thin and short terminal fibers, directed toward the photoreceptor synaptic bodies. The thin terminal fibers end in a small cluster of two to four knobs. These knobs are located below the short axon cell and axonless type I endings, at the intermediate row of the outer plexiform layer [33].

Preliminary Golgi EM studies have shown that the terminal knobs penetrate into the synaptic complex of the "straight" cones containing the red oil droplets [10].

REPTILES

The two basic types of horizontal cells found in mammals and birds have also been described in the reptile retina: the short axon horizontal cell, found by Cajal [2] and named "brush" and "stellate" horizontal, and the axonless horizontal cell described by Gallego and Pérez Arroyo [14] in the turtle retina.

Cajal's initial description of the short axon horizontal cell included two different types, "brush" and "stellate," which are the same names applied by him to the two structures he described in the avian retina. As we have previously seen, the "stellate" horizontal in birds is not an independent cell but the axon terminal of the "brush" horizontal cell [31]; on the contrary, in reptiles Cajal's "stellate" cell is actually an individual cell. According to Cajal both cell types have an axon whose endings he was unable to stain. The axon terminal of the "brush" cell has been described with the help of neurofibrillar and Golgi staining techniques [14] and in our opinion, Cajal's "stellate" cell has no axon and, therefore, it can be identified with the recently described axonless horizontal cell [14].

Recent studies with the Golgi technique applied to the entire retina have shown [14, 35] that the turtle retina, as in birds, has three types of horizontal cells: A short axon horizontal cell and two axonless horizontal cell types.

The short axon horizontal cell. This cell (Fig. 5A) is similar to the short axon cell of the avian retina. The soma, dendrites, and beginning of the axon of this cell were described by Cajal [2] as a "brush" horizontal cell. He was not able to follow the axon to its terminal nor to stain it.

The axon terminals were first seen in silver impregnations of whole flat mounted turtle retinas [14]. They form a plexus located between the photoreceptor synaptic bodies and the horizontal cell bodies. EM studies clearly showed this disposition and also abundant membrane-to-membrane contacts between the axon terminals.

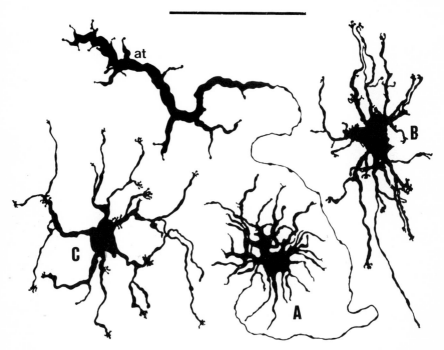

Fig. 5. Horizontal cells of the reptiles retina [35], Golgi method. (A) short axon horizontal cell; (at) axon ending; (B) axonless horizontal cell probably of type I; (C) axonless horizontal cell type II. (The bar length is 20 μm.)

The axon, after a usually straight course of 300 to 400 μm without branching, ends in a large, elongated cylinder-like structure, which gives out short and thick processes leading to thin fibers directed toward the photoreceptor synaptic bodies. Each terminal fiber shows at its tip one or two small knobs.

This "brush" cell soma is located at the outer row of cells of the inner granular layer with a diameter of 10 μm. The outer pole cell gives out several short and thick dendrites directed toward the photoreceptors. Each dendrite ends in a small group of knobs.

This cell type's morphology varies with its location in the retina: It is a small cell near the "foveal line" and its dendrites, packed together, cover areas of the order of 30 μm in diameter. The peripheral cell dendrites spread more horizontally and cover larger areas of the retina, about 50 μm in diameter.

Preliminary Golgi EM studies have shown that the dendrites connect with double cone, and perhaps single cone, synaptic bodies, its axon terminals connecting with rod synaptic bodies as well as with some single cones.

Axonless horizontal cells.   As in the avian retina, two types of axonless horizontal cells have been found.

Axonless horizontal cell type I.   This cell (Fig. 5B), similar to the axonless type I in the avian retina, has not been easily stained. In Golgi stainings [35] it appears as a "bitufted" cell with a round body (7–9 μm in diameter) which gives out, in a horizontal plane, several processes, from three to five, at each opposite pole. Thin terminal fibers come out from the processes running toward the photoreceptors. These fibers end in a cluster of small knobs. In the turtle retina, the distinction between the short axon cell and the axonless type I is not as clear as in the avian retina. Nevertheless, the stained cells obtained allow to consider the axonless cell type I as an independent cell type, similar to the axonless type I cell of the avian retina. Further studies on the reptile retina are needed to determine its connections with the photoreceptors.

Axonless horizontal cell type II.   This cell (Fig. 5C) is similar to the axonless type II horizontal cell of the avian retina and has been clearly seen in Golgi-stained whole turtle retina preparations [14], probably being the "stellate" cell of Cajal's ([2], plate III, Fig. 7) who erroneously stated that one of its processes was an axon.

It has a round body, 9 to 12 μm in diameter, which gives out, at its scleral pole, four to five large horizontally extending processes. They split dichotomically into thinner branches which cover approximately circular areas of about 100 μm in diameter. A small number of thin fibers arise from these processes running toward the photoreceptors. These fibers end in a small cluster of three to five knobs.

AMPHIBIANS

Cajal's description of horizontal cells refers mainly to data obtained with Rana temporaria retinas stained by Golgi's method. As in birds, the outer plexiform layer of the frog retina is made of three superimposed plexuses: The outermost, according to Cajal, is made of small fibers arising from the feet of the ordinary rods; the middle zone is formed by the mingling of basal cones filaments; and the innermost plexus is formed by the club-shaped rods basal filament. In the frog retina Cajal found two types of horizontal cells, "outer" and "inner." Both cell types were, according to Cajal, short axon horizontal cells. It is precisely when describing the amphibian retina that Cajal, referring to horizontal cell, makes the statement that "I believe that these cells are neural in nature and that they may be considered as neurons with very short axons since they originate and finish within the retina itself."

The "outer" horizontal cell has a long axon, characterized by the fact that it branches out to short fine ascending processes which end at the photoreceptor synaptic bodies level, the final ending is formed by two or three ascending and varicose branches. The "inner" horizontal cells are larger and their dendrites shorter than those of the "outer" cells. Cajal postulated that one of these processes originating in the soma was an axon which ending he was unable to determine. Dogiel [36] studying the frog retina described a single type of horizontal cell, the "stellate," but this cell does not look like an horizontal cell due to the fact that it has a descending process directed toward the inner plexiform layer. In our opinion, the cell described by Dogiel is a type of "interplexiform" cell that we have seen very clearly in the frog retina.

Our many attempts to stain horizontal cells with several Golgi techniques have succeeded only in staining clearly a type of short axon horizontal cell (Fig. 6A). It is a cell with numerous and closely packed dendrites, running toward the photoreceptor synaptic bodies, and which ends in isolated knobs or a small knob cluster. The axon is very thin and from time to time gives out small fibers also directed toward the photoreceptor synaptic bodies. In the few observations that we consider to have obtained a full axon staining, its endings are small varicose structures, in agreement with Cajal's description of the "outer" horizontal cells.

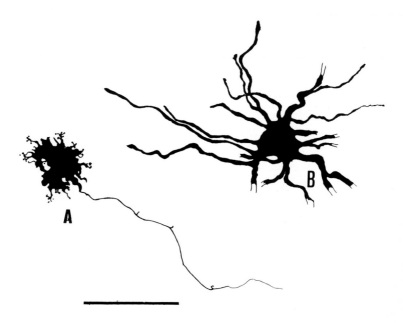

Fig. 6.   Horizontal cells of the amphibian retina, Golgi method. (A) incomplete staining of a short axon horizontal cell; (B) incomplete staining of an axonless horizontal cell. (The bar length is 50 μm.)

In our Golgi-stained retinas, a very rich plexus, of thick fibers crossing in all directions, is detected at the outer plexiform layer level. Occasionally cells with an axonless cells structure (Fig. 6B), described in other tetrapoda, have been seen but not in photomicrographs sufficiently clear to allow us to confirm or describe this cell type in the frog retina. Further studies are needed to clarify the types of horizontal cells existing in the amphibian retina as well as their photoreceptor connections.

DISCUSSION

Since Svaetichin's discovery of the S-potentials [37] and until 17 years later, the sites of their origin were uncertain. Once it was clearly demonstrated that S-potentials were only generated by horizontal cells [38], new problems arose, especially in the tetrapoda retina, due to the insufficient knowledge of the functional structure of the outer plexiform layer. The new types of horizontal cells found in the past 15 years, and their connections with the photoreceptors, were ignored in many electrophysiological studies; as a consequence, the interpretation of the intracellular recordings was incomplete or, in many cases, misleading.

Due to the large size of the horizontal cell in the fish retina, its different types have easily been impaled with microelectrodes, making it possible to identify the cell being recorded, on the basis of a good understanding of the outer plexiform layer structure and the knowledge of the horizontal cell types found in the particular retina under study. In tetrapoda retina, the situation has been different because the electrophysiological studies were made, in many cases, without a good knowledge of the outer plexiform layer functional structure. In interpreting the intracellular recordings, when working with the tetrapoda retina, we have to keep in mind the existence of two clearly different horizontal cell types, the short axon and the axonless cells with different connections with the photoreceptor–bipolar synapse. Also the chances to blindly impale a short axon horizontal cell are scarce because of their scanty distribution in the outer plexiform layer as well as the small size of their cell body.

S-potentials from large horizontal cells in the fish retina are graded responses and we can postulate that the same type of responses will be recorded from all the axonless horizontal cells in tetrapoda retinas, but in the case of the short axon horizontal cells, especially in those species with axon lengths of 1000 μm or longer, the possibility of recording spikes instead of graded potentials cannot be excluded.

As a consequence of the recent studies on the structure and connections of the horizontal cells in the tetrapoda retina, the existence in their retinas of two systems of functionally different horizontal cells may be postulated: The short axon horizontal system which relates the cone–cone bipolar to the rod–rod bipolar synapses and the axonless horizontal cell system which connects only cone–cone bipolar synapses. There is also a fundamental difference between these two systems: The axonless horizontal cells show membrane-to-membrane contacts among them, suggesting electrical coupling, also forming plexuses, at least in low mammals, which extend all over the retina. On the contrary, the short axon horizontal cells do not show these kinds of contacts among them at their soma or dendrite levels, but membrane-to-membrane contacts have been observed up to now only between large axon endings in the bird retina.

There has been some confusion in the nomenclature of the horizontal cells since their discovery last century and especially with the recent description of new cell types. It seems convenient to follow some rules when giving names to the new cells, based not only on their morphology but also on their functional connections.

In our opinion [1], in all tetrapoda retinas we can consider: First, the division of horizontal cells into short axon and axonless types. In the retinas where more than one type of each basic horizontal cell is found, they can be named "short axon horizontal cell, type I, type II . . ." or "axonless horizontal cell, type I, type II . . ." instead of using descriptive names as "stellate," "brush," "tufted," . . . or names indicating situations as "inner" or "outer" which have been misleading in the past.

The evidence we have up to now shows that the short axon horizontal cell is found in all tetrapoda retinas and that the axonless horizontal cell has also been found in low mammals, birds, and reptiles.

Primates appear to be an exception among mammals because the axonless horizontal cell has not been detected in their retinas, two types of short axon horizontal cell having been described instead.

The neurofibrillar methods, which stain the axonless horizontal cell in low mammals, have failed to demonstrate it in the monkey retina, but with Golgi's method we have been able to show [10, 32] the existence of axonless cells at the sclerad level of the inner granular layer, which on a first approximation, could correspond, on the basis of their morphology, to the axonless horizontal cells found in low mammal retina. Nevertheless, in Golgi EM studies we have never been able to show their connections with the photoreceptors synaptic bodies. If this connection is not demonstrated, we have to reach the conclusion that probably these cells are microgliocytes whose processes spread horizontally in one plane at the outer plexiform layer level.

The short axon horizontal cell type I relates the cone–cone bipolar synapse through its dendrites with the rod–rod bipolar synapse through its axon terminals (Fig. 7). In the parafoveal area, six to nine cones are related to 300–400 rod located between 1500 and 2000 μm away. The short axon horizontal cell type II contacts only with cones both by its dendrites and by its axon terminals. The functional connections of this cell type are similar to those of the axonless cell in low mammals.

In low mammal retina (Fig. 8), especially in cats, the two basic types of

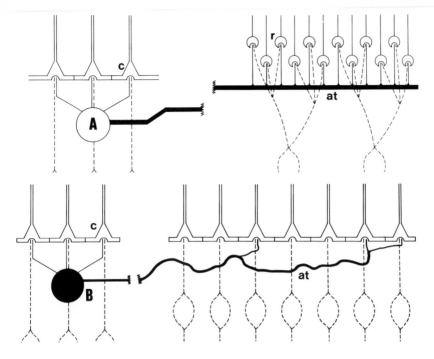

Fig. 7.   Connections of the short axon horizontal cells in the monkey retina; (A) type I cell; (B) type II cell; (at) axon ending; (c) cones; (r) rods.

horizontal cells have been widely studied. The short axon horizontal cell corresponds to the type I of the primate retina. In cat, dog, and rabbit, it has been demonstrated that this cell type relates the cone–cone bipolar synapse through its dendrites with the rod–rod bipolar synapse through the axon terminal, at a distance varying between 200 and 500 μm. The number of cones contacted by one cell's dendrites is of the order of 30 to 40 and the number of rods contacted by the axon terminal, in the cat, is of the order of 3500 to 4000 rods.

One exception among low mammals seems to be the squirrel retina, in which only one type of short axon horizontal cell has been described [39], similar to the type II cell of primates and also having the same connections: cones through the dendrites and cones through the axon terminals.

Very characteristic of the low mammal axonless horizontal cells is that they form a single layer plexus which extends all over the retina. This observation has only been made using the neurofibrillar staining methods which allow counting the number of cells to study their morphological differences between the central area and the periphery of the retina. There are some differences in size

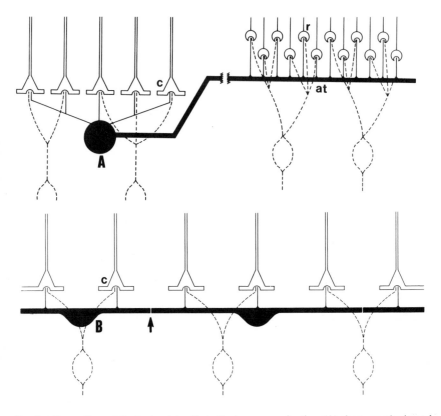

Fig. 8. Connections of the horizontal cells in the low mammal retina; (A) short axon horizontal cell; (at) axon ending; (B) axonless horizontal cell, (arrow) tight junction; (c) cones; (r) rods.

among various species but in all cases the cell processes thin terminal fibers form the lateral component of the cone triads.

To understand the connections of horizontal cells in the bird retina (Fig. 9) we must bear in mind that the outer plexiform layer is made of three different strata: the external (sclerad) row formed by the synaptic bodies of the rods and those of the double cones ("main" and "accessory") and probably some synaptic bodies of single cones. The intermediate row is formed by scattered synaptic bodies of the single straight cones with a red oil droplet and the internal (vitread) row consisting of the oblique cone synaptic bodies.

The short axon horizontal cell dendrites penetrate into the cone triads and the axon terminals into the rod synaptic complex and probably into some single cone synaptic complex too. In the "falconidae" retina the axon length varies between

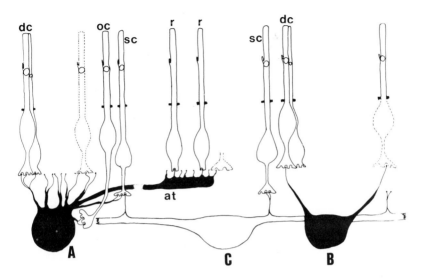

Fig. 9. Connections of the horizontal cells in the bird retina [10]; (A) short axon horizontal cell; (at) axon ending; (B) axonless horizontal cell type I; (C) axonless horizontal cell type II; (dc) double cone; (oc) oblique cone; (sc) straight cone; (r) rod.

200 and 400 μm. The axonless horizontal cell system is formed by two cell types: type I whose connections we have not yet been able to detect and type II which contacts only straight cone synaptic bodies.

We need more information in the synaptology of the horizontal cells in birds as well as in reptiles and amphibians to confirm or rectify the idea of the two horizontal cells system functionally different, generally existing in tetrapoda retinas.

ACKNOWLEDGMENTS

This work has been supported by the "Comisión Asesora de Investigación Científica y Técnica" Grant No. 2796.

I am indebted to Mrs. Rosa Ayllón for continuous technical assistance.

REFERENCES

1. Gallego A: Comparative study of the horizontal cells in the vertebrate retina: Mammals and birds. In Zettler F, Weiler R (eds): "Neural Principles in Vision," Berlín: Springer, p 26, 1976.
2. Cajal S Ramón y: La rétine des vertebrés. La Cellule 9:119, 1893.
3. Gallego A: Description d'une nouvelle couche cellulaire dans la rétine des mammiféres et son role fonctionnel possible. Bull Ass Anat 49:624, 1964.
4. Gallego A: Connexions transversales au niveau des couches plexiformes de la rétine. Actualités Neurophysiol 6e Ser:5, 1965.

5. Polyak SL: "The Retina," Chicago: University of Chicago, 1941.
6. Kolb H: Organization of the outer plexiform layer of the primate retina: Electron microscopy of Golgi impregnated cells. Phil Trans Roy Soc London 258B:261, 1970.
7. Gallego A, Sobrino JA: Horizontal cells of the monkey's retina. Vision Res 15:747, 1975.
8. Kolb H: The connections between horizontal cells and photoreceptors in the retina of the cat: Electron microscopy of Golgi preparation. J Comp Neurol 155:1, 1974.
9. Fisher SK, Boycott BB: Synaptic connexions made by horizontal cells within the outer plexiform layer of the retina of the cat and the rabbit. Proc Roy Soc London 186B:317, 1974.
10. Gallego A: Mecanismos neurales de adaptación visual a nivel de la capa plexiforme externa de la retina. Fundación Juan March, serie universitaria, 1978.
11. Gallego A: Participación de las células horizontales y amacrinas en el procesamiento de la información visual: Correlación morfológica y electrofisiológica. In Fundación Juan March (eds): "Neurobiología." 25:41, Madrid 1977.
12. Mariani AP, Leure-Dupree AE: Horizontal cells of the pigeon retina. J Comp Neurol 175:13, 1977.
13. Genis-Galvez JM, Prada F, Armengol JA: Evidence of three types of horizontal cells in the chick retina. Japan J Ophthalmol 23:378, 1979.
14. Gallego A, Pérez Arroyo M: Photoreceptors and horizontal cells of the turtle retina. The Structure of the Eye III. Edts Yamada & Mishima 311, 1976.
15. Stell WK: Retinal structure in the smooth dogfish. Mustelus canis: Light microscopy of photoreceptor and horizontal cells. J Comp Neurol 148:33, 1973.
16. Stell WK: Horizontal cell axons and axon terminals in goldfish retina. J Comp Neurol 159:503, 1975.
17. Stell WK: The structure and relationship of horizontal cells and photoreceptor-bipolar synaptic complexes in goldfish retina. Amer J Anat 120:401, 1967.
18. Parthe V: Horizontal bipolar and oligopolar cells in the teleost retina. Vision Res 12:395, 1972.
19. Weiler R: "Die Horizontalzellen der Kapfenretina." Doc Thesis: Ludwig Maximilians Universität, Muchen, 1977.
20. Stell WK, Witkovsky P: Retinal structure in the smooth dogfish, mustelus canis: Light microscopy of photoreceptor and horizontal cells. J Comp Neurol 148:33, 1973.
21. Gallego A: Estructura funcional de la retina de los selacios: Fotorreceptores y células horizontales. Morf Norm Pat 3:313, 1979.
22. Kolb H, Mariani A, Gallego A: A second type of horizontal cell in the monkey retina. J Comp Neurol 189:31, 1980.
23. Boycott BB, Dowling JE: Organization of the primate retina: Light microscopy. Phil Trans Roy Soc London 225B:109, 1969.
24. Boycott BB, Kolb H: The horizontal cells of the rhesus monkey retina. J Comp Neurol 148:115, 1973.
25. Dowling JE, Brown JE, Major D: Synapses of horizontal cells in rabbit and cat retinas. Science 153:1639, 1966.
26. Gallego A: Las células horizontales de la retina de los mamíferos terrestres. Trab Inst Cajal Inv Biol 65:227, 1975.
27. Sobrino JA, Gallego A: Células amacrinas de la capa plexiforme de la retina. Actas Soc Esp Cienc Fisiol 12:373, 1970.
28. Gallego A: Horizontal and amacrine cells in the mammal retina. Vision Res Suppl 3:33, 1971.
29. Gallego A: Procedimiento de impregnación argéntica de la retina entera. An Inst Farm Esp II:171, 1953.
30. Orellana JM, Gallego A: Distribución topográfica de las células horizontales de la retina. Actas Soc Esp Cienc Fisiol 5:251, 1959.
31. Gallego A, Barón M, Gayoso M: Horizontal cells of the avian retina. Vision Res 15:1029, 1975a.

32. Gallego A: Las células horizontales de la retina de los vertebrados. Real Acad Nac Med, Instituto de España, 1975b.

33. Gallego A, Barón M, Gayoso M: Organization of the outer plexiform layer of the diurnal and nocturnal bird retinae. Vision Res 15:1027, 1975b.

34. Cajal S Ramón y: Estructura de la retina de las aves. Rev Trim Histol Norm Patol:355, 1888.

35. Pérez Arroyo M: "Estudio topográfico y funcional de la retina de la tortuga." Tesis doctoral. Universidad Complutense. Madrid, 1978.

36. Dogiel A: Über das Verhalten der nervösen elemente in der retina der ganoiden, reptilien, vögel und säugetiere. Anat Anzeiger 3:133, 1888.

37. Svaetichin G: The cone action potential. Acta Physiol Scand 29(Suppl 106):565, 1953.

38. Kaneko A: Physiological and morphological identification of horizontal, bipolar and amacrine cells in goldfish retina. J Physiol 207:623, 1970.

39. West RW: Bipolar and horizontal cells of the gray squirrel retina: Golgi morphology and receptor connections. Vision Res 18:129, 1978.

The S-Potential, pages 31–49
© 1982 Alan R. Liss, Inc., 150 Fifth Avenue, New York, NY 10011

Horizontal Cells in the Teleost Retina

Valentin Parthe

The horizontal cells of teleosts are the retinal elements in which Svaetichin [1] discovered, in 1953, a new and peculiar class of slow potentials. These were recorded intracellularly from what he thought were cone pedicles or myoids, and consequently, he termed them "cone action potentials." Once it became known that the original designation was inappropriate due to the more internal origin of the potentials, they were called S-potentials [2], in recognition of their discoverer.

Horizontal cells (HCs) of the teleost retina were first observed by Heinrich Müller [3,4]. He was able to differentiate in the retinal "Zwischenkörnerschicht," two superimposed layers of morphologically different HCs, and this he did using rudimentary histological methods which could only reveal nuclei and thick nerve cell processes. Müller considered the outer layer as a tight mesh or net ("Netz") formed by large flat cells anastomosed by short and thick expansions. The expansions formed small fenestrations, distributed all along the retina, for the passage of the radial elements. The inner, or deep, layer was considered to constitute a loose cellular net, a sort of continuous membrane, pierced by large spaces. It was formed by small cells, deeply carved and anastomosed with their neighbors by long, fine, and richly ramified protoplasmic bridges. Müller thought he could differentiate a third layer made up of star-shaped cells, smaller and flatter than the preceding ones, which he could not confirm with certainty. He considered that these elements did not represent ganglion cells. In the three decades which followed their discovery they received various denominations— basal, stellate, subreticular, compensatory, and concentric cells. But the descriptive pattern of HCs persisted without substantial modification.

The knowledge of the true organization of HCs and their relation with neighboring retinal elements did not advance until the end of last century. This was due to the limitations of the available analytic means, which did not reveal finer processes and endings, and also the result of the prevailing attachment to doctrines derived from partial and incomplete observations. Schwalbe [5], Hannover [6], Ranvier [7], and Krause [8,9] described two layers of HCs formed by nucleated, flat, star-shaped cells which anastomosed through their expansions to form "continuous networks," "syncitia," "plexii," and "laminae." Reich [10], W. Müller [11], and Retzius [12] observed, in the retinas of certain species of teleosts, a third layer of plexiform aspect, thicker than the first and second layers and formed by long and bulky intermingled fusiform elements. Schwalbe [5] and Schultze [13] considered it as a nervous plexus continuous with the photoreceptors. Krause [9] called it "stratum lacunosum" due to the large vacuoles which he observed in this retinal zone. Schiefferdecker [14] established the lack of nucleus as one of the morphological characteristics of the elements of this third layer, and called them "concentric anucleated cells." Most of the early authors considered that HCs are a variety of supporting elements because of their peculiar morphology, their great development in the teleost retina, and, particularly, because their expansions anatomosed with their neighbors forming a continous concentric reticulum. This functional interpretation reaches its best expression in Schiefferdecker [14], who described HCs as a support system.

In 1887 Tartuferi [15] introduced the Golgi method for the study of the mammalian retina and was the first to see the true morphology of HCs, which he impregnated with silver chromate. He described two classes of HCs whose protoplasmic expansions extended as fine processes to the outer plexiform layer, and mentioned the presence of an axon in some of them. Although these findings pointed to new anatomical realities, he maintained his solidarity with the prevailing syncitial theory. Tartuferi [15] described anastomotic networks between HCs and between their expansions and neighboring retinal elements, ignoring the images which revealed the independence of the cells, the free termination of their processes and the intercellular connections by contiguity.

In contrast to the accepted theories, Cajal [16] showed, with the Golgi method, that in the cerebellum the protoplasmic and axonal extensions terminate freely, and that the interneuronal connections take place by contact of the terminal arborizations. These original anatomical findings, which demonstrated the individuality and independence of the neuron, opened the modern era for the analysis and functional interpretation of the nervous tissue, and determined the decline of the syncitial theory. Cajal [17] performed the most complete study of HCs with the Golgi method, which proved so productive in his hands. He gave the name of "horizontal cells" to the corpuscles disposed transversally to the radial elements in the external zone of the layer of internal grains, which had been known under diverse and ambiguous names until that moment. In the retina of teleosts, he described three superimposed layers of HCs, which he considered to be true neurons with ascending dendrites and horizontally running axons. He classified them as external, intermediate, and internal HC. He found that the dendrites of the external and intermediate HCs enter the external plexiform, where they terminate freely at two different levels. The drawings by which Cajal [17] illustrates these findings imply that HCs from each layer are connected with only one class of photoreceptors. They show that the intermediate HC dendrites terminate externally in the plexiform, in relation to rod spherules, and that the external HC dendrites terminate in the deep zone of the plexiform, where cone pedicles are located. Of the internal HCs, represented by thick fusiform processes, he described two varieties, both bulky at their origin. One is short and rough, with dendritic aspect. The other is thin, has a long course and was considered as an axon. Cajal [17] assumed that both processes, because of their ascending course, terminated in an unknown fashion in the plexiform. Not able to show the termination of the axon, he considered that it ended in the outer plexiform in a similar form to the HC axon in the retina of birds. On the basis of morphological considerations, Cajal [18] suggested the connection of the expansions of HCs and the synapse between the photoreceptor and its specific bipolar cells.

In Cajal's view [19] HCs were not considered association or excitatory-current dispersion elements, but were thought to represent nervous energy stores which could reinforce excitation to allow it to reach the visual centers, a kind of threshold regulation mechanism. In support of this view he referred to the enormous size of HCs of fish and of vertebrates which dwell in low-illumination environments, possessing retinas rich in rods.

The significance and transcendence of the pioneer electrophysiologic work of Svaetichin [1] on the teleost retina constituted the stimulus which opened, in the sixties, the modern era in which, in a massive and systematic way, the study of HCs was undertaken with both classical methodology and new procedures of higher analytical power, particularly the method developed by Stell [20]. The studies were oriented to the analysis of HC structure in an effort to determine the peculiar characteristics which defined their nature and, especially, to establish their precise connections with other retinal cells. For these questions, there were no adequate explanations since Cajal [17,19].

In the Centropomus retina, Villegas [21] showed by electron microscopy (EM) that HCs establish, through their processes, membrane-to-membrane contacts with other HCs forming "a structural unit, like a net." No direct contacts were observed between HCs and photoreceptors. In the same retina Villegas [22] described one layer of external HCs and two subjacent layers of internal HCs. Each cell layer resembles a network. Stripes of dense fibrillar cytoplasm line the first layer of internal HCs, separating it from the others. Villegas and Villegas [23] confirmed these observations and interpreted the stripes of "fibrilose" dense cytoplasm as "bridgelike" interconnecting structures converting the functional network of the first layer of internal HCs into a true syncitium. Invoking the lack of axon in HCs, and other anatomical and functional evidences, the authors maintained the glial nature of HCs and considered the three horizontal layers as the transversal neuroglial system of the retina.

Yamada and Ishikawa [24] reported by EM in the carp retina, two layers of HCs, from which they observed ascending processes that reached the photoreceptor endings. They concluded that both the external and the internal HC establish synaptic contacts with the cone pedicles. Under the internal HC they observed thick anucleated processes in close contact with each other, which they homologated with the anucleated HCs described with light microscopy. Based on the peculiar structure of HCs, they considered them as different from the ordinary neurons. They considered each HC layer as a functional unit formed by independent cells connected laterally by specialized unions covering a large area of the plasma membrane.

In retinas of several species of marine teleosts, Testa [25] described with light microscopical techniques three layers of HCs which were classified as external, middle, and internal, plus a fourth layer formed by star-shaped elements, which were named stellate amacrine cells. All of them have ascending processes, but the methods used did not resolve their contacts. Both horizontal and stellate amacrine cells were considered to possess more properties of glial cells than of neurons and were thought to represent the nervous tissue elements which Svaetichin et al [26] named "controller cells." These cells in which axons were not observed were homologated, functionally, to the short axon neurons which Cajal [18,19] interpreted as accumulators of nervous energy, sort of feedback-control elements.

Stell [20] introduced the Golgi EM procedure, the most successful modification known of the silver-chromate method. By means of such a revealing analytical tool, Stell [20,27,28] clarified the relations between the structures forming the photoreceptor-bipolar-horizontal synaptic complex. He was the first to point out that in fish retinas (initially in the goldfish and later in Centropomus and Squalus) the HC processes end as the so-called synaptic vacuoles. He observed that, in the goldfish retina, dendrites of the external or "sclerad" HC contact cones and end opposite to the synaptic ribbons, while dendrites of the intermediate or "vitread" HC end close to synaptic ribbons of rods. Later, Stell et al [29] demonstrated that HC dendrites can occupy central or lateral positions in the ribbon synaptic complexes, depending upon the class of cone and the type of HC. Of the three layers of HCs of Centropomus, he found [20] that those of the external and middle layers contact cones, and those from the internal layer contact rods. The dendritic terminals have an analogous disposition in the photoreceptors' synapses as in goldfish. Stell [28] concluded that the dendrites of the sclerad HC terminate in endings ramified around the presynaptic ridges of only one cone pedicle, and that dendrites of the vitread HC terminate as lateral processes in numerous rod synaptic complexes. Each cone can contact one or several processes from sclerad HCs, and each rod contacts only with the process of one vitread HC. He considered that the internal HCs of Cajal [17] are not true HCs, and that external HCs of teleosts are homologous to the mammalian ones due to their connections with photoreceptors [27]. He classed them, morphologically, as cells intermediate between neuron and glia [28].

In Mugil, Centropomus, and Eugerres, using the Golgi method and other silver impregnations, Parthe [30] described three superposed layers of HCs (external, middle, and internal) and a layer of stellate amacrine cells. Ascending cell processes of all cell types terminate in the external plexiform layer, in relation with both classes of photoreceptors. Middle and internal HCs emit a process which, after a short horizontal run, reaches the outermost level of the external plexiform layer. Stellate amacrine processes, after contacting analogous processes of neighboring cells, curve and ascend to terminate in the external plexiform. Parthe supposed that HCs are nervous nonconducting elements. In the same teleosts, with the silver chromate method, he showed [31] that ascending processes of external, middle, and internal HCs end at the inner level of the external plexiform in relation with cone pedicles. Processes of stellate amacrines end at the level of, and in relation with, rod spherules. Later, Parthe [32] described HCs according to cell-body shape, position and pattern of division of ascending processes, and recognized that cells previously interpreted as stellate amacrines were true HCs of a distinct type [33]. The form of termination of the ascending processes at the discrete and regular levels at which cone pedicles and rod spherules are located were used as criteria to class them as cone or rod HCs. Parthe concluded that there are three well-defined and -differentiated layers of cone HC in the teleostean retina, and only one type of rod HC, forming one layer [32,34]. In Centropomus, rod HCs are located between the middle and internal layers, forming the third layer. In Mugil, Eugerres, and Lutjanus they are below the internal cone HC, and form the fourth layer. The external cone HC emits a fine descending lateral expansion, similar to a short axon, whose termination was not observed [32,34].

In the carp retina, Witkovsky and Dowling [35] reported with EM the three layers of HCs described by Cajal [17] and admitted, in accordance with Stell's results [28], that the external HC contacts cones while the intermediate HC contacts rods. They reported conventional synapses between HC bodies and between their dendrites, without identifying axons. In the retina of Nannacara anomala, Wagner [36] observed in Golgi preparations two types of HC. The external, d-cells, with short unramified processes which contact both members of double cones, and the c-cells or "radiated stellate horizontals" with ramified processes whose termination in the outer plexiform was not discerned. No axon was found. In the catfish retina, Naka and Carraway [37] described in Golgi preparations three HC types. The external contact cones and the intermediate contact rods. Both cells emit a long lateral process or tail, and the external horizontal occasionally emits two. These processes run through the internal

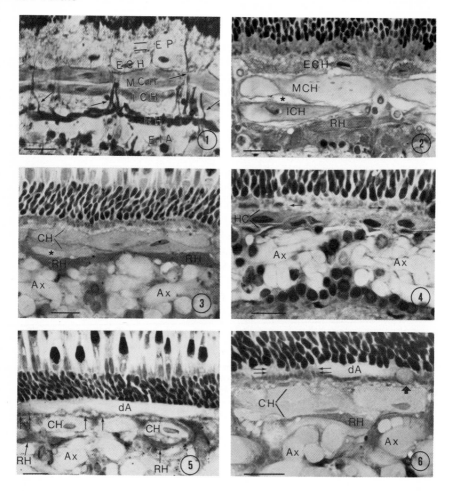

Figs. 1–6. Radial sections of the retina to show the disposition of horizontal cell layers in different teleost species.

Fig. 1. Mugil brasiliensis. Bielschowsky preparation. EP: External plexiform layer. ECH, MCH, ICH: External, middle and internal cone-connected horizontal cell layers. RH: Rod-connected horizontal cell layer. EIA: External intersticial amacrine cell. Arrows indicate ascending branchs of RH. Thickness: 10 μm. Scale: 20 μm.

Fig. 2. Eugerres plumieri. Silver impregnation. ECH, MCH, ICH: External, middle and internal cone-connected horizontal cell layers. RH: Rod-connected horizontal cell layer. Asterisk: Segment from an ECH axon coursing between MCH and ICH. Thickness: 2 μm. Scale: 20 μm.

Fig. 3. Cyprinus carpio. Silver impregnation. CH: Layers of cone-connected horizontal cells. RH: Layer of rod-connected horizontal cells, more intensely stained. Asterisk: Segment from a CH axon coursing between CH and RH.

nuclear layer but their termination was not discerned. The internal HC is different, as it lacks a nucleus and forms several sublayers very close to elements of the inner plexiform. The idea was put forward that these internal HCs might be extensions of the external or intermediate HCs. However, they were drawn as independent cells.

It is Stell's achievement to have demonstrated [38,39] the HC axon in the cyprinid retina and, thus, the elucidation of the nature of the anucleated concentric cells of Schiefferdecker [14], the internal HC cells of Cajal [17], and the cylindrical processes of Stell [28], and of Yamada and Ishikawa [24]. In flat preparations of goldfish Stell and Lightfoot recognized [40] that the layer of sclerad HCs is actually formed by three types of cone-connected cells, which they identified as H1, H2, and H3. Only one type of rod connected cell was found in the layer of vitread HCs. Stell demonstrated [39] that each cone HC emits an axon which follows a descending course to become a robust fusiform mass and suggested as possible synaptic target structures: other axons, bipolar, amacrine, and displaced ganglion cells, rod horizontals, and Cajal's small stellate cells. No axon was seen in the rod HC. HCs were classified as interneurons.

In the carp retina, Mitarai et al [41] differentiated, by means of Procion Yellow injection, three HC layers with ascending processes (external, middle, and internal or rod HCs) and large horizontal processes which form layers under the internal HC. From recordings of S-potentials made prior to injection, they concluded that external and middle HCs are related to cones, while the internal HCs are related to rods. They suggested that the large horizontal processes, from which they recorded time L- and C-type S-potentials as in external and middle HCs, could be their branches, although the anatomical continuity between the two elements could not be demonstrated.

Fig. 4.   Carassius auratus. Silver impregnation. HC: Layer of horizontal cells. Ax: Thick terminal segments of cone-connected horizontal cells axons coursing tangentially in all directions. Arrows: Cone pedicles in which the synaptic complexes are intensely stained. Thickness: 2 μm. Scale: 20 μm.

Fig. 5.   Cyprinus carpio. Silver impregnation. CH: Cone-connected horizontal cells. RH: Rod-connected horizontal cells. Ax: Thick terminal segments of cone-connected horizontal cell axons. dA: Displaced axon from CH, at the level of the external granular layer. Arrows point to photoreceptor endings. Thickness: 2 μm. Scale: 20 μm.

Fig. 6.   Cyprinus carpio. Silver impregnation. CH, RH, Ax, and dA as in Figure 5. A displaced axon, in the external granular layer was cut transversally (arrowhead) and longitudinally; it is partly covered by the descending processes of photoreceptors (double arrows). Thickness: 2 μm. Scale: 20 μm.

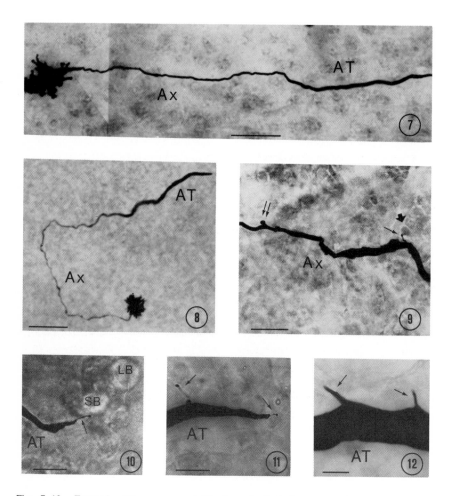

Figs. 7–12. External or H1 cone-connected horizontal cells in flat mounts of Golgi preparations.

Fig. 7. Eugerres plumieri. External horizontal cell. Ax: Axon. AT: Thick terminal segment of the axon. Scale: 50 μm.

Fig. 8. Cyprinus carpio. H1 horizontal cell. Ax: Axon. AT: Thick terminal segment of the axon. Scale: 50 μm.

Fig. 9. Cyprinus carpio. Segment of axon (Ax) from a H1 cell, at the beginning of the thick terminal segment. The arrow indicates a lateral fine process which terminates inside a fenestration as a small spherical mass, close to a bipolar cell body (arrowhead). The double arrow indicates a thick axonal bud. Scale: 20 μm.

Parthe [42] differentiated, in Golgi preparations of the carp retina, three types of cone HC, each of them possessing a descending axon, enlarged into a fusiform terminal segment. Filiform processes with swollen tips emerge from this mass and always terminate inside or contiguous to the fenestrations where bipolar cell processes pass. Displaced axons were seen in the outer nuclear layer. They follow a long course immediately above photoreceptor terminals, and descend to the inner nuclear layer. One rod HC type was observed, without an axon comparable to that of cone horizontals. However, they possess horizontal expansions which follow a short course at the level of the cell bodies and terminate in spherical buds.

Weiler [43], according to the classification proposed by Gallego [44] for HCs in tetrapoda, grouped carp HCs into cells with axon—subdivided in three distinct types—and cells without axon. According to their degree of dendritic ramification they were designated H1, H2, H3, or H4. Cells H1, H2, and H3 each send an axon which terminates in the inner nuclear layer, with an expanded axonal ending whose target cells were not recognized. Cell H4 appears axonless in both Golgi and Procion Yellow preparations. Functionally, H1, H2, and H3 are related to cones, while H4 are related to rods. It was suggested that the role of HCs could be that of transmitting spectral information from photoreceptors to ganglion cells, perhaps via the amacrine cells.

Hassin [45] identified with Procion Yellow injections in the pikeperch retina three HCs—H1, H2, and H3—which form layers, plus two kinds of anucleated cylindrical structures defined as lateral processes. All three types of cells contact cones, H2 with double cones. H2 and H3 have lateral processes. No rod HC was observed. In the same retina, Witkovsky et al [46] found the same cellular types, but established that H1 and H2 contact only double cones, while H3 forms synapses with single cones. They did not visualize axonal processes, but reported large processes separated from cell bodies. No rod HC was observed, but the authors supposed that they exist, intermingled with cone HC bodies.

Fig. 10.   Eugerres plumieri. Terminal segment (AT) of external horizontal cell axon prolonged by a fine ending (arrow) terminated inside a fenestration as a small spherical mass close to a small bipolar cell body (SB). LB: large bipolar cell body. Scale: 10 μm.

Fig. 11.   Cyprinus carpio. Terminal segment (AT) of H1 cone horizontal cell axon. The arrows indicate two fine processes, lateral and terminal, which terminate inside fenestrations, close to bipolar cell bodies. Scale: 10 μm.

Fig. 12.   Cyprinus carpio. Terminal segment (AT) of H1 horizontal cell. Arrows indicate short processes arising from the axon. Scale: 10 μm.

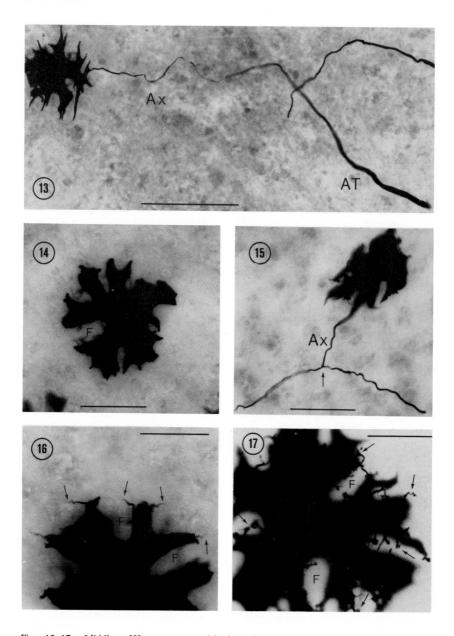

Figs. 13–17. Middle or H2 cone-connected horizontal cells in flat mounts of Golgi preparations.

Fig. 13. Cyprinus carpio. H2 horizontal cell. Ax: Axon. AT: Thick terminal segment of the axon. Scale: 100 μm.

In the retina of Callionymus lira, van Haessendonck and Missotten [47], with the Golgi and Golgi-EM methods, described three types of cone HCs (c-H1,2,3) and one rod HC. The c-H1 cells form the most distal layer, at the outer plexiform, while the others form the proximal layers, at the inner nuclear layer, where the rod HC occupies the outermost level. c-H1 cells contact pale and dark pedicles from double and single cones, while c-H2 cells contact pale pedicles from double cones, and c-H3 send their processes to single cones. At the synaptic complexes, c-H1 endings occupy a lateral position, while c-H2 and c-H3 endings occupy a central position. c-H1 cells emit an axon which terminates at the outer plexiform without contact with photoreceptors. c-H2 and c-H3 cells also possess axons, but their termination was not observed. Rod HCs are only found in the mixed ventral retina and have a large dendritic arborization. The endknobs contact only rods, and seem to always occupy a lateral position in the spherule's triad. No axon was found in rod HCs.

In Eugerres, Parthe [48] confirmed his previous results with Golgi when he demonstrated the whole extension of the lateral expansion "similar to an axon" of the cone external HC, and corroborated the lack of such structure in middle and internal cone HCs. In the latter cells and in the rod HC he described a process which is different from the ascending branches and terminates in a spherical mass always located inside the HC fenestrations, in contact with bi-polars. Such processes from the rod HC contact the large bipolar cell bodies, while those from cone HCs contact the small bipolar cell bodies. This disposition could serve as the anatomical substrate for the horizontal cell function proposed by Svaetichin et al [49–51]. In this view, the horizontal cell represents the negative feedback element ("controller cell"), which at a strategic point in the triad complex regulates the information flow from the receptor to the bipolar, on the basis of delayed information obtained through a sensing device, which is thought to be the terminal button in contact with the bipolar cell body.

Fig. 14. Eugerres plumieri. Middle horizontal cell. Focus at the level of cell body. Ascending processes can be seen out of focus. The thick protoplasmic processes leave spaces which delimit fenestrations (F). Scale: 50 μm.

Fig. 15. Cyprinus carpio. H2 horizontal cell. The axon (Ax) divides in two branches (arrow). Scale: 50 μm.

Fig. 16. Eugerres plumieri. Medial horizontal cell. Focus at the level of cell body with thick protoplasmic processes which delimit fenestrations (F). Arrows indicate fine, short nonascending extensions which terminate inside fenestrations, close to bipolar cell bodies. Ascending branches out of focus. Scale: 30 μm.

Fig. 17. Eugerres plumieri. Medial horizontal cell. Focus at the synaptic level in the outer plexiform layer. Arrows indicate ascending branches and synaptic terminals. F: Fenestrations. Scale: 30 μm.

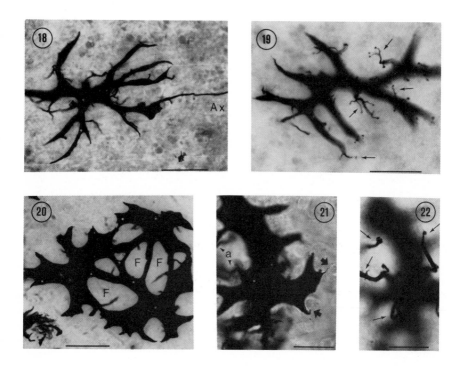

Figs. 18–22. Internal or H3 cone-connected horizontal cells in flat mounts of Golgi preparations.

Fig. 18. Cyprinus carpio. H3 horizontal cell. Focus at the level of cell body with large protoplasmic branches. Ax: Axon. Scale: 50 μm.

Fig. 19. Cyprinus carpio. H3 horizontal cell. Focus at the synaptic level in the outer plexiform layer. Arrows indicate the termination of ascending branches which divide prior to their entrance to the plexiform layer. Scale: 50 μm.

Fig. 20. Eugerres plumieri. Three contiguous internal horizontal cells. Their large protoplasmic branches are in contact and delimit fenestrations (F). Scale: 50 μm.

Fig. 21. Eugerres plumieri. Internal horizontal cell. Focus at the level of cell body with large protoplasmic branches. Ascending processes (a) are partly out of focus. Arrowheads indicate short, fine nonascending processes which terminate inside fenestrations, close to bipolar cell bodies. Scale: 30 μm.

Fig. 22. Eugerres plumieri. Same cell as in Fig. 21. Focus at the synaptic level in the outer plexiform layer. Arrows indicate synaptic terminals of ascending processes. Out of focus in the cell body and thick protoplasmic branches. Scale: 30 μm.

OBSERVATIONS

In the retinas of teleosts HCs occupy zones of different thicknesses in the inner granular layer. They have a tangential disposition and form layers whose number and distinctness vary among species. Members of the Mugiliadae, Lutjanidae, and Gerridae families, such as Mugil brasiliensis (Fig. 1), Centropomus undecimalis, Lutjanus aya, and Eugerres plumieri (Fig. 2), all of estuarine habitat, always have four superposed layers, each formed by a different type of HC. In cyprinids, on the other hand, HC layers are not regularly ordered. Three layers can be usually observed in the retina of the carp (Figs. 3,5,6) and two in that of goldfish (Fig. 4). With the Golgi method it can be seen that the external and middle layers in the carp, and the external layer in the goldfish, are formed by three intermingled and different types of cone HCs.

Two discrete classes of HCs can be recognized in Golgi preparations according to the form and level of termination of the ascending branches at the plane of the photoreceptor endings. M brasiliensis, E plumieri, C carpio, and C auratus all have three types of cone-connected HC and one type of rod-connected HC. The identification of each of the three cone-connected HCs is based on the shape of the cell somata, on the thickness and extension of their lateral processes and ascending branches, and on their pattern of ramification. In retinas with regular layers of cone-connected HCs, these are designated, according to their position in the inner nuclear layer, as external, middle, and internal. On the other hand, in retinas where the three cone-connected HCs form one or two irregular strata, it is convenient to designate them numerically, as H1, H2, H3. The two nomenclatures refer to equivalent cellular types, as they correspond to morphologically individualized and analogous structures. Rod-connected HCs form a single layer usually located under the cone-connected HCs (Figs. 1–3), although on occasions they can be found among the later.

In radial sections of Golgi preparations the external HCs or H1 appear as black rectangular masses with thin and short ascending branches which reach, without dividing, the level of cone pedicles where they terminate in synaptic buttons. An axon can be seen to originate from a side of the cell and to follow a horizontal and descending course (Figs. 30,31). In flat preparations they show a chubby cell soma with few short protoplasmic extensions from which the ascending branches and the axon originate (Figs. 7,8). The axon follows an irregular path. Initially thin and varicous, it descends and enlarges, becoming a long and undulated thick segment (Figs. 7–9) which tapers off. It is prolonged by a thin process with a spherical mass at the tip (Figs. 10,11). These spherical endings terminate in close proximity to the cell body of small bipolars cells (Fig. 10), inside fenestration formed by the lateral processes of HCs. Along its course the axon emits thin filiform apendices, which also end in spherical masses at the proximity of bipolar cells (Figs. 9,11). Thick protusions (Fig. 9) or spiny

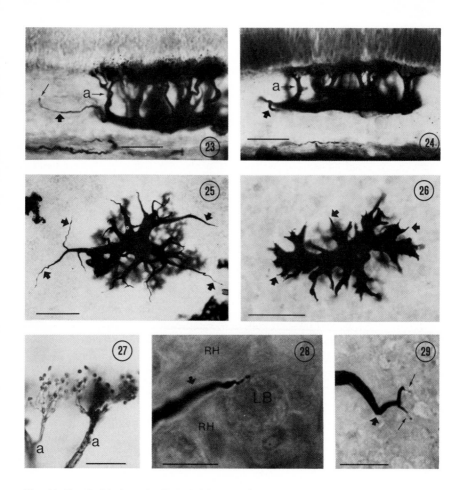

Figs. 23–29. Rod horizontal cells in Golgi preparations.

Fig. 23. Eugerres plumieri. Radial section. a: Ascending branches. Arrowhead indicates a non-ascending, deep extension with an spherical ending (arrow) at the level of the cone-connected horizontal cells. Scale: 30 μm.

Fig. 24. Cyprinus carpio. Radial section. a: Ascending processes. Arrowhead indicates deep extension. Scale: 30 μm.

Fig. 25. Eugerres plumieri. Flat mount. Focus at the level of cell-body and thick protoplasmic processes. Arrowheads indicate deep extensions. Out of focus is the more externally placed synaptic bush. Scale: 50 μm.

Fig. 26. Cyprinus carpio. Flat mount: Details as in Figure 25. Scale: 50 μm.

processes (Fig. 12) can also be seen to arise from the axon, usually from the thick terminal segment. In Eugerres the axons of the external HC's course between the layers of HCs (Fig. 2), while in cyprinids, where all HCs possess axons, their thick terminal segments are conspicuously packed in a large zone of the inner granular layer, between rod HCs and the layer of amacrine cell bodies (Figs. 3–6). In the carp, furthermore, HC axons can be seen displaced at the innermost level of the outer granular layer between rod nuclei and photoreceptor terminals (Figs. 5,6). There they course a variable distance, external to cone pedicles and rod spherules, before they descend toward the inner granular layer.

Cone-connected middle HCs or H2 are the largest cellular elements in the retina of teleosts. In radial sections they appear as large masses which give origin, from their external surface, to numerous ascending branches which divide in two or three processes just before reaching the external plexiform layer (Figs. 32,33). Each process ends in a terminal button at the level of the base of the cone pedicles. These ascending branches are longer and thicker than those of the external HC or H1. While in Eugerres axons have never been observed in middle HCs, in cyprinids an axon can be seen to leave laterally from H2 cells (Fig. 33). In flat mounts (Figs. 13–17) the voluminous cell body is seen to have robust photoplasmic extensions with large spaces between them, and which constitute ample fenestrations with similar spaces from neighbouring cells. From the photoplasmic extensions two types of processes arise, the ascending branches which reach the external plexiform layer and very short fine processes with spherical endings which terminate in the fenestrations at the same plane of the soma (Figs. 16,17), in close proximity to bipolar cell bodies. In cyprinids, not in Eugerres, an axon is seen to originate from one of the large protoplasmic extensions (Figs. 13,15). This axon has the same characteristics as described above for H1 cells, and it is frequently seen to bifurcate (Fig. 15).

Cone-connected internal HCs or H3 cells appear in radial sections as fusiform masses possessing rather thick and long ascending branches which divide at various levels in two or three diverging processes (Figs. 34,35). These enter the external plexiform layer and terminate in synaptic buttons at the level of the base

Fig. 27. Eugerres plumieri. Radial section. Ascending processes (a) illustrating their division and terminal buttons. Scale: 10 μm.

Fig. 28. Eugerres plumieri. Flat mount. Deep extension (arrowhead) terminating in spherical mass close to a large bipolar (LB) in a fenestration formed by other rod horizontal cells (RH) which are seen as nonimpregnated bands of fibrillar material. Scale: 10 μm.

Fig. 29. Eugerres plumieri. Flat mount. Deep extension (arrowhead) which divides in two terminals branchlets (arrows). Scale: 20 μm.

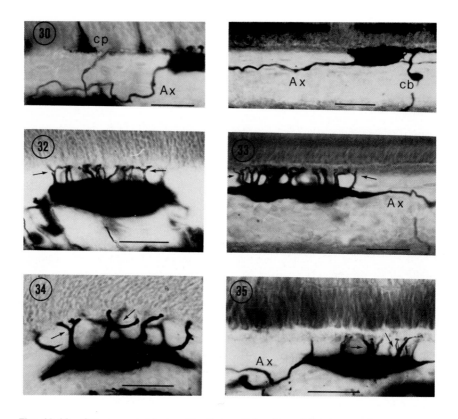

Figs. 30–35. Cone-connected horizontal cells in radial sections of Golgi preparations.

Fig. 30. Eugerres plumieri. External horizontal cell. Ax: Axon. cp: Cone pedicle. Scale: 30 μm.

Fig. 31. Cyprinus carpio. H1 horizontal cell. Ax: Axon. cb: Cone bipolar. Scale: 30 μm.

Fig. 32. Eugerres plumieri. Medial horizontal cell. Arrows indicate the division of ascending branches close to the external plexiform layer. Scale: 30 μm.

Fig. 33. Cyprinus carpio. Two contiguous H2 horizontal cells. Ax: Axon. Arrows as in Figure 32. Scale: 30 μm.

Fig. 34. Eugerres plumieri. Internal horizontal cell. Long ascending branches divide (arrows) far from the external plexiform layer. Scale: 30 μm.

Fig. 35. Cyprinus carpio. H3 horizontal cell. Ax: Axon. Long ascending branches divide (arrows) far from the external plexiforms layer. Scale: 30 μm.

of cone pedicles. The ascending branches of these cells are longer thicker and fewer in number than those of middle or H2 cells. In carp (Fig. 35), not in Eugerres (Fig. 34), an axon is seen, similar to those of H1 and H2. Flat preparations reveal in the carp a slender cell body with long protoplasmic extensions which divide in two or three branches (Figs. 18,19). The axon arises from one of these processes (Fig. 18). In Eugerres, the axonless internal horizontal cells (Fig. 20) have a larger soma and thicker and shorter protoplasmic extensions. In both species the lateral protoplasmic extensions give rise to ascending branches (Figs. 21,22) which reach the external plexiform layer where they contact cones, and to fine deep processes (Figs. 19,21) that end in fenestrations, in the proximity of bipolar cell bodies.

Rod-connected HCs of all the teleostean retinas studied have a characteristics appearance in radial sections, resembling an inverted medusa (Figs. 23,24). They differ from cone-connected HC's in the large number of ascending branches which arise from a soma with the shape of a flattened helmet, and in the dense tuft of terminal processes. In flat mounts they resemble hypertrophic fibrous astrocytes (Fig. 25) or display capricious shapes with an indented irregular contour (Fig. 26). These cells give rise to two types of extensions, ascending branches and deep processes. The ascending branches are numerous, thick, and tortuous; they divide repeatedly, first before entering the external plexiform layer (Figs. 23,24), and then after entering it; here they divide in multiple terminal branchlets which end in synaptic buttons at the level of the rod spherules (Fig. 27). The deep processes (Fig. 25) originate from the lateral protoplasmic extensions and after a short horizontal course terminate in tiny spherical masses in the proximity of large bipolar cell bodies located inside fenestrations (Fig. 28). These deep processes never reach the external plexiform layer, and frequently bifurcate before terminating (Fig. 29). They always run outward from the soma and cover a larger field than that of the ascending branches (Fig. 25).

REFERENCES

1. Svaetichin G: The cone action potential. Acta Physiol Scand 29(Suppl 106):565, 1953.
2. Motokawa K: Physiology of Color and Pattern Vision. Tokyo: I. Shoin, 1970, p 8.
3. Müller H: Zur Histologie der Netzhaut. Z Wiss Zool 3:234, 1851.
4. Müller H: Anatomisch-physiologische Untersuchungen über die Retina bei Menschen und Wirbelthieren. Z Wiss Zool 8:1, 1857.
5. Schwalbe G: Die Retina. In von Graefe, A Saemisch T, eds: Handbuch des gesamten Augenheilkunde, Vol I. Leipzig: W Engelmann, 1874, pp 354–457.
6. Hannover A: La Retine de l'Homme et des Vertébrés. Copenhagen: A.F. Höst et Fils, 1876.
7. Ranvier L: Traité Technique d'Histologie, Paris: F. Savy, 1875–1882, pp 732–759.
8. Krause W: Die Retina. I. Die Membrana fenestrata der Retina. II. Zur Entwicklungsgeschichte der Retina. Int Monatsschr Anat Histol 1:225, 1884.
9. Krause W: Die Retina. II. Die Retina der Fische. Int Monatsschr Anat Histol 3:8, 1886.
10. Reich M: Zur histologie der Hechtretina. Arch Ophthalmol 20:1, 1874.
11. Müller W: Ueber die Stammesentwicklung des Sehorgans der Wirbelthiere. Leipzig: Vogel, 1874.

12. Retzius G: Beiträge zur Kenntnis der inneren Schichten der Netzhaut des Auges. Biol Untersuch 1:89, 1881.
13. Schultze M: Zur Anatomie und Physiologie der Retina. Arch Mikrosk Anat 2:175, 1866.
14. Schiefferdecker P: Studien zur vergleichenden Histologie der Retina. Arch Mikrosk Anat 28:305, 1886.
15. Tartuferi F: Sull'anatomia della retina. Int Monatsschr Anat Physiol 4:451, 1887.
16. Cajal S Ramón y: Estructura de los centros nerviosos de las aves. Rev Trim Hist Norm Pat 1:1, 1888.
17. Cajal S Ramón y: La rétine des vertébrés. Cellule 9:121, 1893.
18. Cajal S Ramón y: Los Problemas Histofisiológicos de la Retina. XIV. Madrid: Concilium Oftalmologicum, 1933, pp 1–8.
19. Cajal S Ramón y: Textura del Sistema Nervioso del Hombre y de los Vertebrados, Vol. 2. Madrid: N. Moya, 1904, p 644.
20. Stell WK: Correlation of retinal cytoarchitecture and ultrastructure in Golgi preparations. Anat Rec 153:389, 1965.
21. Villegas GM: Electron microscopic study of the vertebrate retina. J Gen Physiol 43(6, part 2):15, 1960.
22. Villegas GM: Comparative ultrastructure of the retina in fish, monkey and man. In Jung R, Kornhuber H, eds: The Visual System: Neurophysiology and Psychophysics. Berlin: Springer, 1961, pp 3–13.
23. Villegas GM, Villegas R: Neuron-glia relationship in the bipolar layer of the fish retina. J Ultrastruct Res 8:89, 1963.
24. Yamada E, Ishikawa T: The fine structure of the horizontal cells in some vertebrate retinae. Cold Springs Harbor Symp Quant Biol 30:383, 1965.
25. Testa AS de: Morphological studies on the horizontal and amacrine cells of the teleost retina. Vision Res 6:51, 1966.
26. Svaetichin G, Negishi K, Fatehchand R, Drujan BD, Selvin de Testa A: Nervous function based on interactions between neuronal and non-neuronal elements. In De Robertis EDP, Carrea R eds: Biology of neuroglia. 15. Amsterdam: Elsevier Press, 1965, pp 243–266.
27. Stell WK: Correlated light and electron microscope observations on Golgi preparation of goldfish retina. J Cell Biol 23:89A, 1964.
28. Stell WK: The structure and relationships of horizontal cells and photoreceptor-bipolar synaptic complexes in goldfish retina. Am J Anat 121:401, 1967.
29. Stell WK, Lightfoot DO, Wheeler TG, Leeper HF: Goldfish retina: Functional polarization of cone horizontal cell dendrites and synapses. Science 190:989, 1975.
30. Parthe V: Células horizontales y amacrinas de la retina. Acta Cient Venez 18(suppl 3):240, 1967.
31. Parthe V: Conexiones de las células horizontales y estrelladas de la retina de los teleósteos. Acta Cient Venez 19:13, 1969.
32. Parthe V: Horizontal, bipolar, and oligopolar cells in the teleost retina. Vision Res 12:395, 1972.
33. Parthe V: Clasificación morfológica de las células horizontales de la retina. Acta Cient Venez 21(suppl 1):198, 1970.
34. Parthe V: Morphological classification of the horizontal cells in the teleost retina. Proc In Union Physiol Sci 9:1308, 1971.
35. Witkovsky P, Dowling JE: Synaptic relationship in the plexiform layers of carp retina. Z Zellforsch 100:60, 1969.
36. Wagner HJ: Die Nervösen Netzhautelemente von Nannacara anomala (Cichlidae, Teleostei). Z Zellforsch 137:63, 1973.

37. Naka K-I, Carraway NRG: Morphological and functional identifications of catfish retinal neurons. I. Classical morphology. J Neurophysiol 38:53, 1975.
38. Stell WK: Horizontal Cells in a cyprind fish retina. Abst Annual Meeting A.R.V.O. 1973, p 75.
39. Stell WK: Horizontal cell axons and axon terminals in goldfish retina. Am J Anat 159:503, 1975.
40. Stell WK, Lightfoot DO: Color-specific interconnections of cones and horizontal cells in the retina of the goldfish. J Comp Neurol 159:473, 1975.
41. Mitarai G, Asano T, Miyake Y: Identification of five types of S-potential and their corresponding generating sites in the horizontal cells of the carp retina. Jpn J Ophthamol 18:161, 1974.
42. Parthe V: The horizontal cells in the carp retina. Fourth Panam Cong Anat, Montreal, 1975, p 35.
43. Weiler R: Horizontal cells of the carp retina: Golgi inpregnation and Procion Yellow injection. Cell Tissue Res 195:515, 1978.
44. Gallego A: A comparative study of the horizontal cells in vertebrate retina. I. Mammals and birds: In Zettler F, Weiler R, eds: Neural Principles in Vision. Berlin: Springer, 1976, pp 26–62.
45. Hassin G: Pikeperch horizontal cells identified by intracellular staining. J Comp Neurol 186:529, 1979.
46. Witkovsky P, Burkhardt DA, Nagy AR: Synaptic connections linking cones and horizontal cells in the retina of the pikeperch (Stizostedion vitreum). J Comp Neurol 186:541, 1979.
47. Haesendonck E van, Missotten L: Synaptic contacts of the horizontal cells in the retina of the marine teleost, Callionymus lyra L. J Comp Neurol 184:167, 1979.
48. Parthe V: Horizontal cell processes in teleost retina. J Neurosci Res 6:113, 1981.
49. Svaetichin G, Laufer M, Negishi K, Muriel C: Retinal automatic control mechanisms responsible for Weber's and Steven's laws. Proc Int Union Physiol Sci 8:423, 1968.
50. Svaetichin G, Muriel C: Función retiniana y control automático. Rev Oftal Ven 24:41, 1970.
51. Svaetichin G, Negishi K, Drujan B, Muriel C: S-potentials and retinal automatic control systems. First European Biophysics Congress, Vienna, 1971, p 77.

The S-Potential, pages 51–75
© 1982 Alan R. Liss, Inc., 150 Fifth Avenue, New York, NY 10011

Horizontal Cell Connectivity in Goldfish

William K. Stell, Robert Kretz, and David O. Lightfoot

Detailed structural studies have been useful in clarifying the role of horizontal cells and S-potentials in retinal function. In goldfish, four S-potential types have been described: three photopic (L-type or monophasic, C1-type or biphasic, and C2-type or triphasic) and one scotopic. It has been possible to assign these, respectively, to three types of horizontal cell connected exclusively to cones (CH1, CH2, and CH3) and one type connected exclusively to rods (RH). The connections of CH1, CH2, and CH3, examined by light and electron microscopy, are consistent with a model in which red (R)-, green (G)-, and blue (B)-sensitive cones each act mainly upon one CH type through excitatory or sign-conserving synapses ($\rightarrow$) and CH cells act mainly upon cones through inhibitory or sign-inverting synapses (--$\rightarrow$), thus:

$$R \rightleftharpoons CH1 \text{--} \rightarrow G \longrightarrow CH2 \text{--} \rightarrow B \longrightarrow CH3$$

This paper reviews the light and electron microscopical studies that support our model of horizontal cell connectivity in goldfish.

BACKGROUND

Light microscopical studies of retinal cells, particularly in the bony fishes (teleosts), date back well over a century [1]. It was Svaetichin's awareness of the relatively large dimensions of teleostean cone photoreceptors, revealed by those studies, that led him to attempt the first intracellular recordings from cones in the 1950s. The discovery that the so-called "cone action potentials" were generated by horizontal cells detracts little from the seminal importance of his contribution. Svaetichin's classic work inspired a whole new generation of retinal studies, in which the focus was cellular substructure and function.

The first modern microscopical studies of horizontal cells, undertaken during the 1960s in the aftermath of Svaetichin's astounding observations, began in an atmosphere of wonder and doubt. Data from dye-injection experiments, while suggesting that S-potentials are generated by horizontal cells, were not widely accepted until the pioneering studies of Werblin and Dowling [2] and Kaneko

[3]. The unique physiological characteristics of S-potentials, furthermore, led to persistent speculation that the cells from which they arose might not be real neurons, but neuroglia or some novel intermediate form. In this context, appropriate structural analysis offered promise of new information that might resolve some of the issues of the day. In the main, the early electron microscopical studies of horizontal cells lent credence to the growing belief that they are indeed neurons, that they are influenced by photoreceptor cells through more or less conventional synapses, and that they in turn influence the responses of bipolar cells through their own more or less conventional synaptic outputs.

Now that horizontal cells are seen after all as neurons, certainly unique in personality but not outrageously different, the controversies of 20 years ago sometimes sound rather silly. Gunnar Svaetichin, to his credit, did little to discourage controversy and, indeed, often fanned its flames by championing such heretical notions as the "transferapse." Even 20 years of mainstream efforts, however, have failed to resolve numerous questions concerning the role of horizontal cells and S-potentials in retinal physiology and vision. Detailed structural studies have been particularly useful in addressing such questions. Here we shall review some of the observations on goldfish horizontal cells made during recent years in the first author's laboratory.

OBSERVATIONS

Light Microscopy

Conventional histological sections of goldfish retina reveal only a single layer of horizontal cell bodies, scarcely 5 μm thick, comprising one or two sublayers of flattened nuclei [4, 5]. Scattered throughout the inner nuclear layer are the fusiform, anucleate axonal expansions of some of those cells [6]. The diversity and individual characteristics of these cells can be appreciated only by selective staining of single neurons, as for example by the Golgi method. Application of this method [5] shows that the compact horizontal cell layer in goldfish comprises cells of four types: three that make contact with cones and one that makes contact with rods.

In whole retinas mounted flat it can be seen that cone horizontals of all three types have a single horizontal axon [6]. This axon dips deep into the inner nuclear layer (INL), where it expands to form a long, thick fusiform ending. Cell body, dendrites, and axon alike bear sparse, thin, knobby spines. Rod horizontal cells appear to bear spines but not axons. Cone horizontal cell axons are found at all levels of the INL, some reaching the inner synaptic layer (ISL), and there is evidence that the axons of different HC types form irregular sublaminae in the INL [7]. Apart from this, nothing whatever is known about the neural interconnections of the axons.

Light microscopical analysis of serial semithin (0.5 to 1.0-μm) sections through silver chromate (Golgi) impregnated goldfish cone horizontal cells [5] revealed the chromatic types of cones [8] with which their dendrites make contact. Cells of type CH1 contact all cones within their dendritic field: red-sensitive (R cones, $\lambda_{max} \simeq 625$ nm), green-sensitive (G cones, $\lambda_{max} \simeq 530$ nm), and blue-sensitive (B cones, $\lambda_{max} \simeq 455$nm). Cells of type CH2 contact all the G cones and B zones within their dendritic field, but none of the R cones. Cells of type CH3 contact all the B cones within their dendritic field, but none of the R cones or G cones.

Given these connections, it is obvious that the responses of cone horizontal cells are not to be explained simply by cone-to-horizontal cell synapses, whatever their sign. According to their structural connectivity, the color types in such a system should be $R + G + B$, $G + B$, and B; but the observed functional types are R, $R + G$, and $R + G + B$. An important clue came from studies of temporal transfer functions for the various color components [9], from which a succession of inversion and delay steps could be inferred to yield the following model:

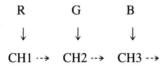

$$\begin{array}{ccc} R & G & B \\ \downarrow & \downarrow & \downarrow \\ CH1 \dashrightarrow & CH2 \dashrightarrow & CH3 \dashrightarrow \end{array}$$

(($\rightarrow$) indicates delay with sign conservation; ($\dashrightarrow$) indicates delay with sign inversion.)

The model was consistent with the observation that the λ_{max} for the major red component of monophasic (L-type) units was 600–625 nm [10–17], the λ_{max} for the green component of biphasic C-type units was 500–550 nm [9–13,15–17], and the λ_{max} for the blue component of triphasic C-type units was 440–480 nm [9, 10, 12, 15–17] in various cyprinid fishes. It had to allow for the possibility of G and B cone inputs to monophasic cells, observed in a few instances [11, 13]. It made no allowance whatever for apparent far-red ($\lambda_{max} \simeq 650$–700 nm) contributions to monophasic cells, in parallel with the standard 625-nm R cone input [13, 15] and to biphasic and triphasic cells [9, 10, 12, 13, 15–17], in which only Orlov and Maksimova [11] found an ordinary R cone input with λ_{max} at 620 nm. It also made no allowance for a similar shift of the λ_{max} for mid-wavelength hyperpolarization in triphasic cells to 560–600 nm, as observed by a number of authors [9, 10, 12, 15–17]. The 680- and 580-nm (pseudo) pigments that might be inferred from such observations appear to be the result of neural interactions [18], perhaps as a result of color opponent action through cone basal processes or telodendria [19, 20].

Electron Microscopy

Our earliest study of silver chromate-impregnated CH1 and RH cells [21–23] by electron microscopy showed that both rod and cone synapses are characterized by clusters of postsynaptic processes opposite presynaptic organelles (synaptic ribbons and arciform densities). Typically a ribbon synapse comprises three postsynaptic processes arranged in a triad opposite the synaptic ribbon. Dendrites of CH1 and RH cells were shown to occupy lateral positions in those triads, whereas dendrites of some bipolars were found to terminate in the center of triads [4].

In a later study [23], we examined Golgi-impregnated cone horizontal cells of all three types in the electron microscope after ultrathin sectioning serially in the plane of the retina, perpendicular to the long axis of the cones. In series of sections through two examples each of CH3 and CH2 and one CH1, a total of 53 cone pedicles were recovered and photographed in their entirety (Table I). Cone types were identified by mapping their position in the cone mosaic and in part by contact with the impregnated cell (eg, CH3 were known already to contact only B cones). The number of synaptic ribbons and ribbon synapses (ribbons with arciform density) in each cone was determined by following ribbons through complete series. These data (Table II) led to the conclusion that, while the number of ribbons tends to be most numerous in R cones and least in B cones, as reported by Scholes for rudd [24], in goldfish only miniature single cones can be distinguished from others by number of synaptic ribbons alone.

In each cone, furthermore, we counted the number of ribbon synapses in which a silver chromate-containing process was present, and identified that process throughout its course within the series as lateral, central, or both in the ribbon synaptic triad. Maps of contacted cones showing the fraction of triads contacting an impregnated process (Figs. 1–5) reveal that the fraction declines as a function of distance from the center of the cell, as shown in other species [25, 26] and as might be expected if the dendritic fields of neighboring homologous cells overlap.

The most interesting and unexpected finding was that horizontal cells of different types contact cones of a given type in different ways, and that horizontal cells of a given type contact cones of different types in different ways (Table III). For example, while the predominantly lateral location of CH1 dendrites reported previously [4, 20, 21] remains valid, the dendritic terminations of CH2 at G cones and CH3 at B cones are mainly in the centers of the triads (Fig. 6). For the most part the horizontal cells seem to care only about cone chroma and not subtype, since contact patterns with R or G cones are the same regardless whether those cones are single or members of a double cone. Contacts with blue-sensitive short and miniature single cones, however, follow a different rule altogether, particularly the contacts of CH3 cells (mainly central in triads of short single but lateral in triads of miniature short single cones).

TABLE I. Cone Horizontal Cells Sectioned

HC type	n	Pedicles recovered
CH1	1	18
CH2	2	25
CH3	2	10
All	5	53

TABLE II. Cone Pedicles Recovered

Cone chroma	Cone type	n	Average number ribbons	Average number ribbon synapses
R	LD	5	16.6 ± 3.1	16.2 ± 2.6
R	LS	4	12.8 ± 1.0	12.8 ± 1.0
G	SD	18	13.3 ± 1.5	13.1 ± 1.2
G	LS	2	12.0 ± 2.8	12.0 ± 2.8
B	SS	17	11.3 ± 1.6	11.2 ± 1.6
B	MS	7	5.9 ± 0.7	5.6 ± 0.5

TABLE III. Patterns of Contact in Cone Triads

HC type	Cone chroma	Cone type	Triads total (no.)	Triads contacted (no.)	Center only	Mainly lateral	Lateral only
					Contacts (%)		
CH1	R	LD	81	53	15	55	30
	R	LS	51	33	9	61	30
	G	SD	54	38	2.5	2.5	95
	G	LS	10	4	0	0	100
	B	SS	17	4	0	0	100
	B	MS	12	10	0	100	0
CH2	G	SD	181	131	83	14	3
	G	LS	21	21	67	28	5
	B	SS	70	47	9	36	55
	B	MS	22	15	13	40	47
CH3	B	SS	103	79	100	0	0
	B	MS	5	5	0	60	40
			627	440			

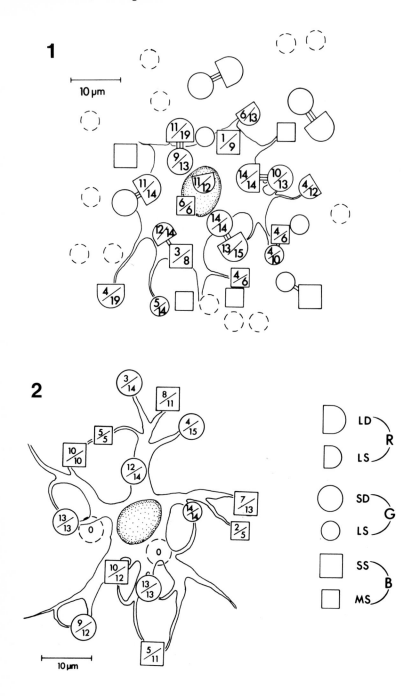

The marked differentiation of horizontal cell contact patterns as a function of cone type suggested a corresponding functional differentiation. Largely because of the polarity of function hypothesized from the light microscopical connectivity data, we assumed the centrally terminating triadic processes to be receptive to input from the photoreceptor and the laterally terminating triadic processes to be mediating output to the next stage of horizontal cell circuitry. Since the lateral processes make extensive contact with cones but in some cases (CH1, CH2 with B cones) appear to receive little or no input from those cones [27], we concluded that their synaptic effect is directed primarily toward the cones. This conclusion is supported by evidence that stimulation of horizontal cells by an annular surround can cause voltage changes in the appropriate cones

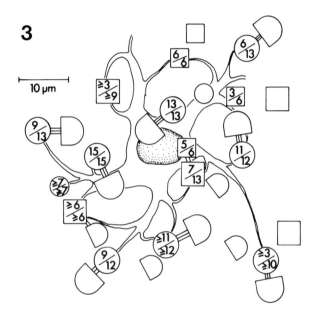

Figs. 1–5. Horizontal planar projections of serially ultrathin-sectioned and reconstructed Golgi-impregnated goldfish cone horizontal cells and their cone contacts. Actual location of nucleus (stippled) and hypothetical outlines typical for cell type are superimposed upon plan of cone pedicles, symbols summarized in Figure 2. Number in cone symbol gives fraction of ribbon synapses (triads) containing at least one dendrite from impregnated cell (≥ indicates number counted in incompletely reconstructed pedicle). Completely enclosed empty symbols: definitely no contacts.

Fig. 1.   Type CH1 cell. Dashed outlines: pedicles located but reconstruction partial and contacts uncertain.

Figs. 2, 3.   Type CH2 cells. Dashed outlines in Figure 2: reconstructed pedicles contacting no impregnated dendrites, tentatively identified as R cones. Other cones not contacted are not indicated in Figure 2.

Figs. 4,5.   See next page.

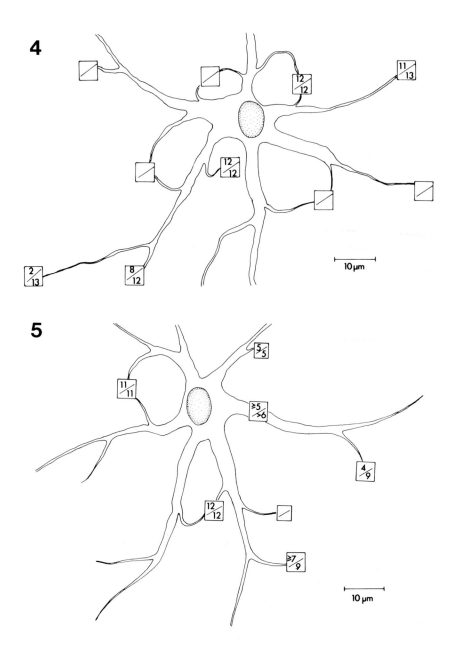

Figs. 4, 5.   Type CH3 cells. Because these cells spread so widely, many of their contacts must have been missed. Empty symbols indicate cones definitely contacted but only partially reconstructed.

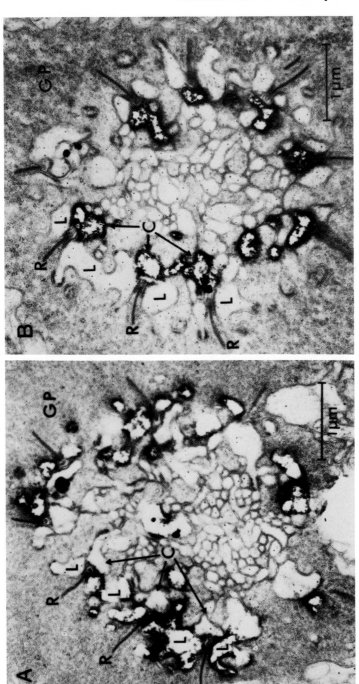

Fig. 6. Electron micrographs of horizontal ultrathin sections through pedicles of G cones (GP) in goldfish retina showing numerous presynaptic ribbons (R) and postsynaptic triads comprising central (C) and lateral (L) cone horizontal cell processes. Dendrites of Golgi-impregnated CH1 cells (A) are predominantly lateral in distribution whereas dendrites of CH2 cells (B) are central. Reprinted, with permission, from Stell et al [23] (Copyright 1975 by the American Association for the Advancement of Science).

[28], and that CH1 cells are GABA-ergic [7] and can modulate cone activity by a GABA-ergic mechanism [29–31]. A diagram summarizing the main pathways is shown in Figure 7.

We undertook further studies of the ultrastructure of horizontal cell membranes in an attempt to characterize their synaptic contacts as to location, direction and mechanism. First, we examined the specializations of membranes revealed by routine fixation, sectioning, and staining [5, 32]. We found the centrally placed cone horizontal cell dendrites (CH1 in R cones, CH2 in G cones, CH3 in B cones) to be very simple in ultrastructure, unspecialized except for a thick undercoat on the membranes nearest the synaptic ridge (Figs. 8–11). The laterally placed dendrites (CH1 in R and G cones, CH2 in B cones, CH3 in miniature B cones) are similarly specialized at the ridge apex and along symmetrical contacts with the central CHC dendrite (Fig. 11A, a and a′). Toward the base of the synaptic ridge there is an almost imperceptible change in the membrane undercoating, opposite a thin amorphous extracellular lamella near the cone synaptic vesicle discharge site (Figs. 8 and 9,b in 11A). Reconstruction from serial sections (Fig. 12) shows that the membrane undercoatings (a, b) are coextensive with the arciform density and its closely related band of vesicle discharge sites, beyond which the synaptic ribbon extends for some distance. This coextension seems to implicate the undercoated CHC membranes in a process related to arciform density and vesicle discharge, such as reception of cone synaptic transmitter or ionic channels controlled by it. The symmetrical

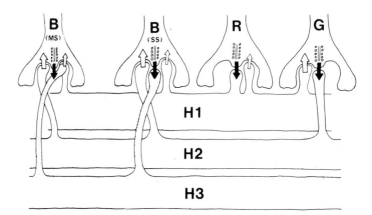

Fig. 7. Cone horizontal cell pathways in goldfish. Filled arrows indicate major sign-conserving (excitatory) synapses whereas clear arrows indicate major sign-inverting (inhibitory) synapses. Not shown are minor sign-conserving synaptic inputs assumed to go from each cell to its postsynaptic horizontal cell dendrites. H1 = monophasic L-type, H2 = biphasic C-type, and H3 = triphasic C-type S-potential. Reprinted, with permission, from Stell [20] (Copyright 1980 by Adam Hilger).

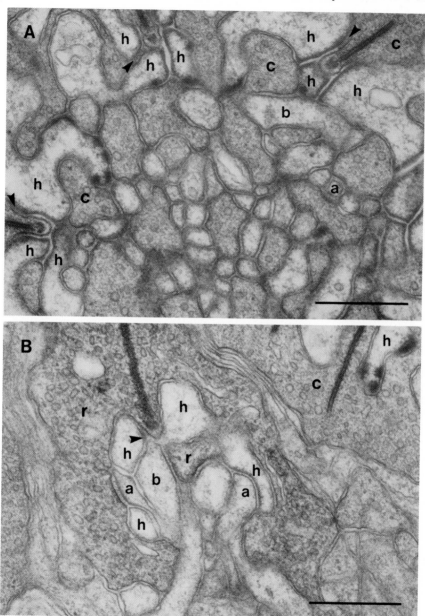

Fig. 8. Electron micrographs of goldfish photoreceptor synapses after conventional fixation, embedding, horizontal thin-sectioning, and staining (Ref. [5]); (A) cone synapse showing three all-HC ribbon synapse triads. c, cone cytoplasm; h, horizontal cell dendrite; a, type a (hyperpolarizing) and b, type b (depolarizing) bipolar cell dendrite. Arrowheads indicate extracellular lamellae; scale marker 0.5 μm; (B) rod synapse; r, rod cytoplasm; other abbreviations, symbols, and scale as in A.

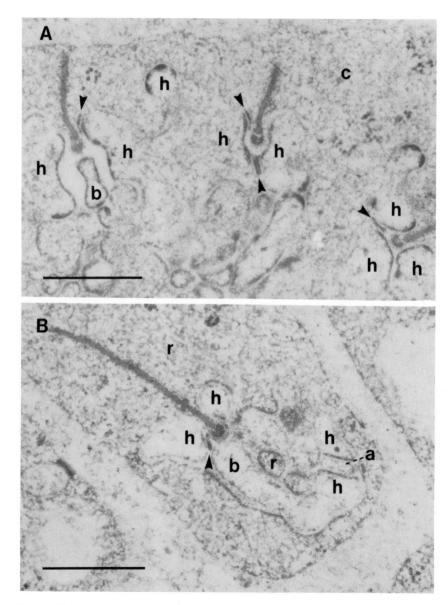

Fig. 9. Electron micrographs of goldfish photoreceptor synapses after aldehyde fixation only, followed by en bloc staining with ethanolic phosphotungstic acid (E-PTA). Abbreviations, symbols, and scale as in Figure 8.

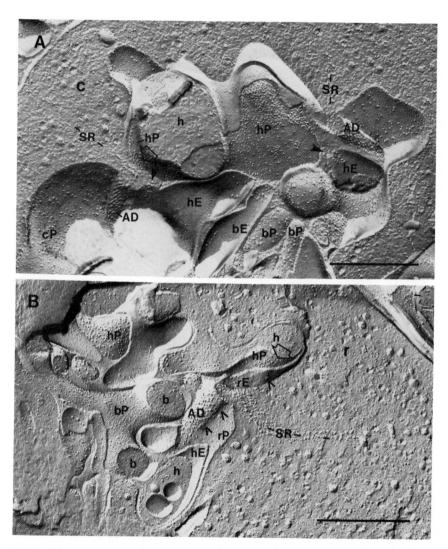

Fig. 10. Electron micrographs of goldfish photoreceptor synapses after aldehyde fixation, glycerol substitution, freeze-fracturing, Pt shadowing (from below), and carbon replication. SR, cross-fractured synaptic ribbon; AD, P-face of synaptic ridge membrane over arciform density; P, P-face (inner leaflet of membrane); E, E-face (outer leaflet of membrane); large clear arrow, patch of P-face particles on horizontal cell membrane opposite photoreceptor vesicle release sites (inverted v). Other abbreviations, symbols, and scale as in Figure 8.

junctions between lateral and central CHC dendrites frequently also include an intermediate, amorphous, extracellular lamella, seen in Figures 8, 10, and 11A, and stained with ethanolic PTA (E-PTA) in Figure 9A. Farther from the ribbon synapse, in light-adapted retinas the lateral CHC processes bear finger-like extensions [4, 32, 33] which contain bar-shaped patches of electron-dense material beneath their membrane (Figs. 8 and 9, c and c' in 11A).

E-PTA, which is often selective for synaptic membrane proteins [34], stains intensely all of the CHC membrane undercoatings (a, b, c) as well as the cone-CHC and CHC-CHC extracellular lamellae (Fig. 9). Freeze-fracture studies [35] show that the undercoated CHC membranes are packed with P-face intramembrane particles (Fig. 10) reminiscent of those thought to represent muscle and electroplax acetylcholine receptors [36, 37]. The CHC membranes bear rows of E-face particles along both types of extracellular lamellae, but are not noticeably specialized at the dense submembrane patches (c) of the finger-like extensions

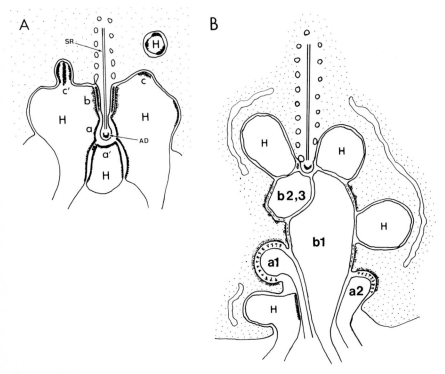

Fig. 11. Diagrams (not to scale) of arrangements in goldfish photoreceptor ribbon synapse. (A) Horizontal cell (H) triad found in cones of all types. (B) Relationships of rod horizontal cell process (H) to dendrites of mixed bipolars (a1, a2, b1, b2, b3). See Figures 8–10 and text. Reprinted, with permission, from Stell [32] (Copyright 1976 by The C.V. Mosby Company).

of lateral dendrites (Fig. 10). We have observed no signs of vesicle attachment in CHC membranes. Studies such as these give further reason to suppose (i) that central and lateral CHC dendrites respond to photoreceptor transmitter, (ii) that central CHC dendrites do not release transmitter in close proximity to either cones or other CHC dendrites at the ribbon contact, and (iii) that lateral CHC dendrites do not release transmitter in close proximity to central CHC membranes. Where the lateral CHC dendrites do release transmitter, and where cones respond to it, remains a complete mystery.

The ultrastructure of RHC membranes is equally interesting and unrevealing. Serial reconstructions [38] show that the (usually) single RH dendritic terminal ends as a pair of lateral processes in the rod ribbon synapse (Fig. 13). The membrane of these processes bears a long, narrow strip of undercoating, readily visible to conventionally prepared (Fig. 8B) or E-PTA-stained material (Fig. 9B), along the apex of the synaptic ridge. Small tufts or lamellae of amorphous, E-PTA-positive material are sometimes seen, not between rod and RH but at the angle between RH, ridge apex, and central bipolar cell dendrite (Figs. 8B, 9B, 11B). Freeze-fracture [35] reveals only modest numbers of P-face particles in RHC dendrites along the ridge apex (Fig. 10B), in contrast with the marked concentration of P-face particles in the presumed postsynaptic region of CHC dendrites. The most noteworthy specialization of RH membranes is found at a distance from the ribbon synapse, where the RH contacts dendrites of type *a* (mixed rod-cone, center-hyperpolarizing) bipolars [32]. According to widely accepted concepts of outer synaptic layer organization such a contact, if functional, might be interpreted as mediating RH-to-bipolar information transfer. The ultrastructure of the contact, however—an unusually narrow cleft, densely undercoated RH membranes (Figs. 8B, 9B), and numerous close-packed P-face particles without signs of vesicle attachment in the RH membrane [35]—is not suggestive of a presynaptic role for RH in a chemical synapse at this contact. We do know, of course, that cyprinid rod horizontals respond to light under scotopic conditions, but apart from this we are in the dark as to their retinal circuit functions.

Intracellular Recording and Marking

The assignment of monophasic responses to type CH1, biphasic to CH2, and triphasic to CH3 cells, was proposed by Stell and Lightfoot [5] as the most economical explanation of their structural connectivity data. Cone horizontal cells had been distinguished from rod horizontals [39, 40], both somata and axon terminals had been identified as sources of S-potentials [39], and some indications of morphological differentiation of the different functional CHC types had been revealed [17, 41] by recording and injection of fluorescent dyes in carp retina. Subsequently, Weiler [42, 43] confirmed conclusively with fluorescent dyes that our structure/function assignments were correct in carp. We decided to attempt a confirmation in goldfish with a marker suitable for electron as well as light

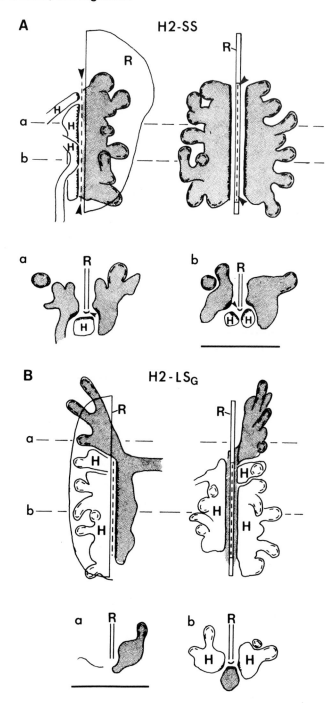

microscopy, so that the contact patterns of functionally identified cells could be examined at high resolution.

We isolated retinas from dark-adapted goldfish 15–25 cm long, mounted them receptor-side up on a Kimwipe pad in a two-sided chamber. The upper chamber received light stimuli (active area ≤ 3mm), a microelectrode, and oxygenated teleost saline flowing 2 ml/min. Retinas prepared this way remain viable for hours and are amenable to both physiological and pharmacological experiments on cells of many functional types [44]. Glass micropipettes of appropriate shape and size (determined empirically) were filled with 3% horseradish peroxidase (HRP, Sigma type VI) in 0.6 M KCl, total resistance 100–350 Mohm measured in fish saline, unbeveled. Responses were recorded to centered circular stimuli

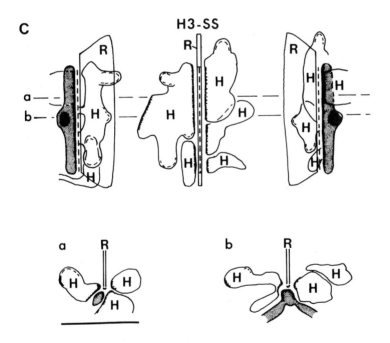

Fig. 12. Graphical reconstructions of serially ultrathin-sectioned goldfish cone ribbon synapses. Golgi-impregnated cone horizontal cell processes are stippled: (A) CH2 in contact with SS blue-sensitive cone; (B) CH2 in contact with LS green-sensitive cone; and (C) CH3 in contact with SS blue-sensitive cone. Upper part of each figure shows orthogonal views of reconstructed ribbon synapse with line-of-sight in the plane of the retina; lower part shows single cross-sections of synapse in planes indicated by a and b; R, synaptic ribbon. Dotted line along R (arrowhead), arciform density. H, unimpregnated CHC processes. Dotted lines in CHC processes, submembrane plaques. Scale marker (bottom), 1 μm.

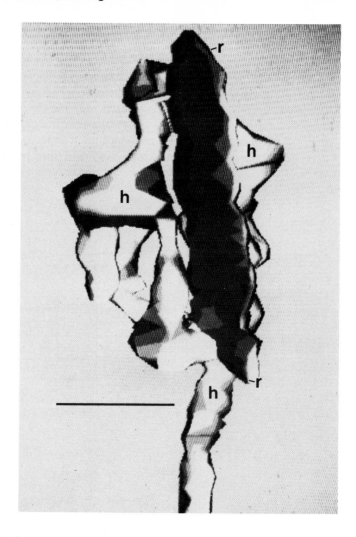

Fig. 13. Computer reconstruction from serial sections of rod horizontal cell dendritic terminal (h) in relation to rod synaptic ribbon (r). Scale marker 0.5 μm.

of various diameters, wavelengths, intensities, and durations. After recording, HRP was injected by passing 0.8- to 2.0-nA current pulses, electrode positive, duration 1 sec, and duty cycle 0.77, for 3–5 min. A small response could still be recorded after injection. The whole retina was fixed with phosphate-buffered 2.5% glutaraldehyde plus 3% sucrose for 12–18 hr at 4°C, reacted histochemically with buffered 0.1% H_2O_2 plus saturated 3.3'-diaminobenzidine for 15 min at 4°C, and examined as an aqueous whole mount to locate marked cells and draw them with the aid of a camera lucida. The retina was then trimmed and postfixed in buffered 1% OsO_4 plus 3% sucrose for 1 hr at 4°C, stained en bloc with uranyl acetate at pH 5, dehydrated, embedded in Epon, and sectioned vertically at 50 μm with a sliding microtome as if it were a Golgi preparation [5]. Serial 50-μm sections were surveyed, stained cells were drawn and photographed, and selected cells were remounted, ultrathin-sectioned, and observed in the electron microscope as described previously [5, 23].

To date we have been able to identify positively CH1 cells as the source of monophasic or L-type cone S-potentials and RH cells as the source of scotopic S-potentials. Commonly recorded S-potentials fell into two classes: hyperpolarizing *rod type,* having $\lambda_{max} \simeq 525$ nm, large amplitude, slow onset and recovery, and high sensitivity; and hyperpolarizing; (monophasic, L-type) *cone type,* having $\lambda_{max} \simeq 621$ nm, small amplitude, rapid onset and recovery, and low sensitivity (Fig. 14). In the light microscope, cells identified functionally as rod horizontals (Figs. 15, 16A) resembled closely those described by Golgi impregnation [4, 6, 45] and did not appear to have axons as did carp rod horizontal cells injected by Lucifer Yellow by Kaneko and Stuart [46]. Electron microscopy (Fig. 17B)

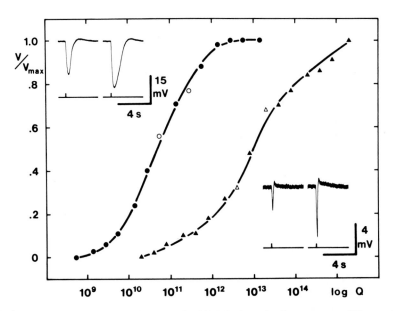

Fig. 14.   Normalized amplitude (V/V_{max}) of goldfish horizontal cell responses to 100-msec light pulses as a function of stimulus intensity (log quanta·cm^{-1}·sec^{-1}). V_{max} for RHC = 31.5 mV, V_{max} for CH1 = 9.8 mV; λ = 525 nm for RHC (circles), λ = 621 nm for CH1 (triangles). Filled symbols show data points only, open symbols give data points for recordings illustrated in insets (RHC upper left, CH1 lower right, with separate calibrations). Curves were fitted by eye.

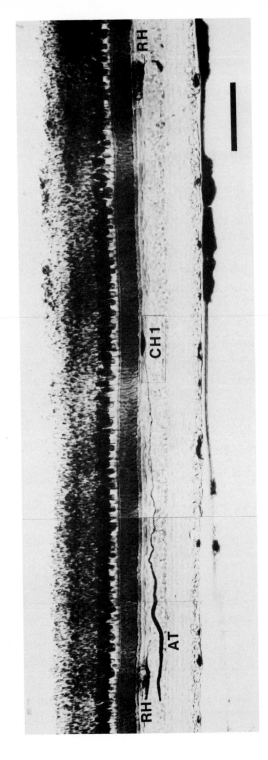

Fig. 15. Light-microscopical survey (montage, different focus levels) of HRP-injected goldfish horizontal cells in 50μm section. Left and right, apparently axonless rod horizontal cells (RH). Center, cone horizontal cell (CH1) with axon and axon terminal (AT) to left. Scale marker 100 μm.

A

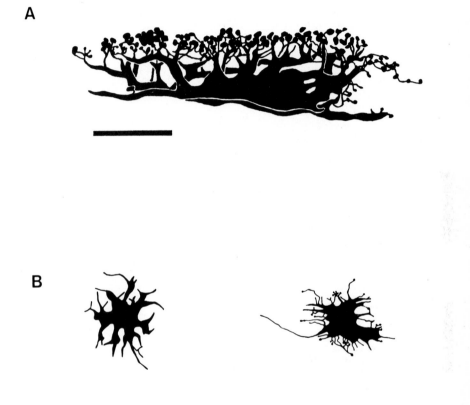

B

Fig. 16.   Camera lucida drawings of HRP-injected goldfish horizontal cells. (A) Vertically sectioned rod horizontal cell showing characteristic candelabra-like dendritic branching pattern and knobby terminals within rod spherules (Refs [4,22]). Scale marker 20 μm. (B) Whole mounted monophasic photopic L-type (CH1) goldfish cone horizontal cells, one with initial portion of axon. Scale marker 50 μm.

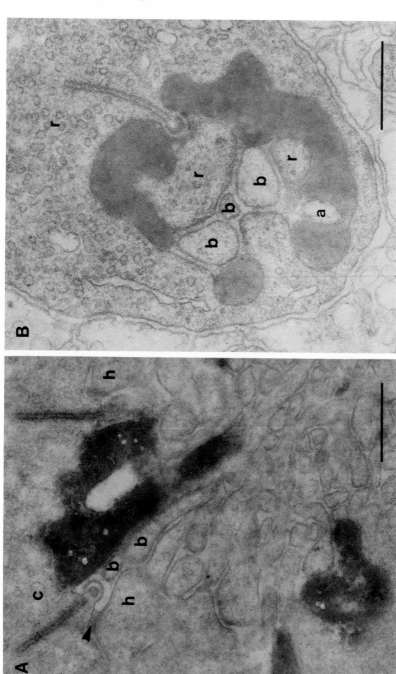

Fig. 17. Electron micrographs of HRP-injected goldfish horizontal cells: (A) Cone horizontal (CH1) in R cone pedicle. (B) Rod horizontal in rod spherule. Symbols and abbreviations as in Figure 8. Scale marker 0.5 μm.

showed that dendrites of these cells terminated in rod spherules, as expected from Golgi-EM studies [4, 21, 22]. Cells identified functionally as photopic L-type (Figs. 15, 16B) resembled closely the cells of type "H1" described by Golgi impregnation [5, 6] and usually could be seen in their entirety (soma + axon) in whole mounts despite the unfavorable optical conditions of aqueous mounting. Electron microscopy of these cells (Fig 17A) showed that their dendrites invaginated the pedicles of cones of all types, specifically R cones, usually ending laterally in ribbon synapses as described by Golgi-EM [4, 5, 21–23].

CONCLUSION

The assignment of photopic monophasic, biphasic, and triphasic, and scotopic S-potentials to CH1, CH2, CH3, and RH cells seems no longer to be in any doubt. Demonstrations of synaptic transmission from CH1 cells to R and G cones as well as details of HC membrane ultrastructure support powerful arguments that the more complex cone S-potentials are generated by a chromatically coded chain of cone horizontal cells acting through cones, as we proposed in 1975. Other actions of cone and rod horizontal cells, most especially their role in modifying bipolar cell responses and the function of their axons, remain to be clarified. The slow potential of Svaetichin, the S-potential, still challenges and fascinates us, like a half-veiled woman, with its beauty and mystery.

ACKNOWLEDGMENTS

We are happy to acknowledge the contributions of Robert Marc, Andrew Ishida, Andre Nagy, Thomas Wheeler, Harold Leeper, and Mel Lockhart to the excitement of our laboratory during the years when this work was taking shape, and to the Medical Research Council of Canada and the Alberta Heritage Foundation for Medical Research for their support at the time this was written. We thank Mary Pollock and Susan Vos for typing the manuscript, and Harold DeC. Clarke for assistance in preparing the figures.

This work was supported by USPHS Research Grants EY 00331 and EY 01190 and a Research to Prevent Blindness—William and Mary Greve International Research Scholarship to W.K. Stell, and by a postdoctoral fellowship of the Swiss National Science Foundation to R.Kretz

REFERENCES

1. Stell WK: The morphological organization of the vertebrate retina. In Fuortes MGF(ed): "Handbook of Sensory Physiology: Physiology of Photoreceptor Organs." Berlin, Heidelberg, New York: Springer-Verlag, 1972, p 111.
2. Werblin FS, Dowling JE: Organization of the retina of the mudpuppy, *Necturus maculosus*. II. Intracellular recording. J Neurophysiol 32:339, 1969.
3. Kaneko A: Physiological and morphological identification of horizontal, bipolar and amacrine cells in goldfish retina. J Physiol 207:623, 1970.
4. Stell WK: The structure and relationships of horizontal cells and photoreceptor-bipolar synaptic

complexes in goldfish retina. Amer J Anat 121:401, 1967.

5. Stell WK, Lightfoot DO: Color-specific interconnections of cones and horizontal cells in the retina of the goldfish. J Comp Neurol 159:473, 1975.

6. Stell WK: Horizontal cell axons and axon terminals in goldfish retina. J Comp Neurol 159:503, 1975.

7. Marc RE, Stell WK, Bok D, Lam DMK: GABA-ergic pathways in the goldfish retina. J Comp Neurol 182:221, 1978.

8. Stell WK, Hárosi FI: Cone structure and visual pigment content in the retina of the goldfish. Vision Res 16:647, 1976.

9. Spekreijse H, Norton AL: The dynamic characteristics of color-coded S-potentials. J Gen Physiol 56:1, 1970.

10. Wagner HG, MacNichol EF Jr, Wolbarsht ML: The response properties of single ganglion cells in the goldfish retina. J Gen Physiol 43 (6, part 2):45, 1960.

11. Orlov OYu, Maksimova EM: S-potential sources as excitation pools. Vision Res 5:573, 1965.

12. Mitarai G: Glia-neuron interaction in carp retina. Glia potentials revealed by microelectrode with lithium carmine. In Seno S, Cowdry EV (eds): "Intracellular Membranous Structure." Okayama: Japan Soc Cell Biol, 1965, p 549.

13. Naka K-I, Rushton WAH: S-potentials from luminosity units in the retina of fish (Cyprinidae). J Physiol (London) 185:587, 1966.

14. Tamura T, Niwa H: Spectral sensitivity and color vision of fish as indicated by S-potential. Comp Biochem Physiol 22:745, 1967.

15. Witkovsky P: A comparison of ganglion cell and S-potential response properties in the carp retina. J Neurophys 30:546, 1967.

16. Norton AL, Spekreijse H, Wolbarsht ML, Wagner HG: Receptive field organization of the S-potential. Science 160:1021, 1968.

17. Mitarai G, Asano T, Miyake Y: Identification of five types of S-potential and their corresponding generating sites in the horizontal cells of the carp retina. Japan J Ophthal 18:161, 1974.

18. Abramov I: Retinal mechanisms of colour vision. In Fuortes MGF (ed): "Handbook of Sensory Physiology: Physiology of Photoreceptor Organs." Berlin, Heidelberg, New York: Springer-Verlag, 1972, p 567.

19. Lockhart ME, Stell WK: Invaginating telodendria: A pathway for color-specific interconnections between golfish cones. Invest Ophthal Vis Sci 18 Suppl:82, 1979.

20. Stell WK: Photoreceptor-specific pathways in goldfish retina: A world of colour, a wealth of connections. In Verriest G (ed): "Colour Vision Deficiencies V." Bristol: Adam Hilger, 1980, p 1.

21. Stell WK: Correlated light and electron microscope observations on Golgi preparations of goldfish retina. J Cell Biol 23:89A, 1964.

22. Stell WK: Correlation of retinal cytoarchitecture and ultrastructure in Golgi preparations. Anat Rec 153:389, 1965.

23. Stell WK, Lightfoot DO, Wheeler TG, Leeper HF: Goldfish retina: Functional polarization of cone horizontal cell dendrites and synapses. Science 190:989, 1975.

24. Scholes JH: Colour receptors, and their synaptic connexions in the retina of a cyprinid fish. Phil Trans Roy Soc London B 270:61, 1976.

25. Kolb H: Organization of the outer plexiform layer of the primate retina: Electron microscopy of Golgi-impregnated cells. Phil Trans Roy Soc London B 258:261, 1970.

26. Wagner H-J: Cell types and connectivity patterns in mosaic retinas. Advan Anat Embryol Cell Biol 55(3):1, 1978.

27. Fukurotani K, Hase H, Hara K-I: Neuronal network in the retina—Interactions between photoreceptors (cones) and horizontal cells. Trans IECE Japan E 60:431, 1977.

28. Burkhardt DA, Hassin G: Influences of cones upon chromatic- and luminosity-type horizontal cells in pikeperch retinas. J Physiol (London) 281:125, 1978.

29. Lam DMK, Lasater EM, Naka K-I: γ-Aminobutyric acid: A neurotransmitter candidate for cone horizontal cells of the catfish retina. Proc Nat Acad Sci 75:6310, 1978.
30. Murakami M, Shimoda Y, Nakatani K: Effects of GABA on neuronal activities in the distal retina of the carp. Sens Proc 2:324, 1979.
31. Djamgoz MBA, Ruddock K: Effects of picrotoxin and strychnine on fish retinal S-potentials: Evidence for inhibitory control of depolarizing responses. Neurosci Lett 12:329, 1979.
32. Stell WK: Functional polarization of horizontal cell dendrites in goldfish retina. Invest Ophthalmol 15:895, 1976.
33. Wagner H-J: Light-dependent plasticity of the morphology of horizontal cell terminals in cone pedicles of fish retinas. J Neurocytol 9:573, 1980.
34. Pfenninger KH: Synaptic morphology and cytochemistry. Progr Histochem Cytochem 5:1, 1973.
35. Nagy AR, Stell WK, Lightfoot DO: A freeze-fracture study of photoreceptor synapses in goldfish retina. Submitted for publication.
36. Nickel E, Potter LT: Ultrastructure of isolated membranes of Torpedo electric tissue. Brain Res 57:508, 1973.
37. Heuser JE, Salpeter SR: Organization of acetylcholine receptors in quick-frozen, deep-etched and rotary-replicated Torpedo postsynaptic membrane. J Cell Biol 82:150, 1979.
38. Stell WK, Lightfoot DO: Computer-aided reconstruction and analysis of goldfish rod synapses. Seitai no Kagaku 30:173, 1979.
39. Kaneko A: Physiological studies of single retinal cells and their morphological identification. Vision Res Suppl 3:17, 1971.
40. Kaneko A, Yamada M: S-potentials in the dark-adapted retina of the carp. J Physiol (London): 277:261, 1972.
41. Hashimoto Y, Kato A, Inokuchi M, Watanabe K: Re-examination of horizontal cells in the carp retina with Procion Yellow electrode. Vision Res 16:25, 1976.
42. Weiler R: Horizontal cells of the carp retina: Golgi impregnation and Procion Yellow injection. Cell Tiss Res 195:515, 1978.
43. Weiler R, Zettler F: The axon-bearing horizontal cells in the teleost retina are functional as well as structural units. Vision Res 19:1261, 1979.
44. Ishida A, Fain GL: D-aspartate potentiates the effects of L-glutamate on horizontal cells in goldfish retina. Proc Nat Acad Sci, in press, 1981.
45. Cajal SR: La rétine des vertébrés. La Cellule 9:121, 1892.
46. Kaneko A, Stuart AE: Coupling between horizontal cells in the carp retina examined by diffusion of Lucifer Yellow. Biol Bull 159:486, 1980.

The S-Potential, pages 77–104
© 1982 Alan R. Liss, Inc., 150 Fifth Avenue, New York, NY 10011

Horizontal Cells in Turtle Retina: Structure, Synaptic Connections, and Visual Processing

Harold F. Leeper and David R. Copenhagen

A heightened interest in turtle horizontal cells was sparked by the discovery by Baylor et al [1] that signals generated in these cells oppose the normal light-induced potentials in cones. Thus horizontal cells play an important role in a complex set of synaptic interactions in which cones are driven summatively through direct interactions with neighboring cones and antagonistically through feedback from horizontal cells. Such feedback interactions are a common feature of neuronal processing throughout the nervous systems of many classes, the turtle horizontal cell-to-cone feedback synapse being one of the best characterized feedback circuits in any vertebrate nervous system. In addition to providing knowledge of the mechanism and role of feedback in sensory processing, the rather extensive studies involving turtle horizontal cells have contributed substantially to our knowledge of the morphology and physiology involved in the initial stages of color processing in vertebrate retinas. These studies have investigated in great detail the high specificity of connections between horizontal cells and photoreceptor cells, the pattern of which appears to be intimately involved in the generation of color-coded responses of horizontal cells. The purpose of this chapter, then, is to review the morphology and physiology of turtle horizontal cells with an interest in understanding their role in color coding and neuronal processing, as well as to point out certain problems and paradoxes which reflect our current level of knowledge.

BACKGROUND

Turtle horizontal cells were observed in histological preparations as long ago as 1857 by Heinrich Müller [2], and since that first description, the identity and classification of these cells often has been contradictory and confused. Much of this confusion centered on the identity and nature of a class of anucleate, tuberous structures adjacent to the more conventional stellate cells at the outer margin of the inner nuclear layer. Both Müller [2] and Schiefferdecker [3] noted the lack of nucleus, but each called the structure a cell. Since that time, additional turtle horizontal cell types have been described periodically, with the anuclate, tuberous structures generally considered to be cells [4–8]. The most complete of these investigations reveals four morphological classes of turtle horizontal cells, and that the anuclate, tuberous structures are horizontal cell axon terminals [8]. Figure 1 summarizes these cell types and their common names.

Electrophysiologically, both luminosity- (L-) and chromaticity- (C-)type horizontal cell responses have been recorded from turtle retina. As in teleosts, L-type cells are those cells which hyperpolarize to light stimuli of any wavelength, whereas C-type cells hyperpolarize or depolarize to light stimuli depending upon the wavelength [9–11]. Simon [5] first distinguished between two classes of turtle L-type responses (L1 and L2) and determined that these responses arose from morphologically distinct structures. Miller et al [6] reported C-type turtle horizontal cells which depolarized to red stimuli and hyperpolarized to green stimuli; therefore, these cells were designated R/G C-type according to tradition [9–11]. Fuortes and Simon [12] reported a second class of turtle C-type cell which depolarized to green stimuli and hyperpolarized to blue stimuli (G/B). Yazulla [13] studied both L- and C-type responses in the turtle; he reported that the chromatic inputs to some L-type horizontal cells were more complex than originally thought and concluded that the G/B cells of Fuortes and Simon also hyperpolarized to red stimuli and may be considered G/BR cells. These names are also included in Figure 1.

Primarily two species have been used in investigations which bear on the subject of turtle S-potentials. The red-eared slider, Pseudemys scripta elegans, is a docile, fresh water turtle whose photoreceptors are primarily cones, with less than 10% rods [4]. There are three chromatic classes of Pseudemys single cones; their spectral sensitivity peaks, determined by intracellular recording, are 630, 550, and 460 nm [14]. All visual pigments in this retina are vitamin A2-based with spectral absorbance maxima at 620, 518, and 450 nm [15]. The differences between absorbance and sensitivity peaks reflect the filtering action of colored oil droplets in turtle cones [14]. In addition to single cones and rods, Pseudemys retina contains double cones which appear to be electrically coupled pairs of red- and green-sensitive cones; such cells have very broad spectral sensitivity curves [16]. Pseudemys rods apparently contain the same 518-nm pigment as green-sensitive cones [15,17]. The most commonly studied of the turtles, Pseudemys has been used in most work in which photopic and chromatic responses were of primary interest. The common snapping turtle, Chelydra serpentina, is an aggressive fresh water turtle whose rods make up 25 [Leeper, unpublished observation] to 40% [18] of its single photoreceptor population. This species also contains single and double cones, as well as rods with a spectral

Names   Contacts

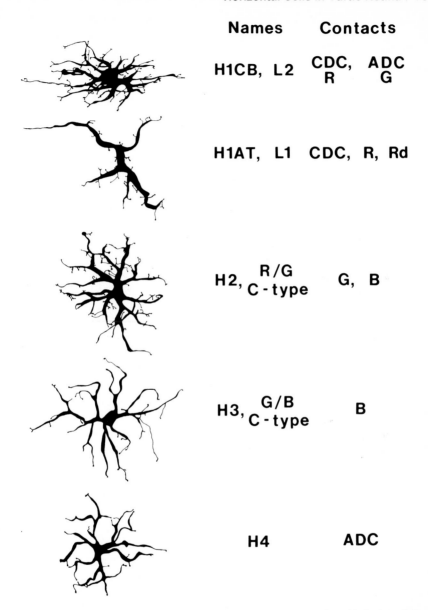

H1CB, L2   CDC,   ADC
                R   G

H1AT, L1 CDC, R, Rd

H2, $\begin{array}{c}R/G\\C\text{-type}\end{array}$ G, B

H3, $\begin{array}{c}G/B\\C\text{-type}\end{array}$ B

H4   ADC

Fig. 1.   Summary figure giving, for each horizontal cell type, a representation of its horizontal view morphology, its name in the morphological scheme of Leeper [8], the type of response it generates (and thus its "name" in the physiological literature), and a summary of the types of photoreceptor cells it contacts: (R) red-sensitive cone; (G) green-sensitive cone; (B) blue-sensitive cone; (CDC) red-sensitive chief member of double cone; (ADC) green-sensitive accessory member of double cone; (Rd) rod. Reprinted, with permission, from Leeper [8] (Copyright 1978 by Alan R. Liss, Inc.).

sensitivity peak at 520 nm [19]. Chelydra has been used primarily to study scotopic responses and interactions between rods.

HORIZONTAL CELLS AND FEEDBACK

Baylor et al [1] found that light responses of Pseudemys cones depend not only upon the photons absorbed by the outer segment of the recorded cell, but also upon photons absorbed by neighboring cones. These effects were found to be of two kinds: neighboring cones interacting directly to sum responses over short distances; and cones separated by larger distances interacting antagonistically. The summation of cone signals occurs over a distance of about 70 μm [1,20], is mediated by electrical rather than chemical synapses [1,20,21], is limited to interactions between cones of the same chromatic class [14], and is believed to result from direct electrical coupling of neighboring cones [4,20, 22,23]. The antagonistic interaction is seen as a depolarizing inflection on the hyperpolarizing cone response induced by a large (eg, 600-μm radius) spot (Fig. 2). These antagonistic interactions increase in magnitude with increasing area of stimulation [1,21], are mediated by chemical rather than electrical synapses [1,24], are not restricted to cones of the same chromatic class [12,25], and are highly labile and particularly susceptible to anoxia [1,22,26]. Three lines of evidence lead to the conclusion that such intractions are mediated by horizontal cells feeding back onto cones:

(1) Depolarizing inflections in cone responses occur only to relatively large stimuli [1,21,25] which are known to be effective stimuli for horizontal cells [5,27–29]. Figure 2 illustrates that feedback occurs only when horizontal cells are strongly activated [1].

(2) Under stimulus conditions which elicit these antagonistic interactions, the response waveforms of cones and horizontal cells are closely matched [21,24]. Note in Figure 2 that the depolarizing inflection in the cone coincides approximately with the peak horizontal cell response, and that this depolarizing inflection in the cone response is in turn reflected in the horizontal cell response.

(3) Most importantly, extrinsic hyperpolarization of horizontal cells has been shown to be capable of eliciting these types of responses from cones. Baylor et al [1] injected currents into a horizontal cell while recording from a neighboring cone and found that a step of hyperpolarizing current produced a transient depolarization of the receptor membrane (Fig. 3). Therefore, unlike the summation interactions between turtle cones which result from direct cone–cone contacts, the antagonistic interactions are mediated by horizontal cells and represent true feedback from second-order neurons onto photoreceptors.

Since the polarity of the polarization is reversed during the feedback interaction, the underlying change in conductance most probably is mediated by chemical rather that electrical synapses. This depolarizing feedback synaptic potential in cones is graded with both the intensity and area of peripheral illumination [1,21,24], and may include a large depolarizing transient (Fig. 3) [24–26]. O'Bryan [24] concluded that the change in cone membrane conductance during feedback is not simple, but rather consists of two separate components with different time courses and reversal levels, and that one of these components represents an increase in membrane conductance. Piccolino and Gerschenfeld [26] further investigated feedback spikes and the synaptic events leading to their generation and found that all Pseudemys cones were capable of showing large depolarizing feedback spikes which result from the activation of a regenerative calcium conductance increase. They also demonstrated that these feedback effects are not necessarily transient, but that sustained peripheral illumination can evoke in cones sustained effects associated with an increase in cone membrane calcium conductance [30].

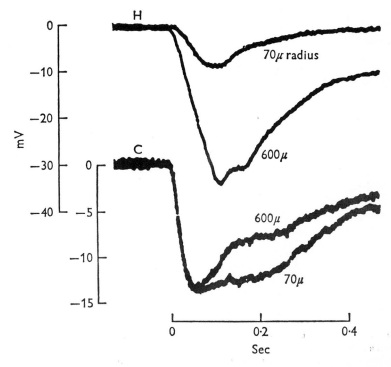

Fig. 2. Simultaneous records from a cone (C) and a horizontal cell (H). Superposed records of responses to stimuli covering different areas. A flash (delivered at time 0) covering a circle of 70-μm radius produced a small response of the horizontal cell and a large, smooth response of the cone. A second flash of the same intensity but covering a circle of 600-μm radius was then given. The response of the horizontal cell was increased. The response of the cone was the same in its initial peak. Later, however, it developed a depolarizing inflection. (From Baylor et al [1].)

The morphological features of the horizontal cell-to-cone feedback synapse have not yet been determined. Horizontal cells make contact with cones by way of small dendritic processes which enter cone synaptic terminals to form "invaginated synapses" characterized by a wedge-shaped synaptic ridge of cone cy-

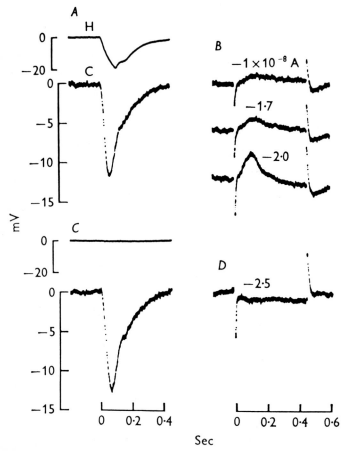

Fig. 3.   Interaction between horizontal cell and cone. (A) Responses evoked by a flash (at time 0) covering a large area (600 μm radius) in a horizontal cell (H) and a nearby cone (C). The response of the horizontal cell develops more slowly and its peak approximately coincides with the inflection in the recovery phase of the cone response. (B) Steps of hyperpolarizing current through the electrode in the horizontal cell produced graded depolarizations in the cone (artifact at make and break of current). The three records correspond to different current intensities through the horizontal cell, as indicated. (C) Recordings after withdrawing the electrode from the horizontal cell. (D) When a hyperpolarizing current was again passed through this extracellular electrode, the microelectrode in the cone picked up a small artifact, but no depolarizing wave. (From Baylor et al [1].)

toplasm which contains a synaptic ribbon (Fig. 5) [4,31]. Adjacent to these ribbons are concentrations of synaptic vesicles which are presumed to contain the chemical transmitter by which cones modify the membrane conductances of the postsynaptic processes; it is concluded that cones are presynaptic to second-order cells at contacts adjacent to the ridge [4,31–34]. While it is generally assumed that horizontal cell-to-cone synapses are also located somewhere in the region of these invaginations, the characteristic morphological features of chemical synapses between neurons are not present to indicate its site; that is, there is no clustering of vesicles in horizontal cell processes [4,31–34]. However, the physiological evidence for the existence of feedback synapses is so compelling that many efforts have been made to correlate other morphological features with this function.

At turtle cone synapses, invaginating processes may distribute themselves to form "dyads" in which two horizontal cell processes are on either side of the ridge, or as "triads" in which a third process is added to the complex at the base of the synaptic ridge (Fig. 5) [4]. The identity of the cell type which gives rise to the central processes has not been established with certainty, although Lasansky [22] considered them likely to be bipolar cell processes. The lateral hor-

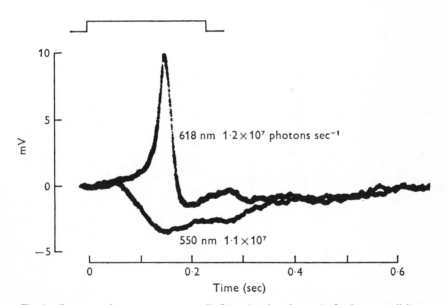

Fig. 4. Response of a green cone to annuli. Steps (monitored at top) of red or green light were applied to an annulus of 1250- to 500-μm radii. The green cone at the center developed a large depolarizing transient for the red stimulus and was hyperpolarized when the light was green. Photon flux over 50 μm² is indicated near each record. (From Fuortes et al [25].)

izontal cell processes engage in two types of specialized contacts with cones; these contacts were classified as "proximal" when the junctions were at the sides of the synaptic ridge (both triads and dyads), or "distal" when the junctions were away from the ridge and at the end of the medial gap between the lateral process (dyads only) (Fig. 5). Lasansky [22] speculated that the proximal junctions might be the site of synapses at which cones are presynaptic, whereas distal junctions are the site of synapses at which the horizontal cells are presynaptic to cones. Freeze-fracturing of the membranes of cones and horizontal cells at invaginated synapses supports the conclusion that proximal junctions are the site of cone-to-horizontal cell transmission, but does not locate with certainty the site of feedback synapses [33,34]. Schaeffer and Raviola [33] found intramembrane particles and synaptic vesicle sites on the cone membrane at proximal junctions; opposite these sites, the horizontal cell membrane contains an elongated aggregate of intra-membrane particles associated with the A face of the plasmalemma. Such features are characteristic of chemical synapses in both central and peripheral nervous systems and indicate that cones are presynaptic to horizontal cells at these sites

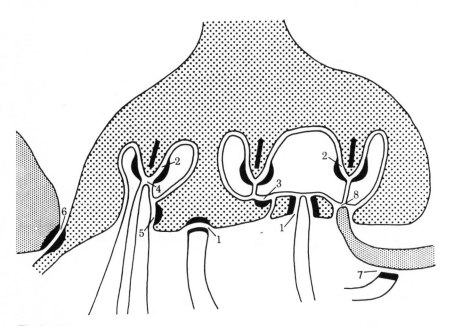

Fig. 5. Diagram illustrating the location of the specialized contacts of a cone pedicle in the turtle retina: (1) basal junctions; (2) proximal junctions of lateral processes (horizontal cell); (3) distal junction of a lateral process; (4) apical junction of a central process in a triad; (5) distal junction of a central process in a triad; (6) junction with an adjacent cone pedicle; (7) en passant junction of a basal process; (8) ending of a basal process. (From Lasansky [4].)

[35–38]. In addition, the horizontal cell membrane contains aggregates of B-face particles either adjacent to the A-face particles or independent of these aggregates and located opposite unspecialized regions of cone membrane [33]. It has not been determined whether these particles correspond to the distal junctions of Lasansky [4]. The lack of sites of interaction between the plasmalemma and the scarce population of horizontal cell vesicles, and the lack of cone membrane specialization opposite the B-face particles, make the function of these particles and the location of the feedback synapses unclear [33]. In the goldfish retina, Stell et al [39] concluded that the position of horizontal cell processes in triadic arrangements might be correlated with synaptic polarity; horizontal cells were thought to be primarily postsynaptic to cones when they occupied the central position of triads, and primarily presynaptic to cones in the lateral positions. Comparable studies of the positions occupied by identified turtle horizontal cell processes in identified cone synaptic terminals might be of great value in advancing our knowledge of the morphology of feedback synapses.

The functional role of horizontal cell feedback onto cones remains speculative, although several possible consequences have been proposed.

(1) Contrast discrimination: The response of turtle horizontal cells under a large spot are larger at the center than at the edge [21,24]. O'Bryan [24] demonstrated that as a consequence the plateau phase of a cone response was decreased less at the edge than at the center of a spot, and concluded that this should lead to a delayed Mach-band effect on the receptor layer. Such an effect may play a role in the enhancement of contrast discrimination, although its role has not been well established.

(2) Adaptation: Bright stimuli initially hyperpolarize and desensitize cones. Negative feedback from horizontal cells acts to depolarize cones, thereby possibly increasing their response range. Thus, feedback may play some role in adaptation, although it is not clear that the effects are large enough to be of major importance [40].

(3) Chromatic processing: Feedback acts to alter the chromatic properties of cones themselves, making their responses wavelength dependent when large stimuli are employed (eg, Fig. 4). Therefore, feedback will affect the processing of chromatic information by the retina. A direct consequence of this effect appears to be the generation of complex, C-type S-potentials in certain horizontal cell types [12,25,41] (see pages 97–99).

CORRELATIONS: L-TYPE UNITS

Sources of Luminosity-type Responses

Simon [5] and Saito et al [7] demonstrated that luminosity responses were generated by two morphologically distinct structures [5,7], and that C-type cells were apparently morphologically different from L-type units [7]. These conclusions were the result of experiments in which the physiological response characteristics of horizontal cells were recorded and then the fluorescent dye Procion yellow was injected to allow the cells to be visualized microscopically. Luminosity responses which had large receptive fields were produced by irregular, tuberous structures for which no clear nuclear region could be demonstrated, and were called L1. Luminosity responses which had smaller receptive fields were called L2 and were generated by stellate cells possessing a distinct soma; the dendrites of these cells often were arranged in an elliptical pattern.

Correlating these morphological features with the structure of Golgi-stained horizontal cells, Leeper [8] concluded that both L1 and L2 luminosity-type responses were produced by the same horizontal cell type which has two distinct parts connected by an axon. Examples of this cell type have cell bodies which possess a dense, often elliptical, array of dendrites, with one of these dendrites giving rise to an axon which courses circuitously across the retina and ends in an irregular, tuberous axon terminal (Fig. 6). These morphological similarities, as well as the nature of the receptor cells contacted by this cell type, led to the conclusion that the axon terminals of this cell type (H1ATs) generate L1-type responses, whereas the cell bodies (H1CBs) generate L2-type responses [8,41]. This conclusion has found strong support by the use of other marker dyes capable of delineating axons and their terminals [42]. Injection of Lucifer yellow into L-type cell bodies resulted in staining of not only the cell body but also (though more faintly) of a nearby axon terminal; the separation between them was an appropriate distance for the separation of an H1 cell body and axon terminal. Similarly, injection of an axon terminal resulted in the staining of a neighboring cell body. Since H1 cells are the only observed turtle horizontal cell type to possess an axon [8], these results support the view that H1 axon terminals are the source of L1-type responses, whereas H1 cell bodies are the source of L2-type responses.

Photoreceptor Contacts of Luminosity-type Units

Simon [5] and Saito et al [7] reported that L1- and L2-type responses were essentially the same except for the sizes of the receptive fields over which they summed their responses; both had similar action spectra and were maximally sensitive to red stimuli. Given these response similarities, one might expect that H1AT and H1CB would contact identical populations of photoreceptors. However, analysis of these contacts reveals this is not to be the case and provides insights into the processing of chromatic information by this retina.

Using a variety of criteria, it is possible to identify not only rods, cones, and double cones in stained sections of retina, but also to distinguish between the chromatic classes of single cone photoreceptors [41,43]. In a morphological analysis of Golgi-stained turtle horizontal cells, Leeper [41] determined that the cell bodies of H1 horizontal cells contacted red- and green-sensitive single cones

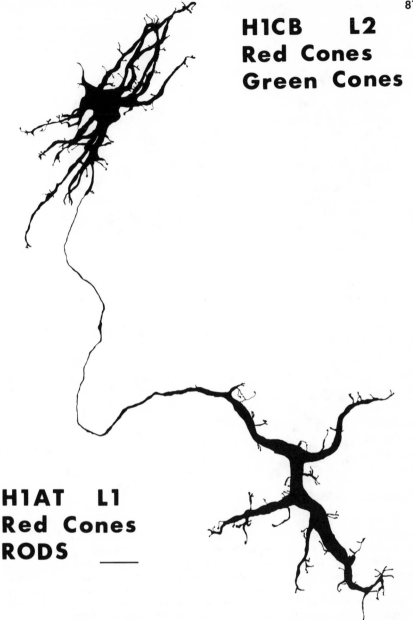

H1CB L2
Red Cones
Green Cones

H1AT L1
Red Cones
RODS ___

Fig. 6.   Camera lucida drawing of a complete H1 horizontal cell from a flat-mounted Golgi-preparation of turtle retina. The H1 cell body (H1CB) and axon terminal (H1AT) are connected by a slender axon. H1CBs contact red- and green-sensitive cones whereas H1ATs contact red-sensitive cones and rods. H1 cells are the only turtle horizontal cells having an axon and H1 axon terminals are the only turtle horizontal cell structures which contact rods. Line = 20 μm. Reprinted, with permission, from Leeper and Copenhagen [44] (Copyright 1979 by Pergamon Press).

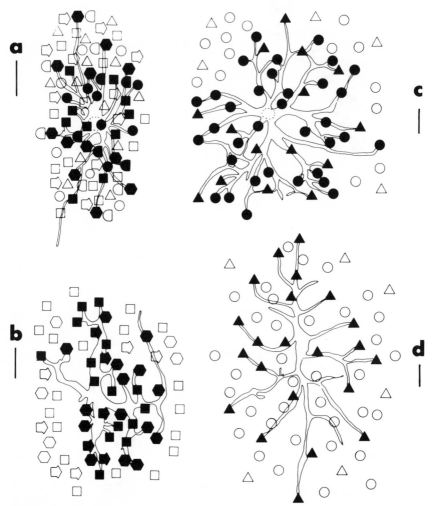

Fig. 7. Receptor cell contacts of an H1CB, H1AT, H2, and H3 determined by analysis of and reconstruction from 1-μm serial sections of Golgi-stained turtle retina. Contacted receptors are represented by filled symbols, whereas noncontacted receptors are represented by open symbols. For the sake of clarity, the locations of certain receptor types have not been included in the cases of H1AT, H2, and H3, since the deleted receptors are clearly not involved in contact with these horizontal cell types. Line next to each cell = 20 μm. (a) H1CB with all receptor cells indicated. (b) H1AT with the location of all red-sensitive single cones, the chief members of double cones and rods indicated. (c) H2 with all green- and blue-sensitive single cones indicated. (d) H3 with all green- and blue-sensitive single cones indicated. □ red-sensitive single cone, ○ green-sensitive single cone, △ blue-sensitive single cone, ◯ chief member of double cone, ◖ accessory member of double cone, ⬠ rod. Reprinted, with permission, from Leeper [41] (Copyright 1978 by Alan R. Liss, Inc.).

and both red- and green-sensitive members of double cones in its dendritic field, whereas the axon terminals of these cells contacted the red-sensitive single and double cones in its dendritic field, but not green-sensitive cones; the axon terminals also contacted rods (Figs. 1 and 7).

The chromatic responses of L1 and L2 have been reported repeatedly to be essentially the same [5,12,25]; in both responses the primary sensitivity is to red-sensitive cones (Fig. 8). However, both response types show some evidence of input from green-sensitive cones, and this input is enhanced in the presence of a red background [12,13,25]. Fuortes and Simon [12] argued that this green impingement was unlikely to come from green-sensitive single cones, since the responses of these cones were slower than the green responses in the horizontal cell. They concluded that this impingement was more likely to come from the green-sensitive members of double cones by way of the red-sensitive members to which they are electrically coupled [16]. The responses of the red-sensitive

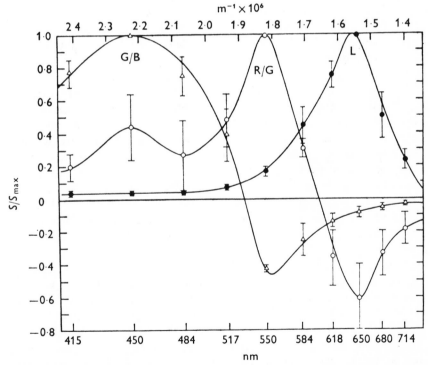

Fig. 8. Spectral sensitivity curves of horizontal cell responses in the linear range. Each point is the mean relative sensitivity measured in 23 L-cells, 16 R/G-cells, and 4 G/B-cells (error bars: standard deviations). Hyperpolarizing responses are plotted up and depolarizing responses are down. (From Fuortes and Simon [12].)

member of such a pair to green stimuli are faster than the responses of green-sensitive single cones, and are matched well to the responses of the L-cells [12]. Thus, neither L1 nor L2 receives substantial input from green-sensitive single cones. This apparent discrepancy between the observation of contacts with green-sensitive cones and the lack of pronounced green sensitivity in L2 (H1 cell body) responses has been explained on the basis of a feedback model for the generation of complex horizontal cell potentials. (This model is presented in more detail below during consideration of the generation of C-type responses.) According to the feedback model, H1CB and H1AT contacts with red-sensitive cones would include both feedforward synapses from cones to horizontal cells to provide the predominant red sensitivity of these responses, as well as to provide the sites of feedback synapses from horizontal cells to cones. H1CB contacts with green-sensitive cones are thought to subserve mainly a feedback function from luminosity cells onto green cones, thereby providing red cone input to certain C-type cells. The results of Yazulla [13], which indicate a pronounced green sensitivity among a small minority of luminosity units, raise the possibility that these contacts may occasionally provide a pathway for feedforward synapses between green-sensitive single cones and H1CBs as well. However, the lack of dye injection markings of the luminosity cells displaying this green sensitivity makes it uncertain whether these responses are, in fact, those of H1CBs or the responses of a cell type which was not observed in Golgi-stained material.

In addition to its contacts with cones, H1ATs contact rods whereas H1CBs do not; this difference provides the most reliable way to distinguish between L1 and L2 responses. The function(s) of these contacts between rods and horizontal cells was at first unclear since neither a feedforward nor a feedback pathway had been established. Copenhagen and Owen [19] looked specifically for the possibility of horizontal cell feedback onto rods and found no evidence to support its existence. Additionally, there was no published evidence of rod input to luminosity-type horizontal cells. This led Leeper and Copenhagen [44] to look specifically for rod input to horizontal cells in well dark-adapted Chelydra serpentina retinas. Their results indicate that the responses of L1 and L2 units differ to dim light stimuli. L1 units (H1ATs) do indeed show a rod-dominated response to dim stimuli, although this rod response never exceeds 2 to 3 mV in amplitude (Fig. 9). To brighter stimuli, the main feature of both L1 and L2 responses is a fast hyperpolarization due to red cone input. Even to bright stimuli, however, L1 responses continue to include a protracted, low-amplitude hyperpolarization due to rod input. The reason why the rod response in H1 axon terminals is of such low amplitude is not yet known. However, it is known that this phenomenon does not result from a gross inequality in the number of rods and cones with which Chelydra H1 axon terminals make contact. Figure 10 shows the distribution of contacted rods and cones for a typical Chelydra axon terminal; this terminal contacts 26 cones and 16 rods. Therefore, it is more likely that this reduced rod input reflects differences in the extent or efficacy of rod and cone synaptic interactions with horizontal cells within the synaptic terminals of these photoreceptors. The ultrastructure of the contacts between turtle rods and horizontal cells has not yet been examined and would perhaps provide some insight into the reasons for the low-amplitude rod input.

Receptive Field Properties of Luminosity-type Units

In many species, horizontal cells of the same subtype are coupled by gap junctions to form an electrical syncytium [31,34,35], and therefore horizontal cells commonly have receptive fields which are much larger than their dendritic

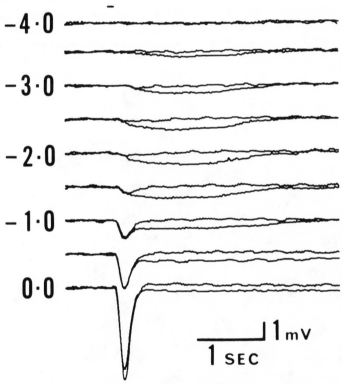

Fig. 9. Superposed responses from two different L-type units recorded from the same *Chelydra* retina. Responses were elicited by a series of 3000-μm diameter spot flashes of 514 nm light of increasing intensity. Waveforms are the computer average of 10 responses at each intensity. Stimulus mark above the −4.0 response. These units were selected to demonstrate the qualitative differences between luminosity-type units showing well-matched fast components. Other units producing mixed responses had slow components with larger saturating amplitude, as well as greater sensitivity. Reprinted, with permission, from Leeper and Copenhagen [44] (Copyright 1977 by Pergamon Press).

fields [27,46,47]. This is also true in turtle retina where horizontal cell receptive fields may be 25 or more times larger than the area covered by the dendritic fields [5,7,28,44]. Simon [5] and Byzov [48] have impaled pairs of turtle L-type cells and demonstrated that L1s and L2s are electrically coupled to other members of the same subtype, but are not coupled to one another. As in other species, this coupling appears to be by way of gap junctions [34].

Simon [5] first proposed that the clearest distinction between the two luminosity-type responses in the turtle was the difference in receptive field size; L1 responses were reported to sum signals over a retinal area approximately six times greater than found for L2 responses. These results were obtained by measuring the magnitude of the response as the size of the stimulating spot was increased. Using a combination of spot and bar stimuli, Lamb [28] also measured horizontal cell receptive field sizes in Pseudemys and found a continuum of sizes without any indication of two groups. This raises doubts about the ability to distinguish reliably between L1 and L2 on the basis of receptive field size alone.

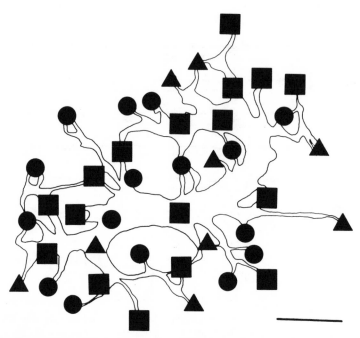

Fig. 10. Receptor cell contacts of a Chelydra serpentina H1 axon terminal determined by analysis of and reconstruction from 1 μm serial sections. Only contacted photoreceptors are indicated. Due to the higher proportion of rods in Chelydra retina, Chelydra H1 axon terminals contact greater numbers of rods than do Pseudemys H1 axon terminals (see Fig. 7). ■ red-sensitive single cone, ▲ red-sensitive chief member of a double cone, ● rod. Bar = 20 μm. [Leeper and Copenhagen, unpublished.]

Leeper and Copenhagen find in Chelydra retina that whereas the receptive field sizes of L1 are larger in general than those for L2 within a limited retinal area, these sizes form a bimodal continuum with considerable overlap between the two types when comparisons are made between retinal regions (Table I). Our results were obtained by using a slit of light as the stimulus and plotting the amplitude of the response as a function of position as the slit was moved across the retina (Fig. 11). This analysis can be used to determine a "length constant" for the cell, and this in turn is proportional to the cell's receptive field [20,28]. In addition, our results were based upon identifying the response type on the basis of dye-injection morphology and/or the presence or absence of rod input, which we find to be a reliable distinguishing characteristic. In Psuedemys, the size of horizontal cells varies greatly, but systematically, over the surface of the

TABLE I. Summary of the Length Constants λ of 24 Chelydra Luminosity Units[a]

H1 Cell body = L2 (λ Avg)	H1 Axon terminal = L1 (λ Avg)
136	
138	
180	
185	
197	
200	
223	225
331	
	462
	480
	500
	540
	560
595	585
	600
690	672
	770
801	
	880
	1215
	1620

[a]Cells were usually located in the superior nasal quadrant, but no attempt was made to restrict precisely the area from which recordings were made. Data were analyzed and plotted as explained in the text and Figure 11. Values of obtained on each side of the center of the field were averaged, and the reported λs are the average of two to six values for each cell [Leeper and Copenhagen, unpublished].

retina (Fig. 12). Because of this variation, which we believe would be reflected in the receptive field properties of these cells, identification of luminosity response types on the basis of receptive field size should be even more difficult in Pseudemys than in Chelydra which does not show such extensive variation of horizontal cell size. We here propose that the most reliable identifying distinction between L1 and L2 responses is the presence of rod input to the L1 responses of H1 axon terminals and their absence in the L2 responses of H1 cell bodies.

The size, shape, and density of Pseudemys photoreceptors is highly, and systematically, variable over the surface of the retina, and strikingly manifested by the presence of a horizontally oriented visual streak which extends across most of the retina [49]. This streak contains the highest density of photoreceptors in the retina, with their size, shape, density, and orientation changing toward the periphery [49–51]. Horizontal cells are also highly variable in size and shape

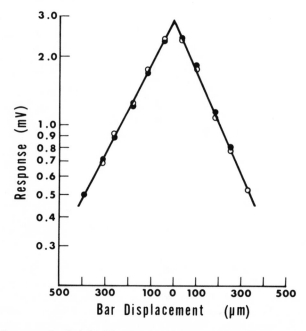

Fig. 11. Response of a Chelydra H1 cell body as a function of the displacement of a stimulus bar. The bar was moved through the field twice. ○ data collected during the first pass of the bar; ● data collected as the bar moved in the opposite direction. Points are the average of three responses at each position; data were collected at points separated by 72 μm. Solid lines were fitted by eye. The bar was produced by passing the light beam through a rectangular slit; the image of the slit on the retina had a nominal halfband width of 50 μm and its length was limited to 3000 μm by an iris diaphragm (Leeper and Copenhagen, unpublished).

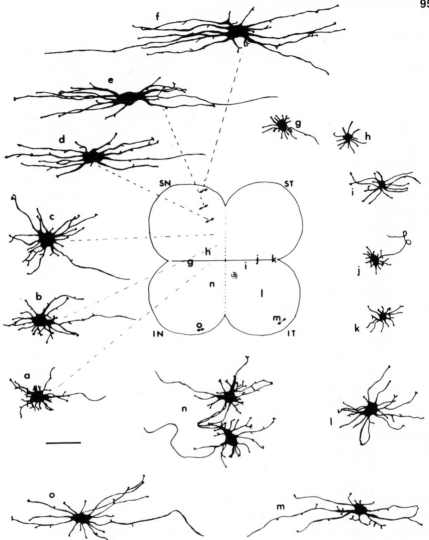

Fig. 12. Camera lucida drawings of 16 H1CBs observed in a single, flat-mounted Pseudemys retina. The illustrated cells, selected from 150 such cells stained in this retina, were chosen to illustrate variations in cell size and shape over the retina. The location of the cells is indicated either by the position of the corresponding cell identification (g–o) or by the position at which the line connecting each drawing with the schematic representation of the retina terminates. The double-headed arrows indicate the orientation of the major axis of some cells with elliptical dendritic fields. The solid horizontal line is drawn through the center of the linear area centralis (which could be clearly observed in this retina by the high density of darkly stained oil droplets) while the vertical broken line represents the separation of the temporal and nasal halves of the retina. The stippled circular area represents the optic nerve head. IT, inferior temporal; IN, inferior nasal; ST, superior temporal; SN, superior nasal quadrants. All drawings at the same scale (except the schematic of the retina); line = 50 μm. Reprinted, with permission, from Leeper [41] (Copyright 1978 by Alan R. Liss, Inc.).

over the retina; Figure 12 illustrates these effects for H1 cell bodies, and similar effects are seen for other types of horizontal cells [8]. Normann et al [52] demonstrated in Pseudemys an interesting correlation between the morphology and receptive field properties of H1 axon terminals in the area of the visual streak. They have shown that these terminals are oriented so that their major axis is parallel to the axis of the streak. The receptive fields of these terminals are found also to be asymmetrical; they are larger in the direction corresponding to the major axis of the cell and the orientation of the streak than in a direction perpendicular to these features. Normann et al [52] conclude that this difference in receptive field characteristics reflects the orientation of the terminals and the pattern of junctional complexes each terminal is capable of making with its neighbors.

The question of the role of the axon in the electrophysiology of horizontal cells remains a point of controversy; do these axons conduct signals between cell bodies and axon terminals, or do they not? In the case of the turtle, we find no evidence that they do. The findings that: (1) the receptive field sizes of L1 and L2 responses in the same retinal area are different [5,6]; (2) L1 responses, but not L2 responses, contain evidence of rod input [44]; and, (3) currents injected into one part of the cell can not be recorded in the other part [5,48] lead us to conclude that functionally, H1 axons do not electrically connect the two parts of the cell. In the cat retina, a similar type of horizontal cell has an axon and a diffuse axon terminal [53–55]; Nelson et al [55] found that the cell body and axon terminal were electrically independent. Further, when length constants of such axons are calculated assuming conventional electrical properties for the cell membranes, the values obtained are not optimistic for conduction [55,56]. Despite these examples and calculations, there are several cases in visual systems where axons of these sorts appear to conduct signals. In the case of teleost horizontal cells, horizontal cell axon terminals are located at the level of the cell bodies of the amacrine cells and make no direct contact with photoreceptors [56,57]. Despite this, some teleost horizontal cell axon terminals produce responses essentially like those of the cell bodies [58,59] and until alternative evidence for the source of these inputs is obtained, it is most reasonable to consider that these potentials are the result of electrical coupling between cell bodies and axon terminals via the axon [56]. In the case of primate foveal cones, Polyak [60] reported that the synaptic terminals of these cells can be separated from their cell bodies by distances of up to 150 μm. To date, there is no satisfactory evidence of regenerative processes to account for signal transmission over such distances in vertebrate photoreceptors. Similar situations occur in the fly retina [61] and the barnacle eye [62]. These cases raise the possibility that the electrical properties of axonal membranes in the retina need not always be those assumed previously, and that in certain cases, axons may play a role in the electrophysiology of horizontal cells by conducting signals between axon terminals and cell bodies.

CORRELATIONS: C-TYPE CELLS

Sources of Chromaticity-type Responses

In addition to the L-type responses and the H1 cell type described previously, two C-type horizontal cell responses and two additional main classes of Golgi-stained horizontal cells (H2 and H3) have been described in turtle retina (Fig. 1). Therefore, it was natural to attempt to correlate the two physiological and morphological classes.

The cell type producing R/G C-type responses has been injected with dye and found to be a class of stellate cells with a dendritic density less than that of H1 cell bodies [7]. Since these cells respond with antagonistic responses to red and green stimuli [7,12] (Fig. 8), it might at first be supposed that these cells make contact with, and receive input directly from, both red- and green-sensitive cones. However, Gouras [63] has proposed that C-type horizontal cells may receive direct input only from the chromatic class of cones responsible for the primary hyperpolarizing responses of the cell, with antagonistic responses being provided by feedback onto this cone class. A general model of this sort is presented in Figure 13. Fuortes and Simon [12] incorporated Gouras' idea into their model of the turtle retina and proposed that turtle R/G C-type cells contact only green-sensitive cones. Leeper [41] found that the class of Golgi-stained horizontal cell which most closely resembled the dye-injected R/G cell type was an axonless stellate cell which contacted all of the green-sensitive single (but not double) cones, and all of the blue-sensitive cones in its receptive field (Figs. 1 and 7). This led to the conclusion that this cell type responds to input from green-sensitive single cones (which includes an antagonistic red-sensitive feedback from L2), and that its contacts with blue-sensitive cones serve to generate further C-type responses. Piccolino et al [64] presented evidence which supports the claim that the red-depolarizing responses in R/G cells are mediated by feedback. They found that in the presence of Sr^{2+} ions, prolonged activation of the feedback mechanism resulted in a repetitive discharge of spikes in cones. Red stimuli, to which green-sensitive cones are photochemically insensitive, produced such repetitive spikes in green cones and trains of depolarizing transient potentials in R/G cells.

There is no documentation for successful dye-injection of cells responsible for generating G/B C-type responses, and therefore direct correlation between the morphology of an identified unit and a class of Golgi-stained neurons has not been possible. Fuortes and Simon [12] proposed that G/B responses would be generated by a horizontal cell receiving input from blue-sensitive cones which in turn received antagonistic feedback from red-sensitive L units; they proposed that these horizontal cells also received input directly from R/G cells and that the lack of a distinct red-sensitive response (Fig. 8) resulted from the cancelling effect of the two red inputs. Leeper [41] proposed that these responses resulted from a class of axonless stellate cells which received input only from blue-

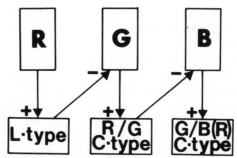

Fig. 13. Diagrammatic representation of the pathways involved in the generation of horizontal cell responses in both turtle and goldfish. This figure emphasizes the cascading manner in which horizontal cell responses become more elaborate without noting the details of the pathways by which this is accomplished (see Fig. 14). R, G, B, red-, green-, blue-sensitive cones; "+", noninverting synapse; "−", inverting synapse.

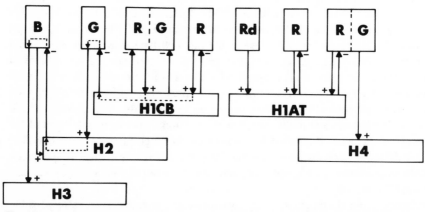

Fig. 14. Diagrammatic summary of the interconnections between horizontal and receptor cells in the turtle retina, including a model for the pathways involved in the generation of horizontal cell responses. R, G, and B in single receptor elements represent red-, green-, and blue-sensitive single cones, respectively. R and G in double elements represent the red-sensitive chief members and green sensitive accessory members of double cones, respectively. Rd represents rods. "+", noninverting synapse; "−", inverting synapse. Figures 13 and 14 reprinted, with permission, from Leeper [41] (Copyright 1978 by Alan R. Liss, Inc.).

sensitive cones, and that the antagonistic feedback from R/G cells onto blue-sensitive cones would account for the observed green- [13,41] and red-sensitivities [13].

Figure 14 shows a detailed model of the proposed interactions between turtle photoreceptors and horizontal cells. This model proposes that one of the primary consequences of horizontal cell feedback is the generation of complex, chromaticity S-potentials. This type of model adequately explains the known morphology and physiology of horizontal cells in the turtle retina [41] and is consistent with the morphology and physiology of the horizontal cells of the goldfish retina [43].

A fourth type of horizontal cell (H4) was observed in Golgi-stained turtle retina. This cell type stained infrequently and was an axonless stellate cell with a dendritic field smaller than H2s and H3s in the same retinal area [8]. The physiological response characteristics of this cell type are not known.

HORIZONTAL CELLS AND BIPOLAR CELL RESPONSES

In a number of species, including turtle, bipolar cells exhibit receptive fields with concentrically arranged center and surround regions which are antagonistically organized [65–70]. The surround response is generally believed to be mediated by horizontal cells, whereas central responses are produced by direct connections with photoreceptors [65,68,71–73]. The best argument for horizontal cell mediation of the surround derives from data correlating the diameter of the surround responses in bipolar cells with the receptive field size of horizontal cells. Richter and Simon [71] showed that center-hyperpolarizing, red-sensitive turtle bipolar cells had surrounds of various diameters but concluded that the largest could be mediated only by the large field axon terminals of H1 horizontal cells. In support of this notion linking horizontal cells and bipolar surrounds are the results of Marchiafava [74] in which currents injected into turtle L-type horizontal cells produced responses in both center-hyperpolarizing and center-depolarizing bipolar cells which were of the same polarity as responses produced by illumination of the surround in these cells. Yazulla [72] concluded that in addition to luminosity cells, R/GB C-type cells also might contribute to the surround of certain bipolars, although the role of C-type cells in the generation of bipolar cell receptive fields has not been well studied in any species. Indeed, C-type horizontal cells appear to be missing from mammalian retinas studied to date [75,76], and their role in retinal functions in lower vertebrates remains a mystery.

Some experimental results call into question the notion that horizontal cells alone mediate the surround responses of bipolar cells. Gerschenfeld and Piccolino [77,78] found that bathing turtle retina in atropine eliminated L-type horizontal cell responses but did not eliminate the surround responses of bipolar cells. Additionally, Marchiafava's results show that there is a significant delay in the current induced polarization of the bipolar cell membrane potential [74]. These results suggest that perhaps the surround responses of bipolar cells are comprised of multiple, perhaps multisynaptic pathways which involve other neurons in addition to horizontal cells.

The mechanism by which horizontal cells influence bipolar cells is not well understood. An appealing possibility is that horizontal cells exert their influence through feedback onto receptor cells rather than by direct synapses onto bipolar cell dendrites. In this way, horizontal cells could influence the responses of bipolar cells by modulating the release of transmitter at the cone synaptic terminal. In the case of turtle, however, the available data suggest a direct horizontal to bipolar cell synapse. Yazulla [72] observed that some bipolar cells exhibit a sustained independent response to the presentation of an annulus alone, a phenomenon never observed in red-sensitive cones. Furthermore, an annulus superimposed upon a spot can drive the bipolar potential beyond the resting potential, again a sustained response property never observed in cones [72]. Richter and Simon [71] demonstrated that the surround and central responses behave differently to polarization of the bipolar cell membrane potential with intracellularly injected currents. Additionally, they show that there is a difference in the linear range responses to large and small diameter spots of light. These results are inconsistent with the surround being mediated strictly via feedback to the cones.

CONCLUSION

Studies of turtle retina have been remarkably fruitful in providing data relevant to the processing of visual stimuli by vertebrate retinas. As regards horizontal cells, these data include the first evidence that vertebrate photoreceptors do not function autonomously of second-order neurons, but rather are subject to feedback influences. These data provide one of the most complete bodies of information on both the morphology and physiology of horizontal cells for any species. Despite this, much work remains, for we do not yet know precisely what horizontal cells do. While these data implicate horizontal cells in, for example, the processing of chromatic information and the formation of bipolar cell receptive fields, it remains to be determined exactly how the morphology and physiology of horizontal cells affect the functioning of ganglion cells which provide the common pathway to the brain for all visual information.

ACKNOWLEDGMENTS

The authors would like to thank Laury Belzer for her excellent photographic services. This work was supported by research grants EY 02962 to HFL, EY 01869 to DRC, and EY 00468 to Dr. K. T. Beown, from the National Eye Institute, National Institutes of Health, United States Public Health Service.

REFERENCES

1. Baylor DA, Fuortes MGF, O'Bryan PM: Receptive fields of cones in the retina of the turtle. J Physiol (London) 214:265, 1971.
2. Müller H: Anatomisch-physiologische Untersuchungen über die Retina bei Menschen und Wirbelthieren. Z wiss Zool 8:1, 1857.
3. Schiefferdecker P: Studien zur vergleichenden Histologie der Retina. Arch mikrosk Anat 28:305, 1886.
4. Lasansky A: Synaptic organization of cone cells in the turtle retina. Philos Trans R Soc Lond (Biol) 262:365, 1971.
5. Simon EJ: Two types of luminosity horizontal cells in the retina of the turtle. J Physiol (London) 230:199, 1973.
6. Miller WH, Hashimoto Y, Saito T, Tomita T: Physiological and morphological identification of L- and C-type S-potentials in the turtle retina. Vision Res 13:443, 1973.
7. Saito T, Miller WH, Tomita T: C- and L-type horizontal cells in the turtle retina. Vision Res 14:119, 1974.
8. Leeper HF: Horizontal cells of the turtle retina. I. Light microscopy of Golgi preparations. J Comp Neurol 182:777, 1978.
9. Svaetichin G: Spectral response curves from single cones. Acta Physiol Scand 39:17, 1956.
10. Svaetichin G, MacNichol EF: Retinal mechanisms for chromatic and achromatic vision. Ann NY Acad Sci 74:385, 1958.
11. MacNichol EJ, Svaetichin G: Electrical responses from the isolated retinas of fishes. Amer J Ophthalmol 46:26, 1958.
12. Fuortes MGF, Simon EJ: Interactions leading to horizontal cell responses in the turtle retina. J Physiol (London) 240:177, 1974.
13. Yazulla S: Cone input to horizontal cells in the turtle retina. Vision Res 16:727, 1976.
14. Baylor DA, Hodgkin AL: Detection and resolution of visual stimuli by turtle photoreceptors. J Physiol (London) 234:163, 1973.
15. Liebman PA, Granda AM: Microspectrophotometric measurements of visual pigments in two species of turtle, Pseudemys scripta and Chelonia mydas. Vision Res 11:105, 1971.
16. Richter A, Simon EJ: Electrical responses of double cones in the turtle retina. J Physiol (London) 242:673, 1974.
17. Liebman PA: Microspectrophotometry of photoreceptors. In Dartnall HJA (ed): "Handbook of Sensory Physiology. VII/1 Photochemistry of Vision." Berlin, Heidelberg, New York: Springer–Verlag, 1971, p 105.
18. Underwood G: The eye. In Gans C, Parsona TS (eds): "Biology of Reptilia." New York: Academic Press, 1970, p 1.
19. Copenhagen DR, Owen WG: Functional characteristics of lateral interactions between rods in the retina of the snapping turtle. J Physiol (London) 259:251, 1976.
20. Lamb TD, Simon EJ: The relation between intercellular coupling and electrical noise in turtle photoreceptors. J Physiol (London) 262:257, 1976.
21. Fuortes MGF: Responses of cones and horizontal cells in the retina of the turtle. Invest Ophthalmol Vis Sci 11:275, 1972.
22. Lasansky A: Cell junctions at the outer synaptic layer of the retina. Invest Ophthalmol Vis Sci 11:265, 1972.
23. Raviola E, Gilula NB: Gap junctions between photoreceptor cells in the vertebrate retina. Proc Nat Acad Sci 70:1677, 1973.
24. O'Bryan PM: Properties of the depolarizing synaptic potential evoked by peripheral illumination in cones of the turtle retina. J Physiol (London) 235:207, 1973.
25. Fuortes MGF, Schwartz EA, Simon EJ: Colour-dependence of cone responses in the turtle retina. J Physiol (London) 234:199, 1973.

26. Piccolino M, Gerschenfeld HM: Characteristics and ionic processes involved in feedback spikes of turtle cones. Proc R Soc Lond (Biol) 206:439, 1980.
27. Naka K-I, Rushton WAH: The generation and spread of S-potentials in the fish (Cyprinidae). J Physiol (London) 192:437, 1967.
28. Lamb TD: Spatial properties of horizontal cell responses in the turtle retina. J Physiol (London) 263:239, 1976.
29. Kaneko A: Electrical connexions between horizontal cells in the dogfish retina. J Physiol (London) 213:95, 1971.
30. Gerschenfeld HM, Piccolino M: Sustained feedback effects of L-horizontal cells on turtle cones. Proc R Soc Lond (Biol) 206:465, 1980.
31. Stell WK: The morphological organization of the vertebrate retina. In Fuortes MGF (ed): "Handbook of Sensory Physiology. VII/2 Physiology of Photoreceptor Organs." Berlin, Heidelberg, New York: Springer–Verlag, 1972, p 111.
32. Raviola E, Gilula NG: Intramembrane organization of specialized contacts in the outer plexiform layer of the retina. J Cell Biol 65:192, 1975.
33. Schaeffer SF, Raviola E: Ultrastructural analysis of functional changes in the synaptic endings of turtle cone cells. Cold Spring Harbor Symp Quant Biol 40:521, 1976.
34. Raviola E: Intercellular junctions in the outer plexiform layer of the retina. Invest Ophthalmol Vis Sci 15:881, 1976.
35. Pfenninger K, Akert K, Moor H, Sandri C: The fine structure of freeze-fracture presynaptic membranes. J Neurocytol 1:129, 1972.
36. Heuser JE, Reese TS, Landis DMD: Functional changes in frog neuromuscular junction studied with freeze-fracture. J Neurocytol 3:109, 1974.
37. Landis DMD, Reese TS: Differences in membrane structure between excitatory and inhibitory synapses in the cerebellar cortex. J Comp Neurol 155:93, 1974.
38. Landis DMD, Reese TS, Raviola E: Differences in membrane structure between excitatory and inhibitory components of the reciprocal synapse in the olfactory bulb. J Comp Neurol 155:67, 1974.
39. Stell WK, Lightfoot DO, Wheeler TG, Leeper HF: Goldfish retina: Functional polarization of cone horizontal cell dendrites and synapses. Science 190:989, 1975.
40. Byzov AL: Role of horizontal cells in the mechanism of retinal adaptation. Neirofiziologiia 1:210, 1969. (In English translation, Neurosci Transl 14:63, 1970–71).
41. Leeper HF: Horizontal cells of the turtle retina. II. Analysis of interconnections between photoreceptor cells and horizontal cells by light microscopy. J Comp Neurol 182:795, 1978.
42. Stewart WW: Functional connections between cells as revealed by dye-coupling with a highly fluorescent naphthalimide tracer. Cell 14:741, 1978.
43. Stell WK, Lightfoot DO, Color-specific interconnections of cones and horizontal cells in the retina of the goldfish. J Comp Neurol 159:473, 1975.
44. Leeper HF, Copenhagen DR: Mixed rod-cone responses in horizontal cells of snapping turtle retina. Vision Res 19:407, 1979.
45. Yamada E, Ishikawa T: The fine structure of the horizontal cells in some vertebrate retinae. Cold Spring Harbor Symp Quant Biol 30:383, 1965.
46. Tomita T, Tosaka T, Watanabe K: The fish EIRG in response to different types of illumination. Japan J Physiol 8:41, 1958.
47. Norton AL, Spekreijse H, Wagner HG: Receptive field organization of the S-potential. Science 160:1021, 1968.
48. Byzov AL: Interaction between horizontal cells of the turtle retina. Neirofiziologiia 7:279, 1975 (in Russian).
49. Brown KT: A linear area centralis extending across the turtle retina and stabilized to the horizon by nonvisual cues. Vision Res 9:1053, 1969.

50. Granda AM, Haden KW: Retinal oil globule counts and distributions in two species of turtles: Pseudemys scripta elegans (Weid) and Chelonia mydas mydas (Linnaeus). Vision Res 10:79, 1970.
51. Baylor DA, Fettiplace R: Light path and photon capture in turtle photoreceptors. J Physiol (London) 248:433, 1975.
52. Normann RA, Kolb H, Hanani M, Pasino E, Holub R: Orientation of horizontal cell axon terminals in the streak of the turtle retina. Nature (London) 280:60, 1979.
53. Kolb H: The connections between horizontal cells and photoreceptors in the retina of the cat: Electron microscopy of Golgi preparations. J Comp Neurol 155:1, 1974.
54. Boycott BB, Peichl L, Wässle H: Morphological types of horizontal cell in the retina of the domestic cat. Proc R Soc Lond (Biol) 203,229: 1978.
55. Nelson R, Lutzow AV, Kolb H, Gouras P: Horizontal cells in cat retina with independent dendritic systems. Science 189:137, 1975.
56. Stell WK: Horizontal cell axons and axon terminals in goldfish retina. J Comp Neurol 159:503, 1975.
57. Naka K-I, Carraway RG: Morphological and functional identifications of catfish retinal neurons. I. Classical morphology. J Neurophysiol 38:53, 1975.
58. Kaneko A: Physiological and morphological identification of horizontal, bipolar and amacrine cells in goldfish retina. J Physiol (London) 207:623, 1970.
59. Marmarelis PZ, Naka K-I: Spatial distribution of potential in a flat cell. Application to the catfish horizontal cell layers. Biophys J 12:1515, 1973.
60. Polyak SL: "The Retina." Chicago: University of Chicago Press, 1941.
61. Zettler F, Järvilehto M: Decrement-free conduction of graded potentials along the axon of a monopolar neuron. Z vergl Physiologie 75:402, 1971.
62. Shaw S: Decremental conduction of the visual signal in barnacle lateral eye. J Physiol (London) 220:145, 1972.
63. Gouras P: S-potentials. In Fuortes MGF (ed): "Handbook of Sensory Physiology. VII/2 Physiology of Photoreceptor Organs." Berlin, Heidelberg, New York: Springer–Verlag, 1972, p 513.
64. Piccolino M, Neyton J, Gerschenfeld HM: Synaptic mechanisms involved in responses of chromaticity horizontal cells of turtle retina. Nature (London) 284:58, 1980.
65. Werblin FS, Dowling JE: Organization of the retina of the mudpuppy, Necturus maculosus. II. Intracellular recording. J Neurophysiol 32:339, 1969.
66. Matsumoto N, Naka K-I: Identification of intracellular responses in the frog retina. Brain Res 42:59, 1972.
67. Kaneko A: Receptive field organization of bipolar and amacrine cells in the goldfish retina. J Physiol (London) 235:133, 1973.
68. Schwartz EA: Responses of bipolar cells in the retina of the turtle. J Physiol (London) 236:211, 1974.
69. Naka K-I, Ohtsuka T: Morphological and functional identifications of catfish retinal neurons. II. Morphological identification. J Neurophysiol 38:72, 1975.
70. Werblin FS: Synaptic interactions mediating bipolar responses in the retina of the tiger salamander. In Barlow HB, Fatt P (eds): "Verbetrate Photoreception." London, New York, San Francisco: Academic Press, 1977, p 205.
71. Richter A, Simon, EJ: Properties of centre-hyperpolarizing, red-sensitive bipolar cells in the turtle retina. J Physiol (London) 248:317, 1975.
72. Yazulla S: Cone input to bipolar cells in the turtle retina. Vision Res 16:737, 1976.
73. Werblin FS: Control of retinal sensitivity: II. Lateral interactions at the outer plexiform layer. J Gen Physiol 63:623, 1974.

74. Marchiafava PL: Horizontal cells influence membrane potential of bipolar cells in the retina of the turtle. Nature (London) 275:141, 1978.
75. Nelson R: Cat cones have rod input: A comparison of the response properties of cones and horizontal cell bodies in the retina of the cat. J Comp Neurol 172:109, 1977.
76. De Monasterio FM: Spectral interactions in horizontal and ganglion cells of the isolated and arterially perfused rabbit retina. Brain Res 150:239, 1978.
77. Gerschenfeld HM, Piccolino M: Muscarinic antagonists block cone to horizontal cell transmission in turtle retina. Nature (London) 268:257, 1977.
78. Piccolino M, Gerschenfeld HM: Lateral interactions in the outer plexiform layer of turtle retinas after atropine block of horizontal cells. Nature (London) 268:259, 1977.

The S-Potential, pages 105–122
© 1982 Alan R. Liss, Inc., 150 Fifth Avenue, New York, NY 10011

Membrane Mechanisms of the Activity of Horizontal Cells

Alexey L. Byzov and Yu A. Trifonov

The discovery by Gunnar Svaetichin in 1953 [1] of S-potentials in the carp retina was a very significant event. However, its real importance has been cleared up gradually. The understanding passed through several stages: astonishment aroused by the unusual shape and sign of the light response, long debates about identification of the S-potential sources, and the recording, after some unsuccessful attempts, of light responses in cones and rods, as well as in bipolars. It became clear, along with the accumulation of experimental data, that the absence of spikes in S-potential sources is not the result of cell damage by the recording microelectrode or of some other possible factors, but is a specific feature of most retinal cells. However, the nonspike activity of retinal neurons continued to be considered as an exception to the rule, as a unique feature of the visual system. Only recently data have appeared which show that the nonspike transmission and processing of signals in different parts of the nervous system is much more widespread than it was thought previously [2]. It was even supposed that such an "electrotonic" processing of information plays a main role in brain activity [3].

The retinal studies seem to be of a special interest, in view of the ideas mentioned. Nowadays the retina, in particular its distal region, where none of the cellular elements (photoreceptors, horizontal cells (HC), and bipolars) generate spikes, is one of the nervous centers studied in more detail.

This paper summarizes the results of our studies in the last years, which concern the membrane mechanisms of HC activity. The experiments were carried out mostly on L-cells of fish and turtle retinas. The following questions are considered: (a) synaptic mechanism of HC responses to input signals from photoreceptors; (b) participation of the cell membrane (nonsynaptic membrane) of HCs in the generation of electrical response to light; (c) the "output" of HCs— what is the nature of the output signals, where and by what mechanism are they transmitted? The last question is connected with the attempt to estimate the role of HCs of L-type in the processing of signals in the external plexiform layer of the retina.

SYNAPTIC MECHANISM OF LIGHT RESPONSES IN HORIZONTAL CELLS

The nature of S-potentials, ie, of light responses of HCs, was a subject of long discussions. They were even supposed to be of a glial origin [4,5]. The attempts to find, by analogy with neurons, the equilibrium potential of the light response by means of polarization of HCs through an intracellular microelectrode yielded such contradictory results [6–9] that it was impossible to reach definite conclusions. Now we know the reasons of these failures. The first one is the strong electrical coupling between HCs [10–12]. Because of this coupling the point polarization of the HC layer through the microelectrode is noneffective. As shown by theoretical analysis [13], the input resistance of a syncytium depends very weakly on the membrane resistance of individual cells. The second reason is the voltage-dependent properties of the HC membrane, which distort the changes of input resistance caused by synapses.

More fruitful results were obtained in another group of experiments, based on attempts to change the release of transmitter from photoreceptor terminals. It is known that depolarization of the presynaptic membrane results, in all chemical synapses, in an increase of release of transmitter, whereas hyperpolarization has the opposite effect. It was shown that depolarization of presynaptic terminals of photoreceptors by means of pulses of current passed radially through the retina evokes depolarizing responses in HCs of the turtle [14,15] and carp retina [16]. In darkness the photoreceptors are depolarized [17] and, accordingly, the HCs of L-type are depolarized. On the other hand, all factors which decrease the release of transmitter, such as hyperpolarization of the presynaptic membrane by radial current [15,18], the suppression of the release of transmitter by Mg^{2+} ions [19], by Co^{2+} ions, or by the decrease of Ca^{2+} ion concentrations [20], result in the hyperpolarization of HCs. Therefore, the hyperpolarizing light response of HCs is the result of a decrease of liberation of depolarizing transmitter from the photoreceptors.

This conclusion was confirmed when we finally succeeded in effectively depolarizing the HC membrane by extrinsic current. The syncytial structure of the HC layer, which, as mentioned previously, hindered the effective polarization of the cell membrane through an intracellular microelectrode, became a basis of a new method. This method, applied in three somewhat different modifications, was described in detail elsewhere [21–25].

The general feature of all three modifications is that the current was driven into the HC layer by means of an extracellular electrical field caused by current passed tangentially through the retina from low resistance ($< 100\text{-}\Omega$) electrodes. It is of worth to note that in one modification of the method [24,25] the membrane of the HC layer was polarized uniformly over an area of several millimeters along the preparation. This made it possible not only to measure more exactly the reversal potential of the light response, but also to apply the method of potential clamp to the study of the membrane properties of HCs (for more details see [26]). An important feature of the method of uniform polarization of a syncytial structure is that the density of current which crosses the membrane does not depend on membrane resistance and is proportional to the intensity of the extracellular current.

Experiments with uniform polarization of HC membrane are illustrated in Figure 1a and b. The hyperpolarizing light response of L-type HC decreased

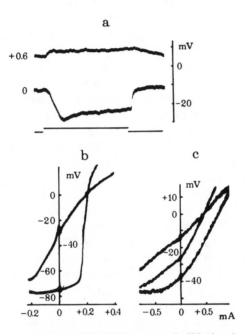

Fig. 1. Measurement of reversal potential of light response in HC of turtle and pike retina. (a) Reversion of light response of L-type HC in the turtle retina with depolarization above zero level of membrane potential. Numbers at the left show the intensity of longitudinal current passed through the preparation. The shift of the curve with current corresponds to the change of membrane potential. The light stimulus is a spot 115 μ in diameter for 1.3 sec. Polarization is not uniform. (b) Stationary voltage-current curves of HC membrane of pike retina, taken with uniform polarization. The abscissae here as well as in Figures 1c, 2a and b, and 5a and b are the intensities of longitudinal depolarizing (at the right) and hyperpolarizing (at the left from zero) current (in milliamps), which is proportional to the density of current crossing the membrane. The upper curve was taken in darkness, the lower one in supersaturating light. The curves intersect slightly above zero potential. (c) Stationary voltage-current curves of HC membrane in turtle retina (in the same cell as in Fig. 1a, ie, with nonuniform polarization). The upper curve was taken in darkness, the middle curve with a constant light spot of small diameter (115 μ), and the lower curve with a constant large spot (2 mm diameter). One can see the apparent shift of equilibrium potential upward with the increase of area illuminated.

with depolarization up to zero level of membrane potential, and reversed its sign with further depolarization (Fig. 1a). Figure 1b shows one example of voltage-current curves of HC membrane in the pike retina. The curves were taken directly from an oscilloscope where the vertical displacement of the sweep was controlled by the membrane potential, and the horizontal displacement by the current passed through the retina. One can see that the slope of the curve in darkness is much less steep (ie, the resistance is lower), than in the light, at the same levels of potential. The conclusion follows from this that the resistance of the subsynaptic membrane decreases in darkness. This is in agreement with the fact that the curves intersect near zero level of membrane potential.

Similar results were obtained in the HCs of L-type in the turtle retina. For technical reasons, we could not perform, in these experiments, the uniform polarization of HC membrane over a large area. The correct estimation of the equilibrium potential of light responses requires, under these conditions, a small light spot centered on the microelectrode. The increase of light spot size leads to overestimation of the reversal potential, as seen in Figure 1c (see also [22,23]). Nevertheless, this overestimated reversal potential was usually not very much higher than zero membrane potential (Fig. 1c), being similar in L_1 and L_2 cells. Probably the same conclusion fits also to HCs of Necturus retina [27]. It should be noted that Werblin [27] failed to reverse the light response by polarization, and the equilibrium potential estimated by him was much higher than zero level (sometimes up to $+50$ mV). However, the point polarization of the HC layer through the microelectrode, used by Werblin, gives even more overestimated values than our method. Therefore, his figures of equilibrium potential in HCs are strongly overestimated, especially because of large-area illumination.

As to the ionic mechanism of postsynaptic responses in HCs of the L-type, one can assume that it is similar to that of excitatory synapses, ie, the transmitter acts to increase mainly the sodium conductance of the subsynaptic membrane. This assumption was confirmed experimentally by Waloga and Pak [28]. The proximity of the equilibrium potential to zero indicates the possible participation of K^+ ions in the response. Another way to explain this fact is to postulate a relatively high intracellular Na^+ concentration. Both assumptions need direct experimental examination.

VOLTAGE-DEPENDENT PROPERTIES OF THE CELL (NONSYNAPTIC) MEMBRANE OF HORIZONTAL CELLS

The cell membrane and synaptic membrane of HCs are in parallel to the extrinsic current passed through the syncitium (see Fig. 6a). In darkness, when the HCs are depolarized, the conductance of the subsynaptic membrane is much higher than that of the rest of the cell membrane. Therefore, the voltage-current curve has a small slope and is more or less linear (Fig. 1b and c). With a bright light the conductance of the subsynaptic membrane drops strongly, and the total conductance is determined mainly by the cell membrane. In the range of low membrane potentials, the slope of voltage-current curve (ie, the resistance of the HC membrane) is high in comparison with that in darkness. However, with very negative membrane potentials the resistance drops sharply to values lower than those seen in darkness. Therefore, the resistance of the HC membrane is strongly voltage dependent.

If the resistance of the subsynaptic membrane in bright light is high enough, the voltage-current curve seen under these conditions reflects the properties of the cell membrane only. In the retina of both fish and turtle, the resistance of the cell membrane drops with hyperpolarization by a factor of 10 or more (Fig. 1b and c). The voltage-current curves of Figure 2a and b, taken on HCs of the ide retina under voltage-clamp conditions [25,26] even have regions with negative slope resistance, in the middle range of membrane potentials. This means that the HC membrane is able, under some conditions, to produce regenerative potentials. In experiments [21] with polarization of the HC layer (without voltage clamp), this regenerative property looks like a "spontaneous" shift of membrane potential from one level to another, when a constant depolarizing current of a "threshold" intensity is passed (Fig. 2c).

The voltage-current curves of Figures 1 and 2 can be considered as stationary, because they show the steady states of membrane potentials without interference by capacity distortions and transients. This was achieved by a slow change of intensity of the current (or of a command potential in voltage-clamp experiments). For example, the curves of Figures 1 and 2 were taken in the course of 4–8 sec. However, sometimes the membrane potential of HCs changed, in response to a long rectangular pulse of current, so slowly (see Fig. 2c) that one could suppose a strong time dependence of nonlinearity. One should mention, however, that theoretically this last assumption is not necessary, because even with the instantaneous nonlinearity the constant current can evoke, due to the existence of a membrane capacity, any slow changes of membrane potential (provided that the slope resistance of the membrane is high enough). Therefore, special experiments are needed to decide how rapidly the mechanism of membrane nonlinearity works and whether it is possible to attribute the slow changes of membrane potential, as in Figure 2c, to the time dependence of membrane nonlinearity. The problem was settled, to some extent, in experiments with voltage-clamp of the HC membrane.

As mentioned previously, the method of polarization developed enables the shift of the membrane potential of the HC layer uniformly over a large area. For experiments with voltage clamp, a special powerful current generator was constructed, capable of generating for short periods of time high potential drops across the extracellular resistance of the preparation [26]. Due to some technical difficulties, the time resolution of the system was restricted to about 15 msec.

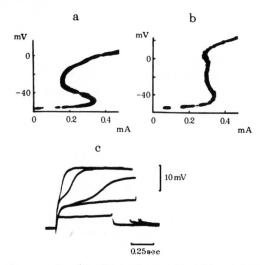

Fig. 2. Regenerative properties of the HC membrane. (a) and (b) are examples of voltage-current curves of ide HCs taken during continuous bright diffuse light under voltage clamp conditions [26]. Curve a has one, and Curve b two regions with negative slope resistance. (c) is the shift of membrane potential in HCs of pike retina, evoked by constant currents of different intensities passed along the retina [21]; intensity of currents from the bottom: 35, 45, 48, 50, and 60 μA.

Figure 3a illustrates an attempt to measure the delay (if it exists) in the conductance changes of the HC membrane in the pike retina, when the holding potential was changed by two instantaneous depolarizing steps (lower curve). The upper curves show currents generated under these conditions. It can be seen that, after initial transients, due to recharge of the membrane capacitance, the current is stabilized at different levels: For the right step the increase of current is much less than for the left one. This corresponds to a higher resistance with depolarization (see the voltage-current curves in Figs. 1 and 2). However, in both cases the new levels of current (and therefore of membrane resistance) are attained in less than 20 msec (a more exact appreciation cannot be given at present). Therefore, the voltage dependence of the HC membrane is a relatively fast process.

The experiments with voltage clamp have also confirmed the previous conclusion on the reversal potential of HCs light response, which is near zero. Figure 3b shows the current response of a HC to light stimulation, recorded at three different levels of holding potential indicated on the left. It is seen that the light responses recorded as changes of current required to hold the potential (lower curve) decreased when the holding potential approached the zero level (middle curve) and reversed when the potential was shifted over this level (upper curve).

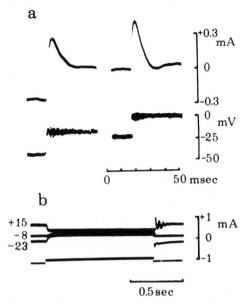

Fig. 3. Voltage clamp experiment in pike retina. (a) The change of longitudinal current (upper traces) passed through the preparation during two instantaneous depolarizing steps of holding potential (lower traces). The transient peaks in the current traces reflect the recharge of membrane capacitance. It is seen that the right potential step evokes a much lower change of constant current than the left one, because the resistance of the HC membrane is considerably higher in the depolarized state. (b) This shows the current responses of HCs to light with different levels of holding potential in HC membrane (indicated by numbers at the left, in millivolts). The lower trace is the light monitor.

CHANGES OF IONIC CONDUCTANCE UNDERLYING THE NONLINEARITY OF THE HC MEMBRANE

A priori, the form of the voltage-current curve of the HC membrane (ie, of the curve taken in bright light) can be interpreted in two ways. According to the first interpretation, which seems to be more natural, the decrease of the slope of voltage-current curve with hyperpolarization is the result of an increase of K^+ conductance. The equivalent electrical circuit of such a membrane is shown in Figure 4a. The K^+ channels activated by hyperpolarization within the working range of membrane potentials are unusual for neurons, but have been described in the membrane of starfish eggs [29].

However, an alternative interpretation of the nonlinearity of the HC membrane is possible. Although the membrane potential in bright light (when the synapses are completely closed) is determined mainly by K^+ ions, the increase in the slope of the voltage-current curve (formally, the increase of membrane resistance) may be the result not of an decrease of K^+ conductance, but of an increase of

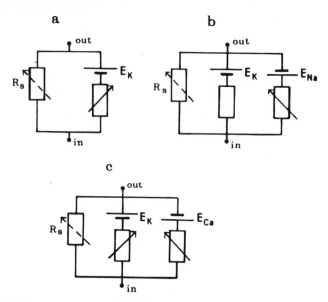

Fig. 4. Equivalent electrical circuits illustrating different hypotheses on the ionic mechanism underlaying nonlinearity of the HC membrane. R_s is the resistance of the subsynaptic membrane, which is controlled by light (it is very high in bright light or after Co^{2+}). (a) Nonlinearity is based on voltage-dependent K^+ channels, the conductance of which is high with hyperpolarization and is decreased with depolarization. (b) In bright light K^+ conductance predominates, but depolarization increases Na^+ (or Ca^{2+}) conductance. (c) Nonlinearity is based on K^+ channels, as in (a), but Ca^{2+} channels activated by depolarization also take some part.

conductance to other ions (Na^+ or Ca^{2+}) whose equilibrium potential is more positive than the membrane potential in the light. This is the mechanism for generation of action potentials in electrically excitable membrane of nerve and muscle fibers. The equivalent circuit corresponding to this hypothesis is shown in Figure 4b. The choice between these alternatives can be made in experiments with different ionic composition of the superfusion fluid, and by adding specific inhibitors of ionic channels.

The combination of polarization of the HC layer by means of an extracellular electrical field and perfusion of the preparation by a salt solution led to some new technical difficulties. As a consequence we gave up, in most experiments, the uniform polarization of HC membrane over a large area. Therefore, the voltage-current curves shown below are somewhat distorted, as compared with real ones, but this is not of great importance for the main results.

The experiments have shown that from the two alternatives mentioned previously, the first is nearer to the truth. The decrease of extracellular K^+ concentration (from 4 mM to 0) was accompanied by a small hyperpolarization of

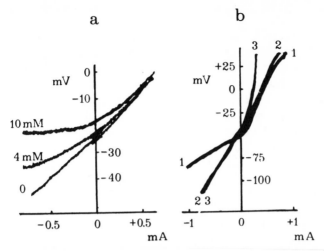

Fig. 5. (a) Voltage-current curves of HC membrane of turtle retina in bright light with different K$^+$ concentrations in perfusion solution (values near the curves). All curves were taken from one and the same HC successively (starting from the upper one) with 12-min intervals, during which the solution with indicated K concentration was flowing. Decrease of K$^+$ concentration led to hyperpolarization of HC and to the increase of the slope of hyperpolarizing part of the curve. (b) Effect of Ba^{2+} and Ca^{2+} ions on the voltage-current curve of goldfish HCs. Curve 1 is the control after blocking the synaptic transmission with Co^{2+} (0.5 mM); curve 2 was obtained 5 min after addition of 3 mM Ba^{2+}, curve 3 was obtained 7 min after change to a solution with 20 mM of Ca^{2+} (instead of Na$^+$). All curves were taken in one and the same cell successively and are superimposed photographically.

HCs and by a noticeable increase of the slope in the hyperpolarizing half of the voltage-current curve (Fig. 5a). On the other hand, with the increase of K$^+$ concentration up to 10 mM the HCs were depolarized, and the slope of the hyperpolarizing part of voltage-current curve decreased. At the same time, the depolarizing part of the curve was little changed (Fig. 5a). Depolarization of the membrane with the increase of K$^+$ concentration indicates that the membrane potential is determined by potassium ions, when the synapses are closed. Moreover, judging by the changes in the slope of the hyperpolarizing part of the voltage-current curve, K$^+$ ions are the main carriers of transmembrane current during hyperpolarization of HCs. We tried also to see the effect of Ba^{2+}, which is known to be a specific inhibitor of K$^+$ channels [30], also effective for K$^+$ channels in the membrane of starfish eggs [29]. The addition of Ba^{2+} (1–5 mM) in the solution increased the slope of the hyperpolarizing part of the voltage-current curve in the retina of both goldfish (Fig. 5b, curve 2) and turtle. Therefore, Ba^{2+} ions actually blocked the K$^+$ channels. All these effects remained after interruption of synaptic transmission by Co^{2+} ions. Hence, they cannot be explained by the action of the agents on photoreceptors or synaptic transmission between them and HCs. Tetraethylammonium, which is known to inhibit voltage-dependent K^+ channels in different membranes including the membrane of vertebrate rods [31], had no effect on the voltage-current curve. However, this result does not contradict the conclusion reached previously, because K^+ channels of the HC membrane differ from those of the nerve membrane in their activation with hyperpolarization and not with depolarization.

On the other hand, the substitution of choline or Tris for Na^+ did not change appreciably the voltage-current curve in light. The same can be said about the substitution of SO_4^{2-} for Cl^- (with isotonicity made up by sucrose). Therefore, apparently neither Na^+ nor Cl^- take part in the mechanism of nonlinearity of the HC membrane.

More complicated is the situation with Ca^{2+} ions. On the one hand, such inhibitors of Ca^{2+} channels as 0.05–0.5 mM D-600 [32], up to 5 mM Cd^{2+} [33] and 4mM Co^{2+} had no effect on the shape of the voltage-current curve. On the other hand, the increase of Ca^{2+} concentration in the solution up to 20 mM increased appreciably the slope of the depolarizing part of the curve (Fig. 5b, curve 3) without affecting its hyperpolarizing part. It is unlikely that this effect can be attributed to the influence of Ca^{2+} ions on Na^+ channels, because, as mentioned earlier, the removal of Na^+ from the solution had no effect on the voltage-current curve. Hence, one can assume in accordance with the second alternative that depolarization of the HC membrane actually results in an increase of permeability to Ca^{2+}. In the normal solution, where the concentration of Ca^{2+} is not more than 1 mM, this process probably has only a small effect on the voltage-current curve. It is possible, however, that the changes of Ca^{2+} conductance are responsible for the upper loop of the voltage-current curve, which appeared in some of our experiments (Fig. 2b).

Therefore, the nonlinearity of the HC membrane in the retina of fish and turtle is based mainly on voltage-dependent K^+ channels activated by hyperpolarization. This explanation corresponds to the equivalent circuit of Figure 4a. However, some contribution of Ca^{2+} channels activated by depolarization is also possible. In the equivalent circuit of Figure 4, it can be indicated by the addition of a Ca^{2+} battery with a voltage-dependent internal resistance (Fig. 4c), the minimal value of which is relatively high.

AMPLIFICATION OF GRADED POTENTIALS IN HORIZONTAL CELLS

Because of its voltage dependence, the HC membrane takes part in the generation of electrical responses to light stimulation. In order to imagine what could be the effect of this involvement, it is convenient to consider the model of HC. The model and the method of calculation are described separately [25,34]. Here we will mention only the main properties of the model and the results obtained.

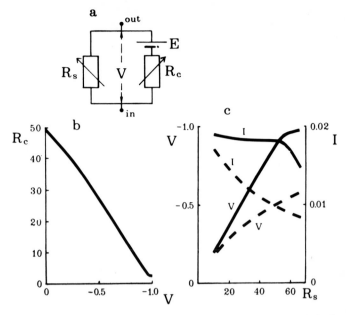

Fig. 6. The model of the HC membrane. (a) Equivalent circuit of the model, R_s is the resistance of the subsynaptic membrane controlled by light, R_c is the internal resistance of the resting potential battery (E) of the cell membrane, V is membrane potential. (b) The function $R_c = f(V)$, R_c in relative units, V in units of E = 1. The curve $R_c = f(V)$ was measured as the chordal resistance on the "light" voltage-current curve of Figure 1b; R_c^{max} (when V = 0) is taken as equal to 50. (c) Calculated membrane potential (V) and synaptic current (I) as functions of the resistance of the subsynaptic membrane (R_s); the increase of R_s corresponds to the increase of light. Solid lines correspond to nonlinear $R_c = f(V)$, dashed lines were calculated for constant R_c ($R_c = Const = 50$). It is seen that nonlinearity of R_c results in amplification of potentials (the slope of curve V is increased) and in stabilization of current (solid curve I) in the range of potentials where R_c is nonlinear.

The model of the HC is shown in Figure 6a. R_s is the resistance of the subsynaptic membrane, which is low in darkness, when the excitatory synapses are opened, and increases in light. No battery is represented here because in the actual HCs its emf (ie, the reversal potential of light response) is near zero. The rest of the membrane (nonsynaptic) is represented by a battery of resting potential E, with its internal resistance R_c. It was shown previously that this battery is mainly a K^+ battery and that the value of R_c depends on the voltage (V) across the membrane: It is low with high membrane potential and increases with depolarization. The function $R_c = f(V)$ is easy to measure experimentally from the voltage-current curve taken in bright light, if one accepts that R_s is infinite (practically, many times higher than the resistance of the nonsynaptic membrane) when the synapses are closed. Function $R_c = f(V)$ (Fig. 5b) was measured as a chordal resistance from the voltage-current curve "in light" shown in Figure 1b. The model is adapted to reproduce only steady states and, therefore, has no capacitances. It also has no resistances which correspond to electrical coupling between HCs. Hence, it can reproduce only the result of uniform illumination over a large area of the retina. For simplicity all numerical values of the model are expressed in relative units.

Let us consider how the nonlinearity of the HC membrane affects the light responses. The lower solid line in Figure 6c shows the calculated membrane potential (V) with the increase of subsynaptic resistance R_s (ie, with the increase of light intensity). The lower dashed line, shown for comparison, was calculated for the case of a linear HC membrane (R_c = Const = 50). One can see that the nonlinearity results in an increase of steepness of the curve in the range considered, ie, in the increase of light responses of HCs. Therefore, the HC membrane is able to amplify the potential changes generated by the synapses.

As compared with the well-known electrogenic membrane of the axon, the HC membrane has some peculiar features. First, its electrogenic properties are based on a quite different ionic mechanism: Instead of an increase of Na^+ permeability with depolarization, K^+ permeability is decreased. Second, membrane potential does not jump, as in the axon membrane, from one level to another, at least under normal conditions. On the contrary, graduality of potentials is preserved, which seems to be an essential property for "electrotonic" processing of signals in the retina.

There is another interesting property of the model, as well as of HCs themselves. As seen in Figure 6a, the resistances of subsynaptic (R_s) and cell membranes (R_c) are in series with respect to the current generated by the battery of the resting potential (E). During the light response, both resistances change in opposite directions: R_s increases and R_c decreases. As a result, the current is stabilized to some extent: It changes relatively little during the light response. This is shown by the solid curve I in Figure 6c, calculated for the nonlinear R_c, in comparison with the dashed curve I, calculated for R_c = Const = 50. If the voltage-current curve has a vertical part in some range of potentials, stabilization of current has to be perfect in this range, because different voltages correspond to one and the same current.

One practical important conclusion can be drawn from what was said previously. The changes of extracellular current generated by HCs in response to diffuse illumination, and recorded as a component of the ERG, can depend upon the intensity of the light in a quite different way than the changes of membrane potential in HCs.

One can try to estimate the functional significance of the nonlinearity of the HC membrane. Three different assumptions were made by us in different papers, and all three seem to be correct. First, because of nonlinearity the conditions for propagation of potentials along the HC layer are maintained relatively constant with different intensities of illumination [23,42]. Indeed, the resistances of subsynaptic and nonsynaptic membranes change in opposite directions with the increase of diffuse illumination. Due to this, the slope (differential) resistance and, accordingly, the space constant of the HC layer for small changes of potential is kept up more or less constant over a wide range of membrane potentials. The second assumption also concerns the propagation of potentials along the HC layer, but from a somewhat different viewpoint. Nonlinearity results in amplification of potentials, and therefore they are propagated along the HC layer to greater distances [22,25]. In nerve structures which function "electrotonically," but have a relatively large size (as the HC layer in retina), such a property should be of great use.

According to the third assumption, nonlinearity of the HC membrane serves to stabilize currents generated by these cells over areas with uniform illumination. The meaning of the last assumption will be clear in the next section.

ON THE OUTPUT SIGNALS OF HORIZONTAL CELLS

As interneurones, HCs receive inputs from photoreceptors and transmit their signals to HCs of other types as well as back to photoreceptors, and to bipolars. This fact is beyond doubt, because it was shown experimentally that polarization of HCs by extrinsic current evoked responses in different retinal structures: It evoked the local ERG [35], the response of ganglion cells [36,37], of cones [38] and of bipolars [39,40]. However, the mechanism of signal transmission is reliably known in only one case: The electrical coupling between neighboring HCs of the same type [12,41,42]. Chemical synapses, which are typical outputs in other neurones, were described between HCs and bipolars; however, they are relatively rare in the retina of the cat and rabbit [43,44] and were not found in monkey retina [45]. It was supposed by several authors that the output of HCs, in particular the mechanism of feedback from HCs to photoreceptors, is localized at the processes of HCs invaginating synaptic terminals of receptors [46,47]. However, no chemical synapses were found between HC processes and receptors, at least of a conventional type [48].

Based on some observations we supposed, some time ago, that the feedback of HCs to photoreceptors is carried out not by chemical synaptic transmission, but in another way—by means of currents generated by the HCs. The hypothesis, as well as experimental data on which it is based, are described separately [25,39,49–55]. Here we will only mention briefly the main idea and some consequences which seem to be of interest for the problem under discussion.

According to the hypothesis, the output signal of HCs is a synaptic current generated when the subsynaptic membrane is activated by transmitter released from photoreceptors. The current, when flowing along the gap between photoreceptor and HC, evokes a potential drop near the synapse, which is practically applied to the presynaptic membrane of the photoreceptor. As a result, a feedback appears which is positive if the synapse is excitatory. The deep invaginations of HC processes into the receptor terminals are in favor of such feedback, because the longitudinal resistance of the gap is higher and, accordingly, the potential drop evoked by synaptic current is higher. It was also supposed that the same feedback mechanism controls the activity of receptor synapses with other HCs and bipolars within the same triad, because all postsynaptic elements in a triad are probably controlled by one and the same presynaptic apparatus.

In attempts to estimate the functional consequences of this hypothesis, we have tried to consider the spatial distribution of outputs of the HC layer in the cases when these outputs are controlled by synaptic currents or by membrane potential (as in usual chemical synapses). The calculations of synaptic currents and membrane potentials in the HC layer with different stimulus configurations were made in a two-dimensional model of the HC layer [56].

The model consisted of a set of elements (HCs) connected with each other through relatively low resistances ("electrical contacts" and resistance of the cytoplasm) in a rectangular net of 40 × 40 elements. Each element was the model of HC shown in Figure 6a. One element corresponded approximately to a square 0.1 × 0.1 mm in the retina. The model was run in a computer. A more detailed description of the model and the analysis of its properties was done separately [56]. Here we reproduce only the results of computation specially repeated by Shura-Bura with the nonlinearity $R_c = f(V)$ shown in Figure 6b.

Solid lines in the lower part of Figure 7a show how membrane potential (V) and synaptic current (I) change along the line crossing the border between the less and the more illuminated parts of retina (see the upper part of Fig. 7a). One can see that membrane potential changes gradually from the lower (left) to the higher (right) levels, and the border between two differently illuminated parts is blurred. On the contrary, in the curve of currents the border is stressed sharply by oppositely directed peaks. It is important to note that over large uniformly illuminated areas on both sides of the border, the synaptic currents are almost equal, in spite of different levels of membrane potential. It was already mentioned (see Fig. 6c) that this is the result of current stabilization by the nonlinearity of the HC membrane, as seen from the comparison with the dashed line (I) in Figure 7a, computed for $R_c = Const = 50$.

Figure 7 also illustrates the distribution of potentials and currents in the HC layer when there is a small dark spot on a bright background (b) or viceversa (c). In both cases one can see relatively small and blurred changes of membrane potential and very sharp and big changes of synaptic currents.

Therefore, the spatial distribution of membrane potential and of synaptic currents in the HC layer, with light stimuli of different configurations, differs very much from each other. One can note that the current distribution resembles,

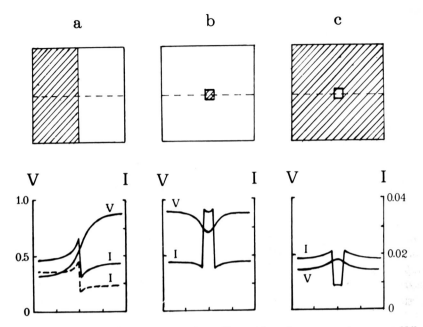

Fig. 7. Two-dimensional model of the HC layer. The model, made as a computer program [56], is equivalent to a set of elements (HCs shown in Fig. 6a) connected with each other through low resistors (2.4, in relative units) in a rectangular net of 40 × 40 elements. These resistors represent the coupling between adjacent cells, as well as the resistance of the cytoplasm. Each element corresponds approximately to a square 0.1 × 0.1 mm in the retina. The computations were specially repeated by Shura-Bura with nonlinearity $R_c = f(V)$ shown in Figure 6b. The upper pictures show the distribution of light in the model: The dashed areas correspond to weak light ($R_s = 20$), the white areas to bright light ($R_s = 50$, in relative units, see Fig. 6). The lower graphs show the distribution of membrane potential (V) and synaptic currents (I) along the dashed lines in upper pictures. V is expressed in fractions of E = 1. (a) The right half of the "retina" is illuminated more brightly than the left half. The dashed trace (I) corresponds to $R_c = Const = 50$; (b) a small dark spot on a bright background; (c) a light spot on a weakly illuminated background.

to some extent, the properties of bipolars: It is known that bipolars give much larger responses to small spots than to diffuse illumination [57,58]. This resemblance could serve as an argument in favor of an important role of "current" outputs of HCs. One has to bear in mind, however, that the "chemical" feedback (ie, the "potential" outputs of HCs), as it is easy to show, also smooths over, at the level of presynaptic terminals of receptors, the differences in signals from large uniformly, but differently illuminated retinal areas.

Thus, the mechanism of output signals of HCs to other retinal neurones is still a problem which needs additional experimental efforts.

REFERENCES

1. Svaetichin G: The cone action potential. Acta Physiol Scand 29 Suppl 106:565, 1953.
2. Shepherd GM: "The synaptic organization of the brain. An Introduction." London: Oxford University Press, 1974.
3. Schmitt FO, Dev P, Smith BH: Electrotonic processing of information by brain cells. Science 193:114, 1976.
4. Svaetichin G, Laufer M, Mitarai G, Fatechand R, Vallecalle E, Villegas J: Glial control of neuronal networks and receptors. In Jung R, Kornhuber H (eds): "The Visual System: Neurophysiology and Psychophysics." Berlin: Springer-Verlag, 1961, p 445.
5. Nelson R: A comparison of electrical properties of neurons in Necturus retina. J Neurophysiol 36:519, 1973.
6. Tasaki K: Some observations on the retinal potentials of the fish. Arch Ital Biol 98:81, 1960.
7. Trifonov Yu-A, Utina IA: Investigation of the mechanism of current action on the L-type cells of the retina. Biophysica 11:646, 1966.
8. Toyoda J, Nosaki H, Tomita T: Light induced resistance changes in single photoreceptors of Necturus and Gekko. Vision Res 9:453, 1969.
9. Maksimova EM, Maksimov VV: On the changes in direct current input resistance in horizontal cells of fish retina during excitation. Neurophysiology 3:210, 1971.
10. Naka K-I, Rushton VAH: The generation and spread of S-potentials in fish (Cyprinidae). J Physiol 193:437, 1967.
11. Maksimov VV: In Kostyuk (edt): "Synaptic Processes." Kiev Naukova Dumka, 1968 p 247.
12. Kaneko A: Electrical connections between horizontal cells in the dogfish retina. J Physiol 213:95, 1971.
13. Minor AV, Maksimov VV: Passive electric properties of the model of flat cell. Biophysica 14:328, 1969.
14. Trifonov Yu-A, Byzov AL: The response of the cells generating S-potentials to the current passed through the eye cup of the turtle. Biophysica 10:673, 1965.
15. Trifonov Yu-A: Study of synaptic transmission between photoreceptor and horizontal cell by electric stimulation of the retina. Biophysica 13:809, 1968.
16. Byzov AL, Trifonov Yu-A: The response to electric stimulation of horizontal cells in the carp retina. Vision Res 8:817, 1968.
17. Tomita T: Electrophysiological study of the mechanisms subserving colour coding in the fish retina. Cold Spring Harb Symp Quant Biol 30:559, 1965.
18. Kaneko A, Shimazaki H: Synaptic transmission from photoreceptors to the second-order neurones in the carp retina. In: F. Zettler and R. Weiler (eds) "Neural Principles of Vision." Berlin: Springer-Verlag, 1976, p 143.
19. Dowling JE, Ripps H: Effects of magnesium on horizontal cell activity in the skate retina. Nature (London) 242:101, 1973.
20. Cervetto L, Piccolino M: Synaptic transmission between photoreceptors and horizontal cells in the turtle retina. Science 183:417, 1974.
21. Trifonov Yu-A, Chailahian LM, Byzov AL: An investigation of the origin of electrical responses of horizontal cells in fish retina. Neurophysiology 3:89, 1971.
22. Byzov AL, Trifonov Yu-A: Electrical properties of subsynaptic and nonsynaptic membranes of horizontal cells in turtle retina. Neurophysiology 5:423, 1973.
23. Trifonov Yu-A, Byzov AL, Chailahian LM: Electrical properties of subsynaptic and nonsynaptic membranes of horizontal cells in fish retina. Vision Res 14:229, 1974.
24. Trifonov Yu-A, Chailahian LM: Uniform polarization of fibres and syncytial structures with extracellular electrodes. Biophysica 20:107, 1975.
25. Byzov AL, Trifonov Yu-A, Chailahian LM, Golubtzov KV: Amplification of graded potentials in horizontal cells of the retina. Vision Res 17:265, 1977.

26. Trifonov Yu-A, Gloubtzov KV, Byzov AL, Chailahian LM: Membrane potential clamping in horizontal cells of the fish retina. Neurophysiology 9:402, 1977.

27. Werblin FS: Anomalous rectification in horizontal cells. J Physiol 244:639, 1975.

28. Waloga G, Pak WL: Ionic mechanism for the generation of horizontal cell potentials in isolated axolotle retina. J Gen Physiol 71:69, 1978.

29. Hagiwara S, Miyazaki S, Moody W, Patlak J: Blocking effect of barium and hydrogen ions on the potassium current during anomalous rectification in the starfish egg. J Physiol 237:167, 1978.

30. Sperelakis N, Schneider MF, Harris EJ: Decreased K conductance produced by Ba^{2+} in frog sartorius fibers. J Gen Physiol 50:1565, 1967.

31. Fain GL, Quandt FN, Gerschenfeld HM: Calcium-dependent regenerative responses in rods. Nature (London) 269:707, 1977.

32. Meech RW: Calcium-dependent potassium activation in nervous tissue. Ann Rev Biophys Bioeng 7:1, 1978.

33. Kostyuk PG, Krishtal OA: Separation of sodium and calcium current in the somatic membrane of mollusc neurons. J Physiol 270:515, 1977.

34. Byzov AL, Trifonov Yu-A, Chailahian LM: Nonsynaptic membrane of the retinal horizontal cells as an amplifier of slow potentials. Neurophysiology 7:74, 1975.

35. Byzov AL: Horizontal cells of the retina as regulators of synaptic transmission. Sechenov Physiol J 53:1115, 1967.

36. Maksimova EM: Effect of intracellular polarization of horizontal cells on the activity of ganglion cells in fish retina. Biophysica 14:537, 1969.

37. Marmarelis PZ, Naka K-I: Nonlinear analysis and synthesis of receptive field responses in the catfish retina. I. Horizontal cell-ganglion cell chain. J Neurophysiol 36:605, 1973.

38. Baylor DA, Fuortes MGF, O'Bryan PM: Receptive fields of cones in the retina of the turtle. J Physiol 214:265, 1971.

39. Trifonov Yu-A, Byzov AL: The interaction in photoreceptor synapses revealed in experiments with polarization of horizontal cells. In Barlow HB, Fatt P (eds): "Vertebrate Photoreception." London: Academic Press 1977, pp 251–263.

40. Toyoda J, Tonosaki K: Effect of polarization of horizontal cells on the on-center bipolar cell of the carp retina. Nature (London) 276:399, 1978.

41. Simon EJ: Two types of luminosity horizontal cells in the retina of the turtle. J Physiol 230:199, 1973.

42. Byzov AL: Interaction between horizontal cells of the turtle retina. Neurophysiology 7:279, 1975.

43. Dowling JE, Brown JE, Major D: Synapses of horizontal cells in rabbit and cat retinas. Science 153:1639, 1966.

44. Fisher SK, Boycott BB: Synaptic connexions made by horizontal cells within the outer plexiform layer of the retina of the cat and rabbit. Proc R Soc B 186:317, 1974.

45. Dowling JE, Boycott BB: Organization of the primate retina: Electronmicroscopy. Proc R Soc B 166:80, 1966.

46. Fuortes MGF, Simon EJ: Interaction leading to horizontal cell responses in the turtle retina. J Physiol 240:177, 1974.

47. Stell WK, Lightfoot DO, Wheeler TG, Leeper HF: Goldfish retina: Functional polarization of cone horizontal cell dendrites and synapses. Science 190:989, 1975.

48. Lasansky A: Organization of the outer synaptic layer in the retina of the larval tiger salamander. Phil Trans R Soc B 265:471, 1973.

49. Byzov AL, Trifonov Yu-A: Hypothesis on the electrical feedback in synaptic transmission between photoreceptors and second-order neurones in vertebrate retina. In Kostyuk (edt) "Synaptic Processes." Kiev: Naukova Dumka 231, 1968.

50. Byzov AL: The model of mechanism of feed-back between horizontal cells and photoreceptors

in vertebrate retina. Neurophysiology 9:86, 1977.

51. Byzov AL, Golubtzov KV: The model of mechanism of feedback by means of electrical current in chemical synapse. Biophysica 22:1081, 1977.

52. Byzov AL, Golubtzov KV, Trifonov Yu-A: The model of mechanism of feed-back between horizontal cells and photoreceptors in vertebrate retina. In Barlow HB, Fatt P(eds): "Vertebrate Photoreception." London: Academic Press, 1977, p 256.

53. Byzov AL, Cervetto L: Effects on applied currents on turtle cones in darkness and during the photoresponse. J Physiol 265:85, 1977.

54. Byzov AL, Golubtzov KV: The model of neurone which acts as a regulator of effectiveness of synaptic transmission. Biophysica 23:119, 1978.

55. Byzov AL: Origin of nonlinearity of voltage-current relationships of turtle cones. Vision Res 19:469, 1979.

56. Shura-Bura TM: Modelling of the reaction of horizontal cell layer to non-uniform illumination. Biophysica 21:566, 1976.

57. Werblin FS, Dowling JE: Organization of the retina of mudpuppy. *Necturus maculosus*. II. Intracellular recordings. J Neurophysiol 32:339, 1969.

58. Thibos L, Werblin FS: The response properties of the steady antagonistic surround in the mudpuppy retina. J Physiol 278:79, 1978.

The S-Potential, pages 123–136
© 1982 Alan R. Liss, Inc., 150 Fifth Avenue, New York, NY 10011

Electrically Evoked Responses (E-Responses) of the Carp Horizontal Cells

Kosuke Watanabe

When a brief electric current is applied through the retina from receptor side to vitreous, a transient depolarizing response is evoked in the horizontal cell (H-cell), the amplitude of which is small in the dark but is large under background light. This phenomenon was first found in the turtle retina by Trifonov and Byzov [1] and later led to a proposal of a hypothetical scheme how S-potential would be generated by light [2]. That is, as is generally accepted, a continuous release of excitatory transmitter from the receptor terminals maintains the membrane potential of a postsynaptic H-cell at a certain depolarized level in the dark and the S-potential is a repolarization of the H-cell membrane following the decrease of transmitter liberation caused by light that hyperpolarizes the receptor membrane. In the carp, similar phenomena were reported by Byzov and Trifonov [3] and were confirmed by Watanabe [4], who similarly concluded that the electrically evoked response (E-response) was a summated H-cell EPSP produced by a transient electrical excitation of the receptor terminals which would probably have properties similar to those of nerve cell membrane. The major reasons for this conclusion are (1) that the E-response is generated only when the stimulating current is passed from receptor side to vitreous but not in reverse direction (Fig. 1A and B); (2) that it is always accompanied with a certain decrease in membrane resistance; and (3) that it possesses absolute and relative refractory periods similar to the action potential of a nerve cell (Fig. 1C). The E-response, however, is not of all-or-none but of graded nature, and its amplitude increases with the increase in stimulating current until it reaches the maximum depolarization. This apparent discrepancy will easily be understood considering the fact that the E-response is a spatially summated EPSP of the H-cell resulting from a number of receptor terminals, each of which may excite in all-or-none fashion but with a different threshold.

All the experimental results described in this paper have been obtained from the eye cup preparation with the blood supply intact of the live carp (Cyprinus carpio). The fish was immobilized with gallamine and was artificially respirated with running water into the mouth and out through the gill. The front half of the eye, including the lens, was removed and most of the vitreous humor was carefully sucked out. Electrical stimuli were applied between a silver eye-holder placed behind the sclera and a spiral-shaped thin silver wire which fitted the curvature of the retinal surface and was dipped in the remaining vitreous humor. Precaution was taken to stimulate the retina as evenly as possible. A two-channel photostimulator using grating monochromators was employed to deliver light stimuli. The recording electrodes were 3 M KCl filled glass micropipettes and the reference electrode was a chlorided silver wire independent of the current electrode and placed into the vitreous humor.

TYPICAL E-RESPONSE AND OTHER ELECTRICALLY EVOKED RESPONSES IN THE H-CELL

As Byzov and Trifonov [3] have already pointed out, the relationship between electrically and light-evoked responses of the H-cell is a very complex one. Since, furthermore, the configuration of E-response is markedly affected by the duration of electrical pulse stimuli, a 1-msec duration has been routinely used, though the optimal range of the pulse width appears to be 0.5–2 msec, within which the waveform of the E-response changes very little.

Figure 1 A and B shows the effects of the polarity and duration of the electrical stimuli on an H-cell response to light and to electricity when other parameters of stimulation are kept constant. When a supramaximal electric current pulse is passed from sclera to vitreous (column A) a typical impulse-like E-response is evoked with 1-msec stimulus (a). On lengthening the stimulus duration, however, it gradually changes its amplitude and shape and finally disappears into a broader depolarization accompanied with an upward shift of the baseline, which is probably caused by stimulus artifact. Traces in column B were obtained when the direction of the current pulses was reversed but with exactly the same parameters as those of the corresponding responses in column A. Against the supramaximal strength of current pulse which produces a typical E-response, only a small dent-like response is observed in the top trace after switching the polarity of stimulation. It must be mentioned that if stimulus duration is less than 0.5 msec no more response can be detected to the vitreous-positive electric current. It must be pointed out, however, that, as stimulus duration is increased, the dent-like response grows up to a hump and then to a long-lasting hyperpolarization which can clearly be distinguished from the stimulus artifact. For example, in the bottom trace in B, the hyperpolarizing response lasts for more than 1 sec against 100-msec stimulus. The nature of this response has not yet been investigated systematically. However, considering the direction of the current flow and the

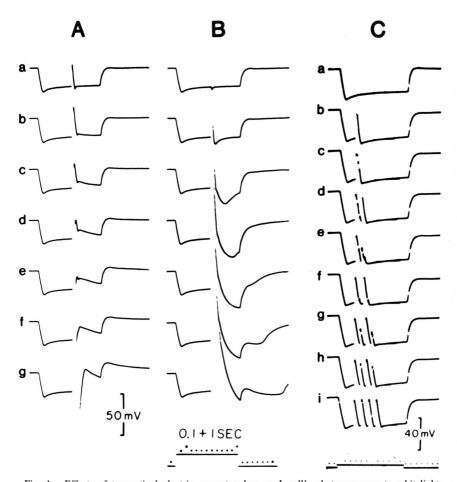

Fig. 1. Effects of transretinal electric current pulses on L-cell's photoresponses to whitelight. Supramaximal current pulses of different duration were passed from sclera to vitreous in A, and in reverse direction in B. Note that a typical impulse-like E-response is evoked by a sclera-positive pulse of 1-msec duration in a. On lengthening the stimulus duration from a to g amplitude and waveform of the response change gradually and finally the response disappears into a broad depolarization accompanied with an upward shift of the baseline probably caused by stimulus artifact. When the polarity of stimulation is switched only a small dent-like response is observable with 1-msec pulse (top trace in B). As stimulus duration is increased the dent-like response grows up to a hump and then to a long-lasting hyperpolarization which may not be an artifact. Stimulus duration: a, 1; b, 10; c, 20; d, 30; e, 40; f, 50; g, 100 msec. Column C indicates absolute and relative refractory periods of E-responses. Trains of four electrical stimuli, each of 1-msec duration are given, sclera-positively, and pulse interval is lengthened from b to i; a, control response without electrical stimulation. Note that only the first stimulus is effective in b and c, and all four pulses are effective with a 150-msec interval in i. Pulse interval: b, 10; c, 20; d, 40; e, 60; f, 80; g, 100; h, 120; i, 150 msec.

structural basis of both receptors and H-cells, it appears that this is not a primary response of the H-cell to the electrical stimulation but a secondary one caused by some unknown event in the receptors resulting in a continuous depression of the excitatory transmitter release.

Notwithstanding that these kinds of response will never occur in natural life of the animal, it is obvious that the system, receptors–H-cells, is able to respond to the electrical stimulation other than its natural stimulus, light. These H-cell responses are rather complicated but, among them, the E-response which can now be defined as a transient depolarizing response evoked by a sclera-positive electrical pulse stimulus appears to be well understood and has been examined as a tool pertinent to the investigation of the synaptic mechanisms between receptors and H-cells.

E-S RELATION AND EQUILIBRIUM POTENTIAL OF THE H CELL

It is obvious from the scheme of S-potential generation that the plateau of an S-potential represents a membrane potential level of the H-cell in the light established by a reduction of the sustained EPSP while an E-response, if elicited, is a transient buildup of EPSP from that level. Accordingly, if E-responses are superimposed on the plateau of S-potentials, sets of paired potential values will be obtained. Thus by plotting the amplitude of E-responses against that of the corresponding S-potentials, a correlation between them can be examined, and if it is linear an equilibrium potential will be estimated by extrapolating the straight line to intersect the horizontal axis. We call such a diagram an "E-S relation," in which the E-response is represented as a function of membrane potential, since, taking the resting dark potential into account, the S-potential represents membrane potential of the cell in the light.

There are three methods to vary the amplitude of the S-potential, that is, by changing the light intensity, the wavelength, and the illumination area. Since, however, a complication exists in the last method because of differences in distribution between receptors stimulated by light and by current, the former two methods are usually employed in combination with a fixed strength of the electrical stimuli to obtain E-S relations for a single H-cell. Generally, straight lines with different slopes are obtained for most cells when the intensity of white light is taken as a variable, and the slope increases its steepness with the increase in stimulating current up to supramaximal. It can be said that, with current stronger than moderate, all the lines drawn intersect the horizontal axis at around a point within the experimental error for a single cell, and the equilibrium potentials thus estimated range from 0 to about 10 mV above the ground (zero potential). Detection of the reversal potential by polarizing the subsynaptic membrane by means of intracellular current injection is difficult because of the electrically coupled syncitium-like property of the cells as pointed by Naka and Rushton [5]. Trifonov et al [6] succeeded in direct measurement of the equilibrium potential by passing polarizing current tangentially through the retina. Values obtained from the E-S relation coincide well with their findings.

DEVIATION FROM THE LINEAR E-S RELATION WITH MONOCHROMATIC LIGHTS

When monochromatic lights are used instead of white light, any deviation from the linear E-S relationship, if present, is more clearly observed in the E-S diagram, and the phenomenon appears to disclose distinct inputs to the H-cell, especially to L-cells. There appears to be no doubt that L-cells in fish retina receive signals from more than two sets of cones [7]. In carp, however, there are contradictory observations; red- and probably green-sensitive [8], red- and far red-sensitive cones [9] appear to be involved. In fact, it is fairly difficult to isolate the contribution of short or middle wavelength cones by means of selective adaptation, especially when that of red-sensitive cones is predominant, because a strong red background light weakens markedly the photoresponse of the cells, resulting in a rather flat spectral response curve from which a definite shift of the peak can hardly be pointed out. Two typical examples of spectral responses to light and to electric current of photopic L-cells are shown in Figure 2A and B. Scanning the wavelength of illumination from 410 to 750 nm in 20-nm steps, equal-quantum monochromatic lights were used to generate S-potentials, and at the plateau of each photoresponse a supermaximal electric current was applied to evoke E-responses. In the case of cell A, the contour of E-responses (crosses) is smooth and almost a mirror image of that of S-potentials (filled circles) with a response maximum at about 620 nm. On the contrary, in the case of cell B, a sharp dip indicating a strong depression at 690 nm is marked in the contour of E-responses while other profiles of the spectral responses show little difference. Figure 2C and D show respective E-S relations taken from the above two cells A and B. While the E-S diagram for cell A indicates a linear relation, that for cell B shows a straight line and several scattered points deviating downward from it, which are all in the deep red region of illumination as indicated by the numbers attached to them. These two cells are extreme examples and there are many cells situated between them with various grades of deviation.

Since, however, the suppression of the E-response is, more or less, a generally observed phenomenon when deep-red illumination is very intense, it appears that such a deviation from the linear E-S relation in the long-wavelength region is one of the characteristics of the photopic L-cells in the carp. In the example shown in Figure 3A and B, the intensity of two monochromatic lights, 530-nm green and 690-nm deep-red, was varied while the electric stimulation was kept constant. Thus two sets of E-S relation for the same cell are indicated, a straight line for green and a curve for deep-red. It is evident that up to moderate intensity deep-red light gives a linear E-S relation, but beyond a certain level of intensity, or when the S-potential exceeds a certain level of the membrane potential, a

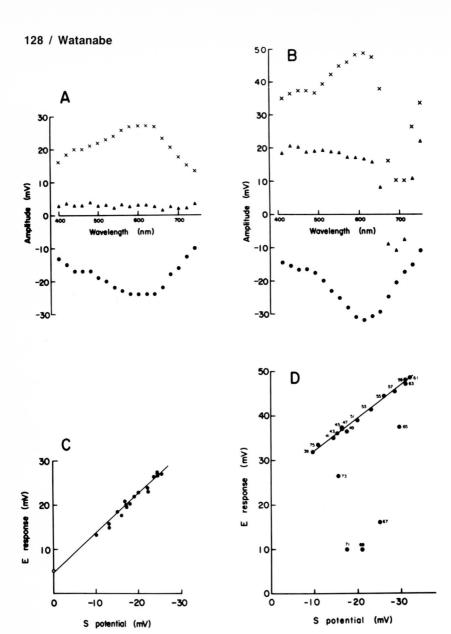

Fig. 2.   (A) and (B) Two examples of spectral response to light (●) and to electrical stimulation (X) of L-cell; (▲) represents peak level of the E-response superimposed on the S-potential. Scanning the wavelength of illumination from 410 to 750 nm in 20-nm steps, equal-quantum monochromatic lights were used to generate S-potentials, and at the plateau of each photoresponse a supramaximal current pulse of 1-msec duration was applied to evoke an E-response. Note that in cell A, the contour of the E-response is almost a mirror image of that of the S-potential, whereas in cell B, a strong depression at 690 nm is seen in the E-response. (C) and (D) Respective E-S relations obtained from cells A and B. Plotting E-responses against corresponding S-potentials produce a straight line in C, and a straight line and some scattered points in D. Note that points deviating from the line are all derived from red illumination as indicated by abbreviated numbers for wavelength.

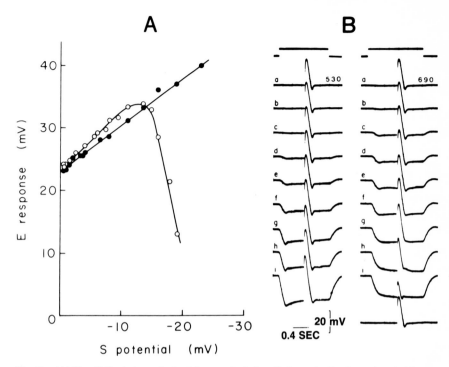

Fig. 3.   (A) Two E-S relations obtained from a single L-cell shown in (B). Intensity of different monochromatic lights, 530-nm green and 690-nm deep-red, was varied while the electrical stimulation was kept constant. Intensity: a, -4; b, -3.5; c, -3; d, -2.5; e, -2; f, -1.5; g, -1; h, -0.5; i, 0 log unit. Note that in (A), up to moderate intensity deep-red light produces a linear E-S relation but when S-potential exceeds a certain level of membrane potential with intense illumination, a strong suppression of the E-response takes place, while green light gives a straight line, suggesting that the L-cell receives inputs from green- and red-sensitive cones. Separation of the two straight lines is probably due to an effect of light adaptation during a sequence of experiments. Note further a striking resemblance between the rising phase of S-potentials and the recovery phase of E-response under each illumination when the S-potential is of moderate size. Slow rising phase of the S-potential with intense deep-red light and an oscillation at the end of the E-response are indications of a recurrent feedback mechanism between red-sensitive cones and the L-cell.

strong suppression of the E-response takes place rather rapidly. From these results it is concluded that L-cells in the carp must receive inputs from at least two sets of cones because the amplitude of the E-response does not depend simply on the membrane potential of the cell but also on the wavelength of illumination, and that the inputs probably come from green-sensitive in addition to red-sensitive cones.

FEEDBACK FROM HORIZONTAL CELL TO RECEPTORS

From the above conclusion a question will arise: Why is the behavior of the E-response under deep-red illumination so different from that in green light? Is it because of the difference between the properties of red- and green-sensitive cones themselves or because of the difference between synaptic connections of those receptors to the L-cell? By comparing carefully the shape of the rising phase of the S-potential with that of the recovery phase of the E-response, a recurrent feedback mechanism at the synapse between L-cell and red-sensitive cones has been proposed in a previous paper [10]. A close similarity of the rising phase of hyperpolarizing S-potential to the recovery phase of the E-response is most clearly observed when an E-response to a constant current pulse is super-imposed on the plateau of each S-potential produced by a large field illumination of different wavelength. Both phases are fairly fast, with a small transient in the range of short wavelengths, but they gradually and equally slow down with increases in wavelength. Such a strong resemblance will lead to a confirmation that both S-potential and E-response are generated from the same subsynaptic membrane, and the mechanism involved in both phases must be the same, that is, inhibition of depolarizing transmitter liberation from the receptor terminals. An example of the most distinctive features of both green and deep-red responses to light as well as to electric pulse will be observed in the bottom traces of Figure 3B. Contrary to the sharp and large green response, a strikingly depressed E-response with an oscillation at the end of recovery phase is superimposed on a slowly going photoresponse to deep-red light.

It has already been pointed out by Byzov and Trifonov [3] that there is an initial depression of the E-response after the onset of white light and that the higher the light intensity, the longer the period of depression. From an examination of a train of E-responses superimposed on the whole course of S-potentials generated by two different monochromatic lights (Fig. 4A), it is evident that this is a phenomenon proper to the red-sensitive cone system and equivalent to a long-lasting relative refractory period mentioned previously. With green light such a depression is also seen in the rapidly rising phase of S-potential and the inhibition is complete as if it is within an absolute refractory period, and the relative refractory period is very short, if present. The characteristic slowing of the rising phase in deep-red light can be explained by the proposal of a recurrent feedback mechanism, assuming the recurrent synapses between red-sensitive cones and L-cell as found in goldfish retina by Stell et al [11] and by Marc et al [12].

In darkness, the L-cell will be depolarized by continuous release of excitatory transmitter from receptor terminals, but this in turn tends to reduce the depolarization of the receptor by recurrent inhibitory synapses. Thus the antagonistic effects of these synapses will determine the level of membrane potential of the

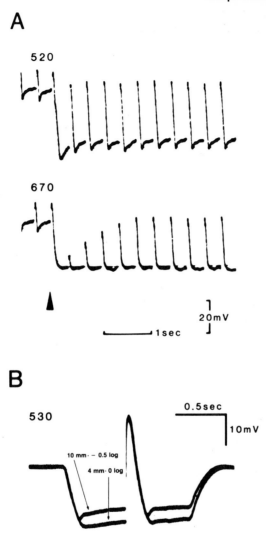

Fig. 4. (A) Difference between properties of green- and red-sensitive cone systems contributing to a single L-cell. Trains of E-responses were superimposed on the whole course of S-potentials generated by different monochromatic illuminations, 520-nm green and 670-nm deep-red. Note that initial depression and gradual recovery of the E-response after the light onset are specific properties of red-sensitive cone system probably equivalent to absolute and relative refractory periods, the latter lasts fairly long under intense illumination. Green-sensitive cone system also shows initial depression of E-response but it is not indicated in this figure. (B) Two photoresponses of a single L-cell to green light showing different waveforms due to difference in spot size; one 10 mm and the other 4 mm in diameter. The intensity and the spot size are adjusted so that the slope of the rising phase of both S-potentials coincide with each other. Apparent waveform of the large field S-potential with on-transient followed by steady depolarization resembles a cone response with feedback from L-cell. Note that light spot of 4 mm in diameter is incapable of producing feedback effect.

receptors and, accordingly, that of the L-cell will be set. When a sudden step-like change is given to this system, for example, by light onset, it will take time to reach a new level, and if an impulse-like depolarizing change such as an E-response is produced, an oscillation may appear during the recovery phase as a result of a transient disturbance in the system. In fact, Murakami et al [13] detected a transient IPSP in cones caused by the E-response.

Feedback from H-cell to receptor has been studied mainly in turtle retina. Direct evidence for this phenomenon was given by Baylor et al [14] who demonstrated that a hyperpolarization of the H-cell by passing current produced a transient depolarization of the receptor membrane and that the photoresponse of the receptor was reduced during the passage of hyperpolarizing current through the H-cell. In the configuration of receptor potential the effect of feedback is generally manifested as a delayed depolarization making the on-transient prominent which is especially marked when a large area is lighted. In the H-cell such an on-transient is also seen with a large spot of illumination, as pointed out in pikeperch retina by Burkhardt and Hassin [15], who suggested the possibility that it might be the consequence of feedback to cones.

In carp S-potentials, on-transient is most common and prominent in C-type cell's response to white light, but it is also observed in L-cells when short or middle wavelength illumination is used as shown in Figure 4 B. In the figure, two responses of a single L-cell to green light are superimposed to show differences in the waveform caused by different spot sizes. The intensity and the spot size are adjusted so that the slope of the rising phase of both S-potentials coincide with each other. Comparing the smooth response to a small spot, the large field response has an on-transient followed by a steady depolarization as if it were resulting from the feedback to cones. However, the illumination area necessary to produce this so-called feedback appears to be too large, so that 4 mm in diameter is still incapable of producing a feedback effect in this cell, whereas 1 mm is sufficient in pikeperch L-cells. Thus it can be concluded that in carp L-cells there are recurrent feedback system to red-sensitive cones but no such a feedback to green-sensitive cones, at least, to whose contributing to generation of luminosity S-potentials.

COMPOSITE E-RESPONSE OF R/G CELLS AND GENERATION OF THE DEPOLARIZING S-POTENTIAL

The E-response of color-opponent R/G cells is characterized by its diphasic shape with a prominent negative peak which is especially marked when superimposed on the depolarizing photoresponse to red light as shown in Figure 5. Furthermore, there is a striking resemblance in behavior after the light onset between the negative component of E-responses superimposed on the positive S-potential of R/G cell and the positive E-responses superimposed on the negative deep-red S-potential of L-cell. In the former an initial depression is observed, followed by a gradual growth (Fig. 5A) which is one of the characteristic features of E-response of L-cells under deep-red illumination, as already described. From analyses of the amplitude of the negative component and of the latency to its

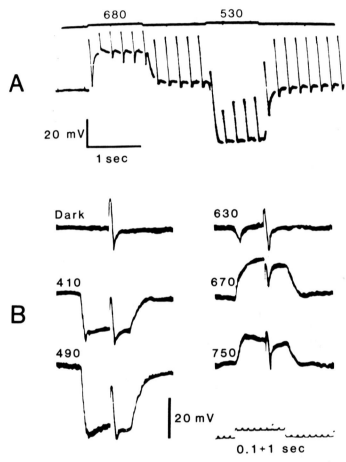

Fig. 5. Two examples of opponent R/G cell. (A) A train of E-responses superimposed on S-potentials generated by deep-red and green lights. Note that the behavior of the negative component of E-responses superimposed on the positive photoresponse resembles remarkably that of E-responses superimposed on deep-red S-potential of L-cell indicated in Figure 4A. (B) Photoresponses of a single R/G cell to different wavelengths, each with an E-response to constant current pulse. Number attached to each response indicates wavelength in nm. 630 nm was a neutral point in this cell. Note that in the response to 670-nm the initial positive E-response does not reach the positive S-potential. Such phenomena occur only when the E-response in darkness does not exceed a large depolarizing photoresponse to red illumination, and suggest that there might be two independent inputs for the R/G cell.

peak as functions of membrane potential, which is varied by changing the intensity of alternate green and deep-red lights, it has been confirmed that the negative component of the E-response and the positive photoresponse to deep-red in R/G cell are both derived from the positive E-response and the negative S-potential of L-cells. Thus it is conclusively stated in the previous paper [10] that the distinct diphasic configuration of the E-response superimposed on the depolarizing S-potential of R/G cells is composed of an initial positive response elicited by direct stimulation of green-sensitive cone terminals together with a delayed response which is generated in L-cells by stimulation of red-sensitive cones and is reversed via synapses between L-cells and green-sensitive cones. It must be pointed out, however, that occasionally the positive peak of the E-response does not reach the maximum depolarization of deep-red S-potential as seen in Figure 5 B at 670 nm, though this phenomenon is observable only when the depolarizing S-potential exceeds the E-response in darkness. Nevertheless, this appears to be negative against the previously mentioned hypothetical scheme that the signal of L-cell is once transmitted to green-sensitive cones via sign-inverting synapses and then conveyed to R/G cell from those cones. What the figure indicates is that there are two independent inputs to R/G cell; one is a positive E-response driven probably by green-sensitive cone terminals, and the other an inverted photo- as well as E-response from the L-cell without passing through the green-sensitive cones. Because if green-sensitive cones had already been depolarized by a red signal from the L-cell, and, accordingly, if they had depolarized the R/G cell, the E-response would start from the level of depolarizing S-potential. However, the figure suggests that the membrane potential of green-sensitive cones stays nearly at the level in darkness. In other words, they are little affected directly or indirectly by deep-red illumination. In Figure 6 a simplified equivalent circuit for an assumed synaptic membrane of the R/G cell is illustrated. The diagram is composed of two subsynaptic membrane components; the one indicated with suffix G is for a green input from green-sensitive cones, and the other with suffix R for a red input from an unknown cell. Under deep-red illumination, e_G is little affected, the value of r_G stays at dark level, and there must be potential drop across r_G produced by a steady current due to a large e_R. When an E-response is evoked at the green synapse, r_G decreases markedly resulting in a transient decrease of the potential drop across it. So that, if e_G of the E-response is not large enough to cover the reduced potential drop, the previously described situation may occur.

The L-cell (H1) in goldfish has been identified as a GABA-ergic neurone, and GABA is considered to be responsible for the negative feedback from L-cell to cones [12]. In carp, according to Murakami and others [13], the depolarizing S-potential in the red region of R/G cell is reversed by application of a large amount of GABA which also abolishes the IPSP generated in cones by the E-response of H-cells. Thus GABA-mediated feedback to cones seems to play an

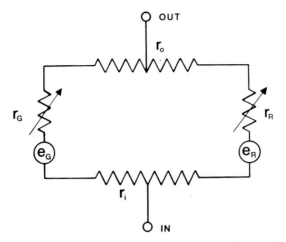

Fig. 6. An equivalent circuit of the R/G cell subsynaptic membrane for two independent inputs. The emf and membrane resistance of green synapse probably activated by green-sensitive cones are indicated with suffix G, and those of red synapse by unknown cell with suffix R. r_i and r_o represent intra- and extracellular resistances, respectively. Under deep-red illumination e_G is affected little and r_G is fixed at a position near the darkness potential. There must be a potential drop across r_G produced by a steady current due to a large e_R. When an E-response is evoked at the green synapse, r_G decreases markedly resulting in a transient reduction of the potential drop across it. If e_G of the E-response is not large enough to cover the decrease of potential drop, the photoresponse to deep-red light may exceed the E-response as observed in Figure 5B, 670 nm.

important role in producing color-opponent C-type S-potentials along the attractive pathways proposed by Stell and others [11] and supported by the author [10]. In fact, recurrent synapses between L-cell and red-sensitive cones have been morphologically identified [12] and appear to operate upon a characteristic slow rising phase of L-cell's photoresponse to deep red light as described previously. However, the structural basis for feedback synapses to cones other than the red-sensitive ones has not yet been established in cyprinid retinas. Similarly, no morphologically distinct synaptic connection has been proven between different types of H-cells, for example, L- and R/G cells. If the L-cell should make GABA-ergic synapses onto the R/G cell, postsynaptic depolarization must be accompanied by a conductance decrease, which contradicts the experimental fact that a decrease in membrane conductance is observed with hyperpolarization, and increase with depolarization irrespective of cell type [16]. Thus there should be some interneurone like the green-sensitive cones in the model of Stell et al [11], or else the L-cell should have some other connection to the R/G cell which fulfills the demands from physiological observations. Burkhardt and Hassin [15] suggested, approving the proposal of Naka and Rushton [17], that independent pathways arising from red- and green-sensitive cones converge upon R/G cell and modulate there the liberation of transmitters which evoke postsynaptic potentials of opposite polarity. In that case, however, it appears to be difficult to explain the phenomenon that artificial polarization of the L-cell by current injection affects the membrane potential of the R/G cell in a similar way to red illumination (Toyoda et al, unpublished). Thus at present more elaborate work is needed to draw an unequivocal conclusion on this problem.

ACKNOWLEDGMENTS

I wish to thank Mr. Y. Katagiri and Mr. Y. Suda for their contribution to much of this work. I also thank Mr. O. Umino for his help in preparing illustrations, Mr. Y. Mayama for the photographic services, and Mr. K. Koike for technical assistance. This work was partly supported by a grant from the Ministry of Education (248114).

REFERENCES

1. Trifonov YuA, Byzov AL: The response of the cells generating S-potential on the current passed through the eye cup of the turtle. Biofisika 10:673, 1965 (in Russian).
2. Trifonov YuA: Study of synaptic transmission between photoreceptors and horizontal cells by means of electric stimulation of the retina. Biofisika 13:809, 1968 (in Russian).
3. Byzov AL, Trifonov YuA: The response to electric stimulation of horizontal cells in the carp retina. Vision Res 8:817, 1968.
4. Watanabe K: S-potential and the electrically evoked responses in the live carp retina. Proc IUPS 9:596. 1971.
5. Naka KI, Rushton WAH: The generation and spread of S-potentials in fish (Cyprinidae). J Physiol 193:437, 1967.
6. Trifonov YuA, Byzov AL, Chailahian LM: Electrical properties of subsynaptic and nonsynaptic membrane of horizontal cells in fish retina. Vision Res 14:229, 1974.
7. Gouras P: S-potentials. In Fuortes MGF (ed): "Physiology of Photoreceptor Organs: Handbook of Sensory Physiology," VII/2 Berlin: Springer-Verlag, 1972, p 513.
8. Orlov OYu, Maksimova EM: S-potential sources as excitation pools. Vision Res 5:573, 1965.
9. Witkovsky P: A comparison of ganglion cell and S-potential response in carp retina. J Neurophysiol 30:546, 1967.
10. Watanabe K, Katagiri Y, Suda Y: Electrically evoked responses (E-responses) of L- and C-type horizontal cells in the carp retina. Sens Proc 2: 326, 1978.
11. Stell WK, Lightfoot DO, Wheeler TG: Goldfish retina: Functional polarization of cone horizontal cell dendrites and synapses. Science 190:989, 1975.
12. Marc RE, Stell WK, Bok D, Lam DMK: GABA-ergic pathways in the goldfish retina. J Comp Neurol 182:221, 1978.
13. Murakami M, Shimoda Y, Nakatani K: Effects of GABA on neuronal activities in the distal retina of carp. Sens Proc 2:334, 1978.
14. Baylor DA, Fuortes MGF, O'Bryan PM: Receptive fields of cones in the retina of turtle. J Physiol 214:256, 1971.
15. Burkhardt DA, Hassin G: Influences of cones upon chromatic- and luminosity-type horizontal cells in pikeperch retinas. J Physiol 281:125, 1978.
16. Tomita T: Electrophysiological study of the mechanisms subserving color coding in the fish retina. Cold Spring Harbor Symp Quant Biol 30:559, 1966.
17. Naka KI, Rushton WAH: An attempt to analyze color reception by electrophysiology. J Physiol 185:556, 1966.

The S-Potential, pages 137–150
© 1982 Alan R. Liss, Inc., 150 Fifth Avenue, New York, NY 10011

Chromatic Properties of S-Potential in Fish

Genyo Mitarai

INTRODUCTION

The intracellular graded potential in the fish retina discovered by Svaetichin in 1953 [1] and called S-potential after him was a distinctive event of great importance, which has brought about an epoch in vision physiology.

In the pioneer work, the potentials were recorded from the isolated retina of the bream and perch and showed a characteristic exclusive hyperpolarization to all wavelength light, showing certain amplitude-wavelength functions. The monophasic spectral response curves thus obtained from many recordings were divided into three subtypes having different spectral maxima at 450, 550, and 600–650 nm, respectively. These curves appeared to correspond well with the action spectra of three different cones predicted by the trichromatic theory, and therefore the potentials were reported originally as the cone action potentials. Based on the measurement of the electrode locations, however, notions of their generating sites were soon revised and then were thought to be the secondary neurons in the outer nuclear layer, and most possible, the horizontal cells [2–6]. At the same time it was found that some of the S-potentials showed color-dependent polarity changes, most of them hyperpolarizing to the short wavelengths and depolarizing to the middle or longer wavelengths, which resulted in the biphasic or triphasic spectral response curves [2,4,7]. The monochromatic curves did not alter their shapes with chromatic adaptation, suggesting that they reflect the action of single type of cones or a linear sum of different cone responses, while the biphasic and triphasic curves showed characteristic phase selective changes, suggesting that they involved the antagonistic actions between different cones [4]. The wavelength-dependent polarity changes of single cell responses were the most attractive, because of the resemblance to the predicted features of the color opponent processes. According to these criteria, the S-potentials were first classified into two main types, ie, the luminosity type, or L-type, and the chromaticity type, or C-type [3,4]. Then, many researchers began to study the generating sites of these potentials by means of injection of dye or reagent from the tip of a micropipette into the recording cells. Crystal violet [2,3], lithium carmine [8–10], Turnbull's blue [12], and AGNO₃ [11] were used in earlier experiments, and the results have been reported over a period of years and described in detail in several papers. Recently, the successful injection of Niagara blue [13] and Procion yellow [14] into all types of neurons, in the Necturus and goldfish retina, respectively, showed that the S-potentials originate in the horizontal cells only. Rod contribution to the S-potentials in the carp retina was suggested by Mitarai and Yagasaki [15], and its existence was confirmed by recording the scotopic luminosity type of spectral response curves in the Centropomus and carp retina. In this case, the generating cells were localized in the most vitread horizontal cell layer [6,16].

On the other hand, three cone types were found by the microspectrophotometry of the cone outer segments [17–19], and the intracellular cone potentials were successfully recorded [20]. These results enabled the further elucidation of a cone-horizontal cell connection which would involve the mechanism converting the trichromatic process into the color opponent process. Thus, the negative feedback from the horizontal cells to cones was demonstrated in the turtle retina as the essential connection to give rise to the C responses [21–24]. Based on these studies in the turtle retina, Fuortes and Simon [24] showed a circuit diagram representing a possible relation between cones and horizontal cells. Stell and his colleagues [25,26], with their morphological studies of the goldfish retina, also presented a "synaptic model" to explain the selective cone-horizontal cell connectivity leading to the C responses.

Throughout the above-mentioned studies, one can see that the spectral response curves and the other chromatic properties of S-potentials have played an important role in discriminating the horizontal cell types and characterizing the neural networks. A number of studies of the cone-horizontal cell interaction explain the chromatic properties of S-potentials, but others remained still unexplained. In this article, some of the remaining problems are discussed based on our recent work with the mugil retina.

REVIEW AND OBSERVATIONS

Photopic L Response

In early stages of the S-potential research, different spectral properties of the L- and C-type S-potentials across fish species were observed by Svaetichin and MacNichol [4] in relation to the inhabiting environment. As regards the L responses of four marine fish species, Lutianidae sp, living at deeper than 30 m, delivered a kind of L response, having the spectral response curve that peaks in the blue green region, Serranidae sp and Centropomidae sp, both of which live near the coast, also delivered a kind of L response but showed different spectral sensitivities from each other, and Mugilidae sp, passing between the freshwater and the seawater, showed three kinds of L responses, the spectral response curves peaking at around 450, 560, and 600 nm, respectively. Tamura and Niwa [27,28], in their comparative studies of 24 fish species, reported that some of these fish living on the coast delivered two kinds of L responses, one having the spectral maxima at green and the other at orange. These results suggested that there were maximally three photopic L responses with different spectral sensitivities, not only across species, but also in a given retina. According to our present knowledge about the photoreceptor to horizontal cell contact, they could be classified into the blue cone-dominated L (L_B), the green cone-dominated L (L_G), and the red cone-dominated L (L_R). However, such coexistence of more than one type of L response in a single retina has not been fully accepted for a long time, not only because of some doubt about a possible misreading of incomplete C response spectral curves as those of L responses but also because of the value of the widely-accepted concept of "luminosity."

In order to criticize this problem, Laufer and Millan [29] examined the spectral sensitivities of the L responses obtained from the retina of Eugerres plumieri, which inhabit the Venezuelan coast, and compared them with the absorption spectra of the cone pigments of the same species. Their results indicated that three L responses, having the different spectral maxima at 476, 568, and 606 nm, could be obtained from different horizontal cells located separately from the scotopic L cells. The shapes of the spectral sensitivity curves, as well as their maxima, were almost identical to those of three cone absorption spectra. This finding of the coexistence of different L responses in a single retina led them to assert the unsuitablesness of the term "luminosity type" for denoting the function of these S-potentials. It is known that the goldfish and carp, common in many retina labs, possess the C-type cells and give only one kind of L response [16,30,31]. This fact favors the concept of "luminosity type" and seemingly has strongly influenced the explanation of the underlying neural network. Taking account of the feedback interaction between cones and horizontal cells [24,25], the L_G and L_B in the strict sense might not exist together with the commonly known C responses in the same retina. Maybe this is why three different L responses found in the mugil retina [5] have not been considered in the S-potential research.

Recently, however, the L_G, in addition to L_R, was found by Hassin [32] in the horizontal cells of the pikeperch. In their most recent study, Mitarai, Usui, and Takabayashi [33] reconfirmed that both L_R and L_G were recorded from the external horizontal cells of the mugil retina (Fig. 4). Our recordings were equally frequent for both types. The results led us to take a second look at the

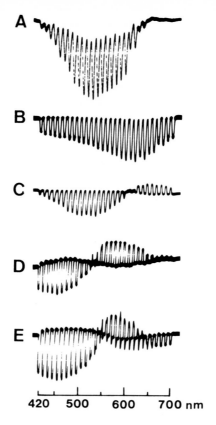

Fig. 1. Five types of specral response curves obtained from the carp retina: Classification of S-potentials into scotopic L (A), photopic L (B), R/G (C), Y/RB (D), and Y/B (E) types.

old papers of the Caracas group [5,29]. In this experiment, we could not record L_B, as described in the previous paper [5], but we can not exclude the possibility because of our small number of samples. We also noticed that the shapes of the spectral response curves were easily changed by an appropriate chromatic adaptation, suggesting that these receive complex cone inputs.

Naka and Rushton [34] have already shown that the L_R found in the tench retina was not univariant with respect to wavelength. Also, many kinds of the complex L-cells, which receive their direct inputs additionally from cones other than the major one, were found in the turtle retina [35]. Even in the photopic L-cells of the goldfish, which have been defined as exclusively red-cone connected, another contact to green and blue cones has been considered possible [36]. It is likely that the three different L responses in Eugerres plumieri are of such complex types.

Summing up, it can be stressed that various photopic L-cells having different action spectra exist in some species in a single retina and that they may belong to the complex types. The exclusive hyperpolarization of these cells may be due to their direct connection to more than a single type of cones. Nevertheless, little is known about the involvement of these different L-types in the cone-horizontal cell circuitry. As discussed later in the description of our results from the mugil retina, a conclusive explanation of the significance of three L-cells coexisting might be obtained by further detailed studies of the functional and morphological identification of these cells in connection with the spectral properties of the C-type cells.

C Responses

Based on the locations of the spectral maxima and the neural points where the signs are reversed on the spectral response curves, the C responses have been subdivided into three, ie, the red green type (R/G), yellow blue type (Y/B), and yellow red blue type (Y/RB) [3,4]. The terms are related to those of opponent color pairs. The abbreviation R/G is used when cells depolarize with red light while hyperpolarizing with green, and similarly for Y/B and Y/RB. So long as the extreme intensity and area of light stimulation, which resulted in the nonlinear features of the response amplitudes, were not used, both spectral maxima and neutral points were reliable features to discriminate these subtypes (Figs. 1, 2).

In their pioneer work, Svaetichin and MacNichol [4] showed that the C responses obtained from many of the shallow water fish were classfied into R/G, Y/B, and Y/RB subtypes. Many subsequent studies showed that in most cases two or three of these subtypes could be recorded in one retina [3-6,28]. The carp [31] and turtle [35] delivered all of the three subtypes, while the goldfish delivered exclusively two, R/G and Y/RB [36]. These results have led us to believe that the C-types are defined, without any exception, as those which hyperpolarize to the short wavelengths and depolarize to the middle or longer wavelenghts. Our present understanding of the color opponent processes in the retina is based on these facts. However, Svaetichin et al [5] reported that the Mugilidae sp showed the reversed type of C responses, G/R and RB/Y, in addition to the above-mentioned common C- and three different L-types. Yet, so far, the reversed C-types have not been obtained from any other fish species used in the retina physiology. Therefore, the early reports have never been discussed till now. If this particular response were a kind of S-potential, it would be a useful clue in the further elucidation of the opponent color mechanisms in the retina. Our recent study of this response is described in the next section.

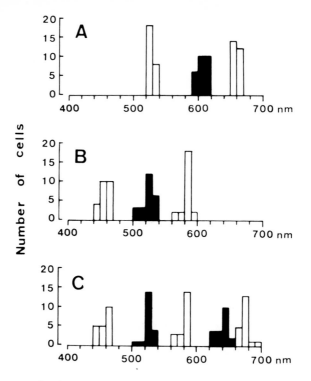

Fig. 2. Histograms showing distribution of the maxima (white column) and the neutral points (black column) of the R/G (A), Y/B (B), and Y/RB (C) types in the carp retina. White columns in the shorter wavelengths indicate the maximum of the hyperpolarization, in the longer wavelengths the depolarization of the spectral response curves, and in the longest wavelength, in C, the second hyperpolarization.

S-POTENTIAL TYPES AND HORIZONTAL CELL ORGANIZATION

In order to elucidate the organization of horizontal cells, the correlation between spectral response types of S-potential and cell types has been studied by applying the procion dye injection method on many of the vertebrate retina. In fish, the successful cell identification was performed with the retina of the goldfish [14], dogfish [38], carp [16,31,39,40], catfish [41], pikeperch [32] stingray [42], and mugil [33].

The horizontal cells in the carp form three superimposed layers and subdivide into the external, the intermediate, and the internal from sclerad to vitread [43,44]. Both the external and intermediate cells extend their long staut

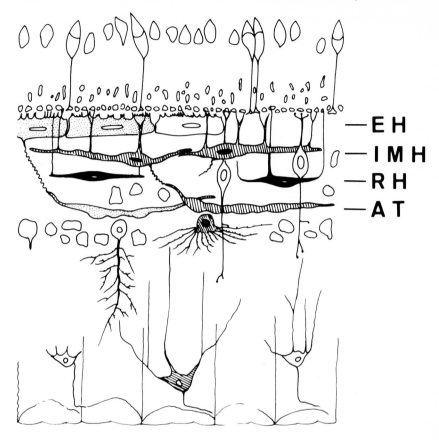

Fig. 3.   Diagram showing the arrangement of external (EH), intermediate (IMH), and rod (RH) horizontal cells, and the axonal processes (AT) of the carp retina, based on the results by procion dye marking.

axons into the most vitread of the inner nuclear layer (Fig. 3). By applying dye injection method on these cells, Mitarai, Asano, and Miyake [31] proved that the external horizontal cells generate exclusively the photopic L responses, the intermediate cells generate the C responses, while the internal cells generate the scotopic L responses, and the axonal processes, forming the fourth layer, also showed that the S-potentials consisted of both photopic L and C responses. These results also emphasized that all of the subtypes of C responses were localized side by side in the same row of the intermediate horizontal cells.

A similar organization was found in the goldfish retina [25,26], but the horizontal cell layers are less distinguishable than those in the carp. This is probably why Stell, for clarity's sake, arranges the cone horizontal cells in three layers in his synaptic model of the goldfish retina, using the abbreviations H_1, H_2, and H_3, respectively for the L, R/G, and Y/RB types [25,36]. The individual response types seems to be more weighted than their localization. Leeper [45,46] described the defined groups of the turtle horizontal cells in a similar way. On the other hand, some researchers use these abbreviations for description of the external, intermediate, and internal cells, corresponding to their stratified arrangements. It has been reported that in the stingray (elasmobranch) retina H_1 generates the L responses reflecting both rod and cone activities, H_2 the scotopic L responses, and H_3 the R/G [41], and in the pikeperch retina H_1 generates the red-sesitive L, H_2 both red- and green-sensitive L, and H_3 the R/G responses [32,47]. There is a large species diversification which would tell us the characteristic functions of horizontal cells so far unknown. Although researchers have difficulty trying to unify these terms, the significance of stratified horizontal cell arrangements can not be overlooked. The horizontal cells of the mugil retina consist of four distinctive superimposed layers [48,49] that add one more layer than those of the goldfish and carp, and the cells of this additional layer were found to generate the reversed C responses.

As described in the preceding section, the C reponses in the mugil retina were divided into the commonly known R/G, Y/B, and Y/RB subtypes and the additional reversed types, G/R and RB/Y [4,5,27]. Based on the electrode depth criterion, and referring to the morphological identification of four layers of horizontal cells in this fish, Drujan, Svaetichin, and Negishi [50] had already noted the reversed C responses generated from the horizontal cells located in the second layer in contrast to the common C types located in the third layer. In spite of numerous recent studies of the spectral properties of the horizontal cells in different fish species and other vertebrates, the reversed C types have been found, so far, only in the mugil retina. One might suppose researchers to have discovered a similar type from the bipolar or amacrine cell responses. However, our most recent recordings of S-potentials in the Mugil cephalus retina reconfirmed that the reversed C responses (G/R, B/Y) do exist among the S-potentials (Fig. 4). Parthe [48] classified the horizontal cells according to their location and photoreceptor connectivity, and proceeding from the distal to the proximal layers called them external, medial, and internal and rod horizontal cells. He found that the cells in the sclerad three layers were cone connected. The Mugil cephalus yielded the same structural profiles at least in the light microphotograph of the iron hematoxylin-stained vertical section. The horizontal cell bodies in the sclerad three layers appeared somewhat rectangularly arranged, very regularly. The horizontal extension of the external horizontal cell was about 25μm, and those of the medial and internal were about 50μm, both making a superimposed pair. The cells in the fourth layer were of a length similar to the medial and internal, but irregularly curved.

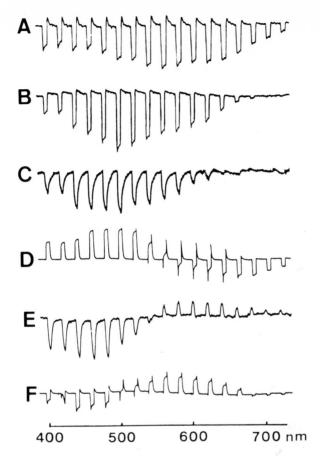

Fig. 4. Six types of spectral response curves obtained from the mugil retina: Classification of S-potentials into L_R (A), L_G (B), scotopic L (C), G/R (D), R/G (E), and Y/RB (F).

Beneath the cells in the fourth layer the large processes which appeared similar to those found in the carp and goldfish retina were also detected. The average thickness of all these cells was about 10μm, and owing to the regular arrangement, the successive recordings could be made easily from the four layers in a single penetration of the electrode.

In order to get the exact correlation between the response types and cell types, we applied the procion dye injection method on the mugil retina. The results indicated that the L_R and L_G, as described in the preceding section, were recorded from the external horizontal cells, the reversed C from the medial (Fig. 5), the common C from the internal, and the scotopic L from the

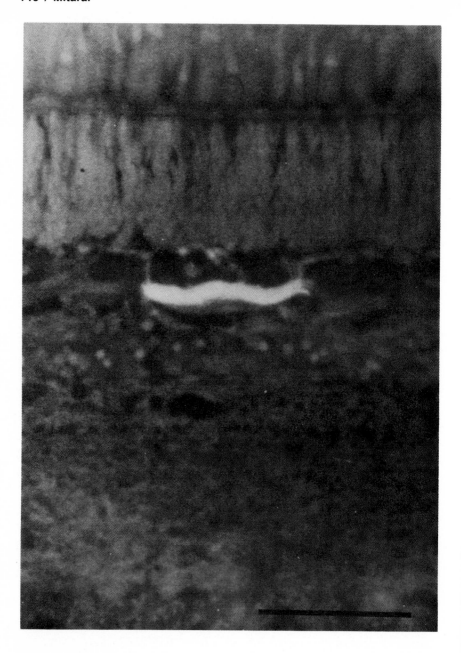

Fig. 5. Fluorescent microphotograph of an medial horizontal cell of mugil retina, forming the second row of horizontal cell layer, from which the reversed C (G/R) was recorded. Just beneath the cell the internal horizontal cell can be seen. Calibration: 50μm.

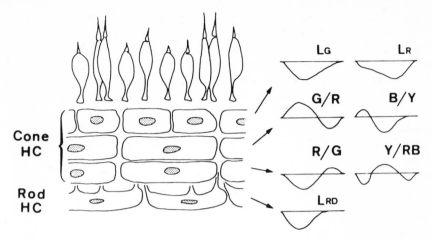

Fig. 6. Diagram showing the arrangement of external, medial, and internal (Cone HC), and rod horizontal cell (Rod HC) of the mugil retina, from sclerad to vitread, and their peculiar spectral response curves.

rod horizontal cell in the fourth layer. Figure 6 sums up the results in a schematic drawing of all horizontal cells and their response types. These corroborate the early results by Svaetichin et al [5] and Drujan et al [50].

It is known that the color opponent cells in the visual pathway consist of four basic types: $+R-G$, $-R+G$, $+Y-B$, and $-Y+B$ [51,52]. In contrast, only two basic types of color opponency are demonstrated in the horizontal cells in most vertebrates. Our recent investigations of the bipolar and amacrine cell responses in the carp retina have shown that there are four basic color channels originating in the bipolar cells [53] and also in the amacrine cells [54]. The results convinced us that the incompletion of horizontal cell color opponency is generally conclusive. However, our present study proved that the incompletion is tied to species diversification. In the mugil retina, the existence of different photopic L cells, as previously described, may have close connection with the existence of their elaborated color types of S-potentials. Probably, the same feedback organization, as established by the study of the turtle and goldfish retina, is involved in the mechanisms, but particular networks should also exists. The Eugerres plumieri from which Laufer and Millan [29] found three photopic L types has a similar horizontal cell arrangement to that in the mugil [48]. It would be interesting to find out whether the reversed C type cells coexist with the common C cells in this fish too.

CONCLUSION

Our recent investigation of the S-potentials in the mugil retina showed the following recording results: 1) two different photopic L responses from the external horizontal cells; 2) the reversed C responses (G/R, B/Y) from the medial (the second layer); 3) the commonly known C responses (R/G, Y/RB) from the internal (the third layer); and 4) the scotopic L responses from the cells in the fourth layer. The results revived faith in the early findings by the research group in Caracas. Comparing the horizontal cell arrangement of the mugil with that of the carp, it seems that the retina having three layers of cone-connected horizontal cells delivers the additional reversed C response and different photopic L responses as well. According to Parthe [49], the retina of several fish species, inhabiting the Venezuelan coast, are also characterized by a neutral organization similar to that of the mugil. Svaetichin opened the new era of retina physiology by his discovery of S-potential and left valuable insight on the color coding process in the retina.

REFERENCES

1. Svaetichin G: The cone action potential. Acta Physiol Scand 299 [Suppl 106]:565, 1953.
2. MacNichol EF Jr, Macpherson L, Svaetichin G: Studies on spectral response curves from the fish retina. In: Visual Problems of Color, Proc of a Symp, Nat Physical Lab 531, 1957.
3. MacNichol EF Jr, Svaetichin G: Electric responses from the isolated retinas of fishes. Am J Ophtalmol 46 [Part 2]:26, 1958.
4. Svaetichin G, MacNichol EF Jr: Retinal mechanisms for chromatic and achromatic vision. Ann New York Acad Sci 74:385, 1958.
5. Svaetichin G, Laufer M, Mitarai G, Fatehchand R, Vallecalle E, Villegas J: Glial control of neuronal networks and receptors. In Jung R, Kornhuber H (eds): Visual System: Neurophysiology and Psychophysics. Berlin: Springer-Verlag, 1961, p 445.
6. Mitarai G, Svaetichin G, Vallecalle E, Fatehchand R, Villegas J, Laufer M: Glia-neuron intersections and adaptational mechanisms of the retina. In Jung R, Kornhuber H (ed): Visual System: Neurophysiology and Psychophysics, Berlin: Springer-Verlag, 1961, p 463.
7. Motokawa K, Oikawa T, Tasaki K: Receptor potential of vertebrate retina. J Neurophysiol 20:186, 1957.
8. Mitarai G: The origin of so-called cone potential. Proc Jpn Acad 34:299, 1958.
9. Mitarai G: Determination of ultramicroelectrode tip position in the retina in relation of S potential. J Gen Physiol 43 [Suppl]:95, 1960.
10. Mitarai G: Glia-neuron interaction in carp retina. Glia potentials revealed by microelectrode with lithium carmine. In Seno S, Cowdry EV (eds): Intracellular Membraneous Structure. Jpn Soc Cell Biol, 1965, p 549.
11. Oikawa T, Ogawa T, Motokawa K: Origin of so-called cone action potential. J Neurophysiol 22:102, 1959.
12. Tomita T, Murakami M, Saito Y, Hashimoto Y: Further study on the so-called cone action potential (S-potential). Its histological determination. Jpn J Physiol 9:63, 1959.
13. Werblin SF, Dowling JE: Organization of the retina of the mudpuppy, Necturus maculosus. II. Intracellular recording. J Neurophysiol 32:339, 1969.
14. Kaneko A: Physiological and morphological identification of horizontal, bipolar and amacrine cells in goldfish retina. J Physiol (Lond) 207:623, 1970.
15. Mitarai G, Yagasaki Y: Resting and action potential of single cone. Ann Rep Res Inst Environ Med Nagoya Univ 2:54, 1955.
16. Kaneko A, Yamada M: S-potentials in the dark-adapted retina of the carp. J Physiol (Lond) 227:261, 1972.
17. Marks WB: Difference Spectra of the Visual Pigments in Single Goldfish Cones. Ph.D. Dissertation, Johns Hopins Univ, 1963.

18. Marks WB: Visual pigments of single goldfish cones. J Physiol (Lond) 178:14, 1965.
19. Liebman PA, Entine G: Sensitive low-light level microspectro-photometer: Detection of photo-sensitive pigments of retinal cones. J Opt Soc Am 54:1451, 1964.
20. Tomita T: Electrophysiological study of the mechanisms subserving color coding in the fish retina. Cold Spring Harbor Symp Quant Biol 30:559, 1965.
21. Baylor DA, Fuortes MGF, O'Bryan PM: Receptive fields of cones in the retina of the turtle. J Physiol (Lond) 214:265, 1971.
22. Fuortes MGF, Schwartz EA, Simon EJ: Colour-dependence of cone responses in the turtle retina. J Physiol (Lond) 234:199, 1973.
23. O'Bryan, PM: Properties of the depolarizing synaptic potential evoked by peripheral illumination in cones of the turtle retina. J Physiol (Lond) 235:207, 1973.
24. Fuortes MGF, Simon EJ: Interactions leading to horizontal cell responses in the turtle retina. J Physiol (Lond) 240:177, 1974.
25. Stell WK, Lightfoot DO: Color-specific interconnections of cones and horizontal cells in the retina of the goldfish. J Comp Neurol 159:473, 1975.
26. Stell WK: Functional polarization of horizontal cell dendrites in goldfish retina. Invest Ophthalmol 15:895, 1976.
27. Tamura T, Niwa H: Spectral sensitivity and color vision of fish as indicated by S-potential. Comp Biochem Physiol 22:745, 1967.
28. Niwa H, Tamura T: Investigation of fish vision by means of S-potential II. Spectral sensitivity and colour vision. Rev Can Biol 28:79, 1969.
29. Laufer M, Millan E: Spectral analysis of L-type S-potentials and their relation to photopigment absorption in a fish (Eugerres plumieri) retina. Vision Res 10:237, 1970.
30. Witkowsky P: A comparison of ganglion cell and S-potential response properties in carp retina. J Neurophysiol 30:546, 1967.
31. Mitarai G, Asano T, Miyake Y: Identification of five types of S-potential and their corresponding generating sites in the horizontal cells of the carp retina. Jpn J Ophthalmol 18:161, 1974.
32. Hassin G: Pikeperch horizontal cells identified by intracellular staining. J Comp Neurol 186:529, 1979.
33. Mitarai G, Usui S, Takabayashi A: Particular type of chromatic responses and arrangement of all the horizontal cell types in the mugil retina. Biomed Res: (in press) 1982.
34. Naka KI, Rushton WAH: S-potentials from luminosity units in the retina of fish (Cyprinidae). J Physiol (Lond) 185:587, 1966.
35. Yazulla S: Cone input to horizontal cells in the turtle retina. Vision Res 16:727, 1976.
36. Stell WK: Photoreceptor-specific synaptic pathways in goldfish retina: A world of color, a wealth of connections. In Verriest G(ed): Colour Vision Deficiencies V. Bristol: Adam Hilger, 1980, p 1.
37. Naka KI, Rushton WAH: S-potentials from colour units in the retina of fish (Cyprinidae). J Physiol (Lond) 185:536, 1966.
38. Kaneko A: Electrical connexions between horizontal cells in the dogfish retina. J Physiol (Lond) 213:95, 1971.
39. Hashimoto Y, Kato A, Inokuchi M, Watanabe K: Re-examination of horizontal cells in the carp retina with procion yellow electrode. Vision Res 16:25, 1976.
40. Weiler R, Zettler F: The axon-bearing horizontal cells in the teleost retina are functional as well as structural units. Vision Res 19:1261, 1979.
41. Naka KI, Nye PW: Role of horizontal cells in organization of the catfish retinal receptive field. J Neurophysiol 34:785, 1971.
42. Toyoda J, Saito T, Kondo H: Three types of horizontal cells in the Stingray retina: Their morphology and physiology. J Comp Neurol 179:569, 1978.
43. Yamada E, Ishikawa T: The fine structure of the horizontal cells in some vertebrate retina. Cold Spring Harbor Symp Quant Biol 30:383, 1965.

44. Witkowsky P, Dowling JE: Synaptic relationships in the plexiform layers of carp retina. Z Zellforsch 100:60, 1969.
45. Leeper HF: Horizontal cells of the turtle retina. I. Light microscopy of golgi preparations. J Comp Neurol 182:777, 1978.
46. Leeper HF: Horizontal cells of the turtle retina. II. Analysis of interconnections between photoreceptor cells and horizontal cells by light microscopy. J Comp Neurol 182:795, 1978.
47. Witkowsky P, Burkhardt DA, Nagy AR: Synaptic connections linking cones and horizontal cells in the retina of the pikeperch (stizostedion vitreum). J Comp Neurol 186:541, 1979.
48. De Testa AS: Morphological studies on the horizontal and amacrine cells of the teleost retina. Vision Res 6:51, 1966.
49. Parthe V: Horizontal, bipolar and oligopolar cells in the teleost retina. Vision Res 12:395, 1972.
50. Drujan BD, Svaetichin G, Negishi K: Retinal aerobic metabolism as reflected in S-potential behavior. Vision Res [Suppl 3]: 151, 1971.
51. Wagner HG, MacNichol EF Jr, Wolbarsht ML: The response properties of single ganglion cells in the goldfish retina. J Gen Physiol 43:45, 1960.
52. DeValois RL, Abramov I, Jacobs GH: Analysis of response patterns of LGN cells. J Opt Soc Am 56:966, 1966.
53. Sakakibara M, Mitarai G: Chromatic properties of bipolar cells int he carp retina. Color Res Appl 7:178, 1982.
54. Mitarai G, Goto T, Takagi S: Receptive field arrangement of color-opponent bipolar and amacrine cells in the carp retina. Sensory Proc 2:375, 1978.

The S-Potential, pages 151–160
© 1982 Alan R. Liss, Inc., 150 Fifth Avenue, New York, NY 10011

The Opponent Color Process and Interaction of Horizontal Cells

Jun-Ichi Toyoda, Toru Kujiraoka, and Masaaki Fujimoto

Horizontal cells in the cyprinid fish retina receive inputs either from cones or from rods. External horizontal cells of Cajal belong to the former type and intermediate horizontal cells belong to the latter type. External horizontal cells are further classified into L-, RG-, and RGB-type cells according to their spectral response pattern. The L-type cells, located most distally in the horizontal cell layer, respond to light with hyperpolarization, irrespective of its wavelength. Morphological studies [1] suggest that they receive direct inputs from three types of cones, blue, green, and red, though mainly from red cones, as is evident from their spectral response maximum near 620 nm. The RG-type cells respond with hyperpolarization to green light and with depolarization to red light. They do not receive direct inputs from red cones but from blue and mainly from green cones. The RGB-type cells respond with hyperpolarization to blue and red light, but with depolarization to green or yellow light. They receive direct inputs only from blue cones.

These spectral responses apparently reflect the opponent color process. They resemble closely three fundamental curves derived from the opponent color theory. For example, they are basically similar to those curves obtained by Hurvich and Jameson [2] from psychophysical experiments on human observers, if differences in the absorption spectra of cone pigments are taken into account.

Spectral responses of cones, in contrast to those of horizontal cells, are monophasically hyperpolarizing with a peak either in the blue, in the green, or in the red region of the spectrum [3]. Thus, the trichromatic theory applies to the responses of photoreceptors. It is apparent that mechanisms of conversion from a trichromatic to an opponent color process take place at the horizontal cell level or at a stage between photoreceptors and horizontal cells. In 1971, Baylor et al [4] reported a negative feedback effect from horizontal cells to cones in the retina of the turtle. A depolarizing response was observed in cones when a neighboring horizontal cell was hyperpolarized by current through a microelectrode. Based on these observations, Gouras [5] suggested that opponent color responses can be explained by such negative feedback effects when there are selective cone inputs to chromaticity-type horizontal cells.

A model proposed later by Fuortes and Simon [6] from their physiological studies on the turtle and by Stell and Lightfoot [1] from their morphological studies on the goldfish actually assumes a specific connection between three types of cones and horizontal cells, including a specific feedback effect between them. In RG-type cells, for example, the hyperpolarizing response to green light is due to direct inputs from green cones, but the depolarizing response to red light is due to a feedback effect from L-type cells to green cones. The transmission from cones to horizontal cells is sign preserving. It is generally accepted that the transmitter, released continuously in the dark by depolarization of cone terminals, acts to depolarize horizontal cells [7]. Therefore, the hyperpolarizing response of L-type cells to red light depolarizes green cones through a feedback pathway and also depolarizes RG-type cells which receive direct input from green cones. The spectral response pattern of RGB-type cells is also postulated as due to the feedback from RG-type cells to blue cones [1]. According to this model, passive hyperpolarization of L- and RG-type cells by current should elicit a depolarizing response in RG- and RGB-type cells, respectively. The present experiments were attempted to test this assumption.

METHODS

The retina was isolated from the excised opened eye of the carp, Cyprinus carpio, and was placed in a chamber, on a piece of filter paper, with its receptor side up. The chamber was placed on the stage of a micromanipulator and two glass micropipettes, one single and the other double-barreled, were inserted into the retina vertically from above. The pipettes were filled with 2.5 M KCl solution and had a resistance of 50–100 MΩ when measured in a Ringer solution. Occasionally, the tips of the double-barreled electrodes were bevelled so as to allow a large amount of current injection into the cell. The two electrodes were set independently on two separate blocks of an electrode holder with their tips as close as possible. For each trial, the single pipette was advanced first until it recorded the response of a horizontal cell and then the double-barreled pipette was advanced to record the response of other horizontal cells.

The light stimulus from a tungsten–halogen lamp was guided onto the retina from above through a lens system. A diffuse white light, attenuated to about 0.4 lm/m^2 by inserting neutral density filters in the light path, was used to confirm intracellular recordings. It was 1.0 sec in duration and was repeated every 5 sec. When the responses of two horizontal cells were recorded simultaneously, their spectral responses were tested to identify their types. Monochromatic lights adjusted to equal quanta were scanned in steps of 30 nm by changing interference filters.

After identification of the type of cells recorded, one of them was polarized by current through one barrel of the double-barreled electrode and its effect on the other was studied. The current applied was 20–30 nA. The voltage drop across the coupling resistance of the electrode, and the field potential due to injected current, were not compensated in the figures presented in this paper. The field potential was recorded at the same electrode depth after deterioration of the response. It often exceeded 2 mV and masked the response. The responses were amplified and monitored on an oscilloscope and at the same time recorded on magnetic tape. These records were later reproduced on an X–Y recorder. Figure 1 illustrates schematically the arrangements of electrodes during experiments and the postulated connections between three types of cones and three types of horizontal cells. The experiments were carried out at room temperature, between 20 and 24°C.

RESULTS

Neighboring horizontal cells are electrically coupled through gap junctions [8,9]. This is the reason why horizontal cells have a large receptive field far beyond their dendritic field [10]. The current injected into a cell polarized the neighboring horizontal cells of the same type. Figure 2 is an example of such an electrical coupling between two RG-type cells. After recording their spectral responses, one of them (trace a) was hyperpolarized and then depolarized by current of 30 nA. It elicited potential changes of the same polarity in the other (trace b). Such an electrical coupling was also observed between L-type cells and between RGB-type cells. The largest coupling ratio observed was about 30% [11]. The electrical coupling was never observed between different types of horizontal cells.

Figure 3 is an example of simultaneous recordings from (a) an L-type and (b) an RG-type cell. Hyperpolarization of the L-type cell by current of 30 nA elicited a depolarizing response in the RG-type cell, and depolarization of the former elicited a hyperpolarizing response in the latter. The polarity of the response precludes the electrical coupling. The effect is probably mediated by a chemical synapse. These effects of polarization of L-type cells on RG-type cells were observed in 15 out of about 100 pairs so far studied. In many of the remaining 85 pairs, the effect was so small that it was masked by the field potential. The effect would become apparent in these pairs when the field potential was subtracted from the recordings. The effect of polarization of RG-type cells on the L-type cells was also tested in many pairs. But the effect was never detectable. This unidirectional effect favors for the synaptic transmission and also supports the view that the current injected into one type will never spread into other horizontal cell types.

Figure 4 is an example of simultaneous recordings from (a) an RG-type and (b) an RGB-type cell. Hyperpolarization of the RG-type cell elicited a depolar-

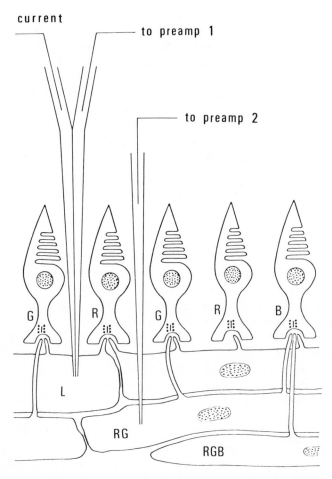

Fig. 1. Schematic drawing of the electrode setting during experiments and of retinal connections between cones and horizontal cells. L-type cells receive inputs directly from red (R), green (G), and blue (B) cones, RG-type cells from green and blue cones, and RGB cells only from blue cones. The gap junction between neighboring L-type cells and RG-type cells is indicated by the thickening of the adjacent membrane.

izing response, and depolarization of the same cell elicited a hyperpolarizing response in the RGB-type cell. Such an effect was observed in about 30 out of 70 pairs studied. Polarization of RGB-type cells, on the other hand, did not elicit a detectable change in the RG-type cells. The responses thus elicited were usually very small.

The difficulty in eliciting a prominent effect is due mainly to the low input resistance of horizontal cells, especially of L-type cells, as a result of the ex-

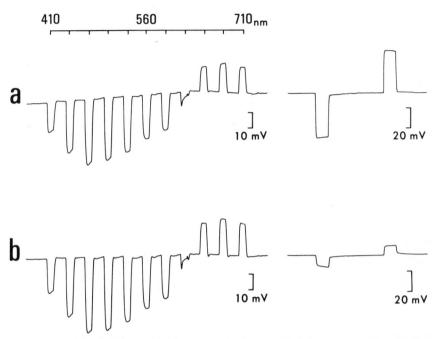

410   560   710 nm

a

10 mV   20 mV

b

10 mV   20 mV

Fig. 2. An example of simultaneous recordings from two RG-type horizontal cells. After recording the spectral response pattern by scanning the monochromatic light from 410 to 710 nm in steps of 30 nm, as shown in the left, one of the cells was hyperpolarized and then depolarized by a current of 30 nA through one barrel of the double-barreled electrode. Its membrane potential was monitored through the other barrel and shown in trace (a) without compensation of the voltage drop across the coupling resistance. Trace (b) shows the membrane potential of the other cell. Duration of both light and current stimuli was 1.0 sec. The traces showing responses to current stimuli are twice as fast as those of spectral responses.

tensive electrical coupling, and to the distance between the two electrodes. Although current injected into a cell spreads to nearby cells, the potential must be rapidly attenuated as a function of the distance between the two cells. The low input resistance of horizontal cells and also the limitation in the amount of current passable through the electrode make it difficult to polarize the cell to a level great enough to elicit a prominent transsynaptic potential in the other cells. Conversely, the response of horizontal cells activated locally by synaptic inputs is greatly attenuated due to the electrical coupling, as is evident from the fact that the response of horizontal cells to a small light spot is hard to detect. The input resistance of RG-type cells is higher, on the average, than that of L-type cells. This may explain the difference in the number of effective pairs recorded in the present experiments. The interaction between horizontal cells would be larger if nearby horizontal cells of the same type were polarized rather uniformly.

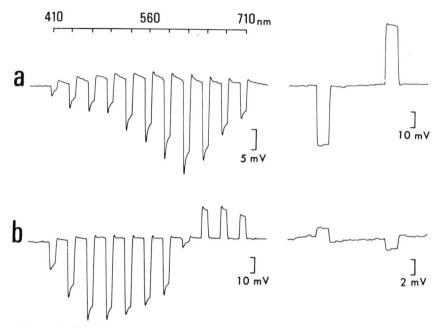

Fig. 3. An example of simultaneous recordings from an L-type and an RG-type cells. After recording the spectral responses, the L-type cell shown in trace (a) was polarized by a current of 30 nA. Its hyperpolarization elicited a depolarizing response in the RG-type cell shown in trace (b). Recording conditions are similar to those of Figure 2.

According to the model proposed, L-type cells have a feedback effect on all three types of cones. The feedback to blue cones should then affect the RGB-type cells. However, no detectable interaction was observed so far between L-type and RGB-type cells in the present experiments.

If the interaction between horizontal cells is mediated by a feedback pathway to cones, polarization of horizontal cells must elicit a depolarizing response in cones. This possibility was tested by simultaneous recordings from cones and L-type cells. Results are still not convincing. Pairs of a green cone and an L-type cell were not recorded stably so far. In a few out of more than 10 pairs of a red cone and an L-type cell, a small effect was detectable when the field potential was subtracted from the response. Hyperpolarization of L-type cells elicited a depolarizing response in cones.

DISCUSSION

Polarization of horizontal cells by current reveals two types of interaction among horizontal cells. One is the sign-preserving electrical coupling and is seen

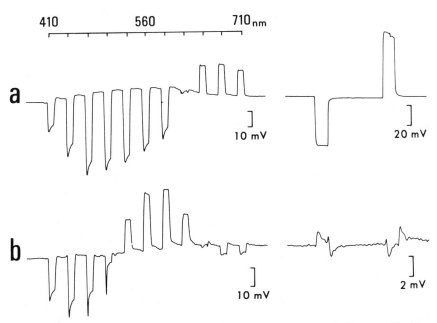

Fig. 4. An example of simultaneous recordings from an RG-type and an RGB-type cells. After recording the spectral responses, the RG-type cell shown in trace (a) was polarized by a current of 30 nA. Hyperpolarization of the RG-type cell elicited a depolarizing response in the RGB-type cell shown in trace (b). In this example there is contamination of transient artifacts in the responses of RGB-type cells at both the on and off of current due to capacitive interference.

between horizontal cells of the same type. The other is sign-inverting. It is seen between L- and RG-type and between RG- and RGB-type cells but the effect is unidirectional, suggesting that it is mediated by chemical synapses. This type of interaction can explain the mechanism of transduction from a trichromatic to an opponent-color process, provided that there are specific connections from each type of cone to corresponding types of horizontal cells. In the goldfish retina, Stell and Lightfoot [1] reported such selective connections between cones and horizontal cells as mentioned already.

There are two possible synaptic pathways that mediate the effect. One is the direct synaptic connection between horizontal cells. The other is the feedback pathway from horizontal cells to photoreceptors.

Conventional synaptic structures between two horizontal cell processes have been reported in the mudpuppy [12] and in the carp [9]. It is possible that these synapses contribute to the lateral interaction observed in these experiments. However, these synapses are often found between neighboring horizontal cells, and it is not certain whether they are sign-preserving or sign-inverting synapses, or whether they explain the unidirectional effect of polarization.

A feedback from horizontal cells to cones first demonstrated in the turtle retina has also been suggested in the fish retina. When the size of a light spot is increased, the later part of the hyperpolarizing cone response of the perch retina is reduced due to a delayed depolarizing phase [13]. The depolarizing phase has been ascribed to the feedback, though the effect of synaptic blocking agents on cone responses has not been systematically studied in the teleost retina. Histochemical studies have shown that L-type horizontal cells in the teleost retina actively take up GABA and this uptake is affected by light [14]. When bicuculline, a specific GABA antagonist, is applied in the bathing medium, the response of horizontal cells of the catfish retina to a large spot of light, which is faster than the response to a small spot of light in the normal solution, becomes as slow as the latter. Since the improvement of the frequency characteristics of horizontal cell responses with an increase in the stimulus diameter has been ascribed to the feedback from horizontal cells to cones, the above results suggest that GABA is involved in the feedback pathway [15]. Recent data by Murakami et al [16] also suggest that GABA acts as an inhibitory transmitter from L-type cells to cones in the carp retina. Brief transretinal current from the receptor to the vitreous side is known to elicit a transient depolarizing response in horizontal cells [7]. Following the depolarizing response of horizontal cells to such current, there appears a small hyperpolarizing response in cones, which is abolished by application of excess of GABA or its antagonists. At the same time, these drugs abolish the depolarizing responses to red light of RG-type horizontal cells, suggesting that the feedback is involved in the opponent color process, although the effect of GABA antagonists by itself does not rule out the direct synaptic interaction between horizontal cells. RG-type cells in the cyprinid fish retina, unlike L-type cells, do not actively take up GABA [14]. The effect of polarization of these cells on RGB-cells, therefore, must be mediated by some other transmitters. Identification of the transmitter will help understanding the mechanisms of interaction among horizontal cells.

The importance of the feedback pathway in the opponent color process is also supported by another physiological experiment on the turtle retina [17]. In this retina, stimulation with diffuse deep-red light depolarizes green cones, which occasionally produces a spike potential. The spike potential is considered to result from a regenerative increase in Ca conductance of the cone membrane as a consequence of a feedback depolarization of the cone terminal. In the presence of Sr ions in the bathing medium, diffuse red light evokes a repetitive discharge of spikes in green cones and at the same time a train of transient depolarizing potentials, probably postsynaptic potentials, in RG-type horizontal cells. The results support the idea that feedback depolarization of green cones is responsible for the depolarizing response of RG-type horizontal cells. The feedback interaction thus takes place probably within a cone pedicle into which the processes of two interacting horizontal cells invaginate. In order to elicit a prominent effect of polarization, the processes of two horizontal cells recorded simultaneously may have to share the same receptor terminal.

Conventional synapses from horizontal cells to cones have been reported in the catfish retina [18]. But such synaptic structures have not been confirmed in most other vertebrate retinas. Difficulty in detecting a depolarizing response of cones to an annular illumination and to hyperpolarization of horizontal cells especially in the cyprinid fish retina led Byzov et al [19] to assume that the feedback effect is mediated by electric current. According to their assumption, the current generated by horizontal cells flows in part through the photoreceptor terminal and elicits a voltage drop across the presynaptic membrane, which in turn causes a change in its ionic permeability.

Whatever the mechanism of the feedback is, the present results on the carp retina are generally consistent with the model of Stell and Lightfoot [1] on the goldfish retina, in which the L-type cells make a feedback connection mainly with green cones and the RG-type cells with blue cones. A minor feedback pathway from L-type cells to blue cones, however, has not been confirmed.

ACKNOWLEDGMENTS

This work was supported in part by Grant EY-02392 from the National Eye Institute, USPHS, and by Grants 448106 and 339016 from the Ministry of Education of Japan.

REFERENCES

1. Stell WK, Lightfoot DO: Color-specific interconnections of cones and horizontal cells in the retina of the goldfish. J Comp Neurol 159:473, 1975.
2. Hurvich LM, Jameson D: Perceived color, induction effects, and opponent response mechanisms. J Gen Physiol 43 Part 2:63, 1960.
3. Tomita T, Kaneko A, Murakami M, Pautler EL: Spectral response curves of single cones in the carp. Vision Res 7:519, 1967.
4. Baylor DA, Fuortes MGF, O'Bryan PM: Receptive fields of cones in the retina of the turtle. J Physiol (London) 214:265, 1971.
5. Gouras P: S-potentials. In Fuortes MGF (ed): "Handbook of Sensory Physiology, VII/2." Berlin, Heidelberg, New York: Springer–Verlag, 1972, p 513.
6. Fuortes MGF, Simon EJ: Interactions leading to horizontal cell responses in the turtle retina. J Physiol (London) 240:177, 1974.
7. Trifonov YuA: Study of synaptic transmission between photoreceptors and horizontal cells by means of electric stimulation of the retina. Biofizika 13:809, 1968.
8. Yamada E, Ishikawa T: The fine structure of the horizontal cells in some vertebrate retinae. Cold Spring Harb Symp Quant Biol 30:383, 1965.
9. Witkovsky P, Dowling JE: Synaptic relationship in the plexiform layers of carp retina. Z Zellforsch Mikrosk Anat 100:60, 1969.
10. Kaneko A: Electrical connexions between horizontal cells in the dogfish retina. J Physiol (London) 213:95, 1971.
11. Toyoda J, Tonosaki K: Studies on the mechanisms underlying horizontal–bipolar interaction in the carp retina. Sens Proc 2:359, 1978.

12. Dowling JE, Werblin FS: Organization of retina of the mudpuppy, Necturus maculosus. I. Synaptic structure. J Neurophysiol 32:315, 1969.

13. Burkhardt DA: Responses and receptive-field organization of cones in perch retinas. J Neurophysiol 40:53, 1977.

14. Marc RE, Stell WK, Bok D, Lam DMK: GABA-ergic pathways in the goldfish retina. J Comp Neurol 182:221, 1978.

15. Lam DMK, Lasater R, Naka KI: Gamma-aminobutyric acid: A neurotransmitter candidate for cone horizontal cells in the catfish retina. Proc Nat Acad Sci 75:6310, 1978.

16. Murakami M, Shimoda Y, Nakatani K: Effects of GABA on neuronal activities in the distal retina of the carp. Sens Proc 2:334, 1978.

17. Piccolino M, Neyton J, Gerschenfeld HM: Synaptic mechanisms involved in responses of chromaticity horizontal cells of turtle retina. Nature (London) 284:58, 1980.

18. Davis GW, Naka KI: Synaptic communication in the catfish outer plexiform layer: Structure and function. In Pinsker H, Willis WD (eds): "Information Processing in the Nervous System: Communication Among Neurons and Neuroscientists." New York: Raven Press, 1980, p 221.

19. Byzov AL, Glolubtzov KV, Trifonov YuA: The model of mechanism of feedback between horizontal cells and photoreceptors in vertebrate retina. In Barlow HB, Fatt P (eds): "Vertebrate Photoreception." London: Academic Press, 1977, p 266.

The S-Potential, pages 161–179
© 1982 Alan R. Liss, Inc., 150 Fifth Avenue, New York, NY 10011

The Feedback Effect From Luminosity Horizontal Cells to Cones in the Turtle Retina: A Key to Understanding the Response Properties of the Horizontal Cells

Marco Piccolino and Jacques Neyton

THE FUNCTIONAL OUTPUT OF HORIZONTAL CELLS

Since the first intracellular recording of electrical activity in the distal retina by Svaetichin in 1953 [1], the horizontal cells (HC) have probably been the retinal neurons most extensively studied with intracellular techniques.

Data obtained during almost three decades of electrophysiological studies have permitted the characterization of most of the response properties of HCs [2]. For a long time, however, these studies have failed in providing any clear indication of the specific role of HCs in the neural operations of the retina. It was well established that HCs participate in the processing of visual information, since the polarization with extrinsic current of their membrane was shown to modify the activity of retinal ganglion cells [3–5]. Anatomical studies, however, did not reveal the synaptic sites where HCs could be identified beyond doubt as presynaptic elements [6]. This lack of a definite morphological evidence for an output of the HCs hindered any precise characterization of the mechanism of transmission from HCs to other retinal cells.

In 1971 Baylor et al obtained evidence that luminosity horizontal cells (L-HC) feedback on cones. In experiments performed in the retina of the turtle, the hyperpolarization of the membrane of a L-HC with a short pulse of inward current was shown to elicit a depolarizing deflection in a cone [7]. A comparison of the light responses of both cones and L-HCs to light spots of different diameters revealed the possible physiological meaning of the feedback synapse. The cones developed smooth hyperpolarizing potentials in response to small light spots which induced small hyperpolarizing responses in the L-HCs. Stimulation of the retina with large light spots induced large hyperpolarizing responses in the L-HCs and resulted in a depolarizing deflection in the cones, superposed to their main hyperpolarizing response. The time course of such depolarizing deflection paralleled the time course of the L-HC light response, and it was, therefore, considered to result from the feedback action of L-HCs on cones, directly revealed in the polarization experiment. Flashing a large spot in the presence of a bright illumination of the center of the cone receptive field permitted the isolation of the depolarizing feedback potential from the main direct hyperpolarizing response. This study opened new perspectives to the understanding of the mechanism of the action of the L-HC and, moreover, revealed an unexpected complexity of the spatial properties of the light response of cones, which had been classically considered to depend only on the light absorbed in their own outer segment [8].

In subsequent years, the properties and the mechanism underlying the generation of the feedback responses have been intensively studied. Fuortes et al [9] showed that the feedback mechanism could affect the response of both red- and green-sensitive cones. In the green cones the feedback depolarizations could be isolated from the direct response using red light stimuli, even in the absence of a central background. This was interpreted as being due to the different spectral characteristics of green cones and L-HCs. Red light is poorly absorbed in green cones, whereas it elicits large responses in red cones. L-HCs receive their main input from red cones and, therefore, they develop large hyperpolarizations in response to retinal illumination with large spots of red light. When such stimuli were flashed on the retina, a pure depolarization was shown to result in green cones, which was interpreted as the consequence of the feedback action of L-HCs. It was also reported that in some green cones, the feedback responses could be large in amplitude and have a spike-like appearance. In other cones, both red and green sensitive, the feedback responses were small and in some cases even undetectable. Fuortes et al suggested that this variability could be the consequence of the injury of the connections between L-HC and cones produced by the microelectrode. O'Bryan studied the membrane mechanism underlying the generation of the feedback potentials, providing evidence that they were associated with a decrease of the input conductance of cones [10]. He reported the occurrence of "feedback spikes" also in red cones in response to bright peripheral illumination and suggested the possibility that these responses could be due to a regenerative process. The properties and the mechanism of generation of feedback responses have been recently studied in our laboratory in Paris by Piccolino and Gerschenfeld [11–12], Gerschenfeld and Piccolino [13] and Gerschenfeld et al [14]. The preparation used was the superfused eyecup of the turtle [15], which allowed the modification of the composition of the retinal extracellular medium, thus permitting the study of the ionic characteristics of feedback responses. In these studies evidence was obtained that feedback spikes are calcium spikes, that is, action potentials due to a regenerative increase of the calcium permeability of the cone membrane. The crucial observation was that these responses were facilitated when the retina was perfused with saline containing a high calcium concentration, or Sr^{2+} or Ba^{2+} ions. Moreover feedback responses were blocked by Co^{2+} and were not affected by tetrodotoxin. Peripheral stimulation was shown to evoke the discharge of feedback spikes in all cones in the presence of Sr^{2+} or Ba^{2+} in the perfusing medium. This suggested that the feedback mechanism could affect all cones, even those which did not show any feedback response in control saline. In the presence of Sr^{2+} or Ba^{2+} ions in the perfusing medium, peripheral stimulation with long periods of light was shown to induce a sustained discharge of spikes, lasting for all the duration of the light stimulus. This finding clearly indicated that the feedback, when activated by a prolonged peripheral stimulation, could affect in a sustained way the cone membrane. Finally, it was shown that the hyperpolarization of the membrane of a L-HC, with pulses of inward current, could elicit the discharge of spikes in cones in the presence of Sr^{2+} or Ba^{2+} in the retina. This was a direct evidence that the spikes induced by peripheral illumination were actually the result of the feedback input from L-HCs.

These results were interpreted as evidence that activation of the feedback circuit leads to an increase of the membrane conductance to Ca^{2+} ions in all cones. In some cones the calcium conductance increase can become regenerative, eventually resulting in the discharge of calcium spikes. In other cones the membrane potential is scarcely affected, but the effect of the feedback input can be revealed by application to the retina of ions which permeate through the calcium channels.

It was also suggested that, through the feedback circuit, L-HCs could modify the flow of the neural message in the forward pathway from cones to second order neurons. It is well established that cones transmit to second order neurons through a chemical synapse [16–18]. Cones release their synaptic transmitter at a great rate in the dark and the release is reduced when the synaptic membrane is hyperpolarized due to the spreading of the hyperpolarization generated in the outer segment following light absorption [19]. As in all chemical synapses, the link between the potential change in the terminal membrane and the transmitter release is the entry of calcium ions across the synaptic membrane, which increases with the depolarization and decreases with the hyperpolarization [20]. If the feedback modulates the calcium conductance of the cone membrane, it is safe to assume that it modifies the release of the cone synaptic transmitter. This is also supported by the consideration that contacts between HC processes and cones are localized at the level of the cone endings, thus being in a strategic position to control the transmitter release. The effects of feedback can be detected even in those cones in which no clear feedback depolarization is recorded in control conditions. This suggests that also in these cones the release of synaptic transmitter can be modified by the feedback. Moreover the finding that the feedback action is sustained, when activated by prolonged light stimuli, suggests that the release of the cone transmitter can be affected in a sustained way by the feedback.

RESPONSES OF SECOND ORDER NEURONS DEPENDING ON THE FEEDBACK CIRCUIT

The Depolarizing Responses of the Chromatic Horizontal Cells

The possibility that the feedback circuit could influence the response of second order neurons in the retina was first proposed by Fuortes and Simon [21] to explain the depolarizing responses of the chromaticity horizontal cells. These cells respond to colored light with either hyperpolarization or depolarization according to the wavelength of the light stimulus [22]. In the turtle retina the more commonly found cells are of the red/green type (R/G-HC), which are hyperpolarized by green light and depolarized by red light. As mentioned previously, green cones are also hyperpolarized by green light and depolarized by red light, and the depolarizing response to red light has been attributed to the feedback circuit. The correspondence between the responses of green cones and those of R/G-HCs led Fuortes and Simon to formulate the hypothesis that the feedback could be responsible for the responses elicited in R/G-HCs by red light. According to this hypothesis R/G-HCs receive their main input from green cones. Green light would hyperpolarize R/G-HCs following the hyperpolarization they induce in green cones. Red light would depolarize green cones through the circuit red cones—L-HC—green cones and this polysynaptic depolarization of green cones would eventually lead to the depolarization of R/G-HCs.

The hypothesis of Fuortes and Simon, although consistent with the results of recent morphological studies [23–24], could hardly be accepted in its original formulation. It required a close correlation between the properties of the depolarizing responses induced by red light in green cones and R/G-HCs, which was not supported by the experimental evidence. The depolarizations induced by red light in R/G-HCs are usually of large amplitude, whereas the feedback depolarizations of most green cones are small. Moreover, whereas prolonged illuminations with red light elicit sustained depolarizations in R/G-HCs, the same stimuli evoke only an initial transient depolarization in most green cones.

These difficulties become less compelling if one assumes that the feedback signal which, through green cones, induces a depolarization in R/G-HCs is not the depolarization, but the calcium conductance increase, and this leads to an increase of the cone transmitter released. If this were the case, one would find that red light stimuli, which depolarize the R/G-HC, lead to the discharge of feedback spikes in the presence of Sr^{2+} in the perfusing medium. This should occur even in those green cones in which no feedback response is detected under control conditions. Moreover, a prolonged red light stimulation would lead to

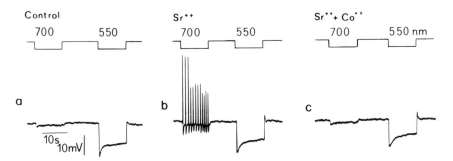

Fig. 1. Responses of a green cone to monochromatic red or green lights (of the indicated wavelength) recorded under different ionic conditions (as indicated). The light stimulus was a spot having an outer diameter (OD) of 3700 μm. The photon flux was about 1.2×10^5 quanta μm^{-2} sec^{-1}. The perfusing medium in (b) contained 5 mM Sr^{2+} ions and in (c) 5 mM Sr^{2+} + 3 mM Co^{2+}

a discharge of repetitive spikes in green cones, lasting as long the stimulus is kept on. Figure 1, which illustrates the results of experiments performed in collaboration with Gerschenfeld [25], shows that this is the case. The responses of a green cone to a large spot of either red or green light were recorded in normal saline (a), during the perfusion with a Ringer solution containing Sr^{2+} ions (b), and in the presence of both Sr^{2+} and Co^{2+} ions (c). This green cone did not show any feedback effect in control saline. Nevertheless, a sustained discharge of large spikes was induced by the prolonged illumination with red light during the application of Sr^{2+}, the green stimulus being ineffective. The spikes were completely blocked by the Co^{2+} ions. In Figure 2 the responses of a green cone to red or green light (a–c) were compared with the responses obtained with the same stimuli in a R/G-HC (d–f). Again only red light elicited spike discharges in the green cone. In correlation with the discharge of the spikes in the green cone, small depolarizing fluctuations appeared in the response of the R/G-HC. These can be interpreted as the responses to the phasic increase of the transmitter release associated with the spike discharge in the green cones. These observations are, therefore, consistent with the hypothesis of Fuortes and Simon and clearly show the sustained character of the feedback action in green cones in the presence of prolonged stimulation with red light.

Does the Feedback Modify the Light Response of L-HCs?

If the feedback affects all cones, it can be supposed to influence the response of all second order neurons in the retina. Working with Gerschenfeld, we have recently considered the possibility that also the response of L-HCs could be modified by the feedback circuit [26]. There is, however, a serious difficulty in trying to distinguish, in the responses of L-HCs, the effects resulting from the

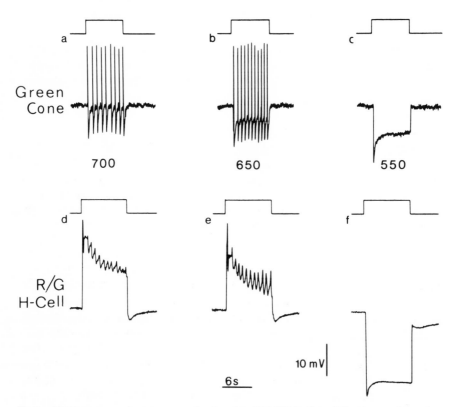

Fig.2. Light responses of a green cone (a–c) and an R/G-HC (d–f) to different monochromatic light recorded in a retina bathed with 6 mM Sr^{2+}. The stimulus was a 3700-μm OD spot and the photon flux was of 1.7×10^6 quanta μm^{-2} sec^{-1}. (From Piccolino et al, Nature 284:58, 1980.)

activation of the feedback loop on the cones impinging on them, from the effects induced by light stimuli through the direct pathway. In the case of R/G-HCs this was possible by using green or red light, due to the difference of spectral properties between the direct pathway and the feedback loop. No comparable possibility is immediately available for the L-HCs if these cells are themselves responsible for the feedback action on cones. Maximal feedback influences on the cones driving the L-HCs could, in principle, be obtained only with stimuli which elicit in L-HCs maximal amplitude responses through the direct pathway.

We tried to overcome this difficulty by confining our study to the analysis of the responses of one of the two L-HC types indentified in the turtle retina, to the small field horizontal cell (L2-HC). These cells were first described by Simon [27] as opposed to the large field type (L1-HC) more commonly impaled.

Simon showed that L2-HCs, as L1-HCs, are mainly driven from red cones. In a preliminary phase of our study, we obtained results suggesting that the cells responsible for the feedback on red cones were of the L1-HC type. On the basis of this finding and of the known spatial properties of the two L-HC types, we formulated the working hypothesis that the effects consequent to the feedback influence on cones should be easily detected in L2-HCs. To justify this hypothesis let us examine Figure 3. Here are illustrated the responses elicited in an L1- and an L2-HC by either light spots of increasing diameter, or annuli of light of a fixed external diameter (3700 μm) and decreasing internal diameter. The amplitude of the responses obtained in the L1-HC with relatively small light spots was smaller than the amplitude of the responses elicited by the same stimuli in the L2-HC. On the contrary, large surface annuli elicited larger amplitude responses in the L1-HC than in the L2-HC. L2-HCs are, therefore, dominated by the input coming from a relatively small population of central cones, whereas the weight of this central cone input is less important for the responses of L1-HCs. This difference is probably the consequence of different degrees of electrical coupling in the cells of the two classes [27]. The different receptive field properties of the two L-HC types permitted us to devise stimulus conditions in which either the primary direct input or the feedback influence could be preferentially activated for the L2-HCs. Small light spots should act mainly through the direct pathway: central red cones—L2-HC, whereas large light annuli should activate

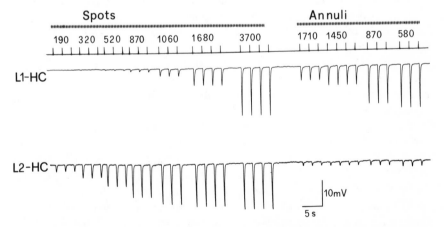

Fig.3.   Light responses of an L1- and an L2-HC simultaneously impaled in a retina perfused with control saline. The light stimuli were either light spots of increasing OD (as indicated in micrometers) or annuli of light of fixed OD (3700 μm) and decreasing inner diameter (ID) (as indicated). In this and the following illustrations, if not otherwise stated, white light was used. The maximum intensity of the unattenuated light at retinal level was about 3×10^5 μW μm^{-2}. In the experiment illustrated in this figure, the light was attenuated by 2.7 log units.

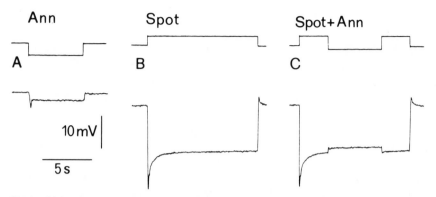

Fig.4. Light responses of an L2-HC to a light annulus (A), to a light spot (B), and to a temporal combination of both stimuli (C) of the same light intensity (3.6 log attenuation). The spot had an OD of 870 μm, while the annulus had an OD of 3700 μm and an ID of 870 μm.

the recurrent loop: peripheral red cones—L1-HC—central red cones—L2-HC. Since the effect of the light-induced hyperpolarization of the central cones is to decrease the release of the cone transmitter and, therefore, to hyperpolarize the L2-HC, the effect of the increase of the cone transmitter, induced by the feedback in the central cones, should be a depolarization of the L2-HC. An experiment intended to verify this hypothesis is illustrated in Figure 4, in which the receptive field of a L2-HC was stimulated with a dim annulus (A), a small spot of the same intensity (B), and a temporal combination of both stimuli (C). The annulus alone elicited a small hyperpolarizing response, whereas it resulted in a small sustained depolarization when applied in the presence of the adapting central background.

By comparing the light responses of L2-HCs with the light responses of red cones, we reached the conclusion that the depolarization induced in L2-HCs by peripheral stimuli was the result of the feedback action on the red cones situated in the central area of their receptive field.

The effects induced in L2-HCs by peripheral stimuli could not, however, be explained only on the basis of the activation of a feedback input to the central cones. For instance, Figure 3 shows that the amplitude of the response induced in L2-HCs by flash illumination with light spots increases monotonically with the increase of the stimulus diameter. This suggests that peripheral illumination could have an agonistic influence on the central response, which was not accounted for by the feedback. We reinvestigated this point and studied the receptive field properties of L2-HCs with light spots of different diameters at different light intensities. Figure 5b shows the responses obtained with a bright light. As for Figure 3 (in which a similar intensity was employed), the peak amplitude of the responses increased monotonically with the increase of the spot size. However, a different behavior was observed with the dim light (Fig. 5a).

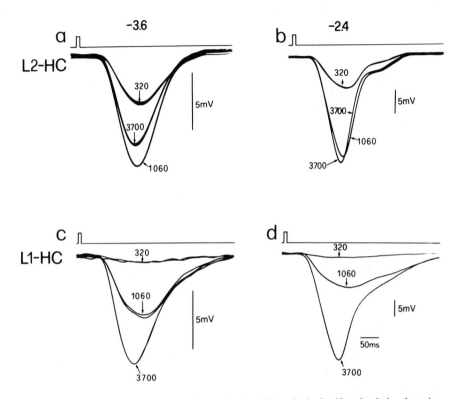

Fig.5.   Light responses of an L2-HC (a,b) and of an L1-HC (c, d) obtained by stimulating the retina with spots of different OD (as indicated in micrometers) at two different light intensities (indicated in relative log units). Notice the different voltage calibration in the different records.

The response amplitude increased when the spot diameter was increased from 320 to 1060 μm but decreased when the illuminated area was increased further. A careful analysis of the responses obtained with the brighter intensity (Fig. 5b) also reveals the possible presence of an antagonistic peripheral influence. The response obtained with the largest spot, although larger in peak amplitude, "crosses" the response to the intermediate size spot, being less hyperpolarized in the recovery phase. These experiments, therefore, suggest that the peripheral illumination could have both an agonistic (hyperpolarizing) and an antagonistic (depolarizing) influence on the response elicited by central illumination. To permit a further examination of these spatial influences, Figure 6 compares the responses elicited in a L2-HC by both a small and a large spot, with the responses induced by an annulus which is the area difference between the two spots. Two different light intensities were used. As in the case of the previous Figure 5, an antagonistic peripheral effect was observed with the dim light, whereas at the

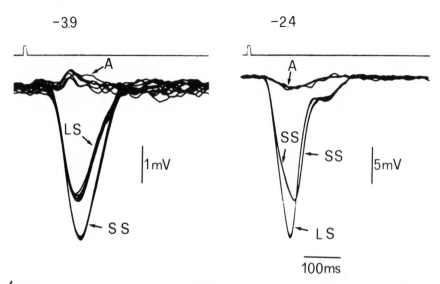

Fig.6. Light responses obtained in an L2-HC by stimulating the retina with a light annulus, (A) 3700 μm OD and 870 μm ID, a small light spot, (SS) 870 μm OD, and a large light spot, (LS) 3700 μm OD, at two different light intensities as indicated in relative log units.

brighter intensity both an initial agonism and a delayed antagonism appeared. The response elicited by the annulus was a very small depolarization with the dim light, and a hyperpolarization with the brighter intensity. Assuming a linear interaction between the central and the peripheral input, one would expect that the response evoked by the annulus would be the difference between the amplitudes of the responses evoked by the large and the small spot, respectively. This is not the case. The depolarization evoked by the dim annulus is too small to account for the antagonistic effect seen at the dim intensity, and the response elicited by the brighter annulus could account neither for the initial agonism nor for the delayed antagonism. It is interesting to note that peak amplitude of the response to the bright large spot is larger than the linear summation of the amplitudes, at the corresponding time, of the small spot and annulus responses. Such complex interaction of peripheral and central input was also revealed in experiments in which a small light spot of various light intensities was combined with a fixed intensity, dim annulus. The same dim annulus could result in either a pure antagonistic effect, or in an initial agonism and in delayed antagonism according to the intensity of the spot.

To explain the spatial properties of the light responses of L2-HCs we assumed that the antagonistic and the agonistic components of the peripheral response result from two different mechanisms, which are differently affected by the illumination of the central area of the receptive field. The agonistic peripheral influence is probably due to a convergence of the input from the more peripheral cones on the L2-HC, and also to the scatter of light from the peripheral illuminated area to the center of the receptive field. The antagonistic effect is likely the consequence of the depolarization of the central red cones, which results from the feedback from the L1-HC. As observed in a previous study [12], the feedback effect on cones can be reduced by a bright central illumination. This was shown to be the consequence of the hyperpolarization of the cone membrane induced by the bright central light (a reduction of the feedback response was also observed if the cone membrane was hyperpolarized with inward current). The reduction of the efficiency of the feedback input to the central cones in correspondence of the peak phase of the response to a bright light spot would unmask in L2-HC the peripheral agonistic influence. This would account for the observed enhancement of the central response. The feedback influence would, in contrast, prevail when the central cones are less hyperpolarized, that is, when the intensity of the central spot is dim, or in correspondence with the recovery phase of the response to a bright spot. Central illumination, by desensitizing the central cones and, thus, reducing their response to the light scattered from the annulus, would also modify the component of the peripheral agonism due to parasite light. The desensitization in the cones does not follow exactly the same time course of their light-induced hyperpolarization [28]. It involves, at least in part, a time-dependent process being particularly developed in the presence of a long lasting central stimulus. This would explain why the peripheral antagonist influence is easily revealed in the presence of such prolonged central illumination (Fig. 4).

Having obtained evidence that the feedback could modify the light response of L2-HCs, we analyzed the spatial properties of L1-HCs looking for the possibility that these cells also could be modified by the feedback. In experiments in which the receptive field of a L1-HC was studied with spots of increasing diameter, no center surround antagonism could be detected, the response amplitude increasing monotonically with the increase of the spot diameter at any light intensity (Fig. 5 c, d). Moreover, a prolonged peripheral illumination in the presence of a central background always resulted in a further hyperpolarization of the L1-HC membrane. This lack of an antagonistic surround effect in L1-HCs must not be, however, considered surprising. Actually, if L1-HCs are responsible for the feedback effect on the cones from which they are driven, one should not expect to find a peripheral antagonism in the L1-HC. Let us see why. Assume, for a moment, that the converse were true, that is, the amplitude of the L1-HC response were reduced following an increase of the stimulus size. If such were the case, the feedback input to cones would be reduced, their responses would increase, and, therefore, also the response of the L1-HC would increase. The absence of a peripheral antagonism in L1-HCs must not lead, however, to the conclusion that these cells are not modified by the feedback. Actually some characteristics of the light responses of L1-HCs could be the

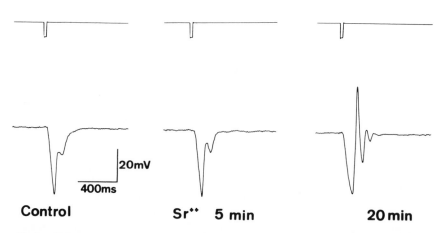

Control   **Sr⁺⁺ 5 min**   **20 min**

Fig.7.   Light responses recorded in an L1-HC in control saline and after the application to the retina of a saline containing 5 mM Sr^{2+}, as indicated. The stimulus was a light annulus (3600 μm OD, 150 μm ID) attenuated by 2.7 log units.

expression of the feedback influence on cones. It has been reported that flash illumination of a large surface of the receptive field can induce in L-HCs of both turtle and fishes [9, 29, 30] responses showing prominent oscillations in their recovery phase. In the turtle, oscillations are observed in both L1- and L2-HCs. The trigger features and the time course of these oscillations indicate that they could be the consequence of the deflections induced by the feedback on cones. The experiment illustrated in Figure 7 supports this hypothesis. The perfusion of the retina with an Sr^{2+}-containing medium, which was shown to increase the amplitude of the feedback responses in cones, resulted in an increase of the amplitude of the oscillations in the transient response of a L1-HC.

Lamb [31] has reported that the value of the space constant which describes the summative interactions in the receptive field of L-HC changes with the light intensity. The effective summation area is found to be larger with brighter light. This effect is evident in Figure 5 for both the L2- and the L1-HC. In the L2-HC the peak amplitude of the response increased by about 1.8 times when the diameter of the light stimulus is increased from 320 to 3700 μm at the dim intensity, whereas it increased by about 3.2 times at the brighter light. In the L1-HC, by comparing the responses to the 1060 and to the 3700 μm (the responses to the 320-μm spot are too small to be taken in account), one finds an increase of about 1.8 at the dim light and an increase of about 3.2 times at the bright intensity. In the case of the L2-HC it is safe to attribute this apparent expansion of the summation area to the decrease of the feedback influence during the peak phase of the response at the bright intensity. By analogy, the same explanation can be proposed for the L1-HC, even if in such case one cannot

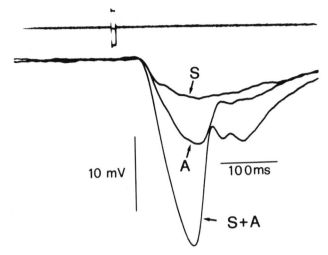

Fig.8. Light responses obtained in an L1-HC by stimulating the retina with a light spot, (S) OD 960 μm, a light annulus, (A) OD 3600 μm, ID 960 μm, and the simultaneous application of both stimuli. The light was attenuated by 2.7 log units.

find a direct evidence of the feedback antagonism. The spatial properties of L1-HCs were further analyzed in the experiment illustrated in Figure 8. Here the receptive field of a L1-HC was stimulated with a small central spot (S), a concentric annulus (A), and with these two stimuli applied together (S + A). The central spot elicited a small amplitude smooth response, whereas the annulus induced a larger hyperpolarization with a rather steep recovery. The combination of the two stimuli elicited a large response with a prominent oscillatory deflection in the recovery phase. The peak amplitude of the response induced by the two simultaneous stimuli was larger than the linear summation of the amplitude of the separate responses at the corresponding time. It was less, however, than the summation of the separate responses during the rapid recovery phase. The enhancement of the central response induced by the peripheral stimulus corresponds to the similar effect observed in L2-HCs. In L2-HCs it was attributed to the existence of different components in the peripheral input. A similar explanation could be, again, offered for the case of the L1-HC. In conclusion, the amplificative character of the interactions between the peripheral and central inputs would be explained in L1-HCs, as in L2-HCs, by assuming the existence of an antagonistic peripheral influence. A somewhat comparable "amplification by lateral inhibition" has been described and discussed at other levels of the visual system [32–34].

Amplificative interactions between the inputs converging on L-HCs have been described in other vertebrates [35–38]. At least in part they could correspond to the similar interactions found in the retina of the turtle. The models proposed to explain such behavior do not take into account the existence of an antagonistic peripheral effect and, therefore, cannot explain most of the properties of the L-HCs of the turtle.

THE OUTPUT OF THE L2-HC

By injecting intracellular dye through the recording electrode, Simon [27] showed that the structures originating the L1- and the L2-HC types of responses have different morphological appearance. On the basis of the recent morphological observations of Leeper [39], there is now reason to believe that L1- and the L2-HCs correspond actually to different regions of the same cell, that is, to the axonal expansion and to the cell body region, respectively. These two regions are connected by a slender fiber, which is probably unable to support a high efficiency electrical conduction. This would explain the difference of the response properties of the two units. Leeper has also shown that only the somatic region contacts green cones and he has, therefore, proposed that L2-HCs are responsible for the feedback depolarization of green cones [24]. We have been prompted by this hypothesis particularly, since our experiments suggested that L2-HCs do not make an important contribution to the feedback on red cones, which is probably the result of the action of only L1-HCs. In collaboration with Gerschenfeld [40], we reinvestigated this point by studying the receptive field properties of the depolarizations induced by red light stimuli in the green cones and by comparing them with the receptive field properties of both L1- and L2-HCs. In both control Ringer and during the perfusion with Sr^{2+} or Ba^{2+} saline, these feedback depolarizations were better obtained with relatively small red light spots than with large red annuli (see Fig. 9). Moreover, the depolarizing responses induced by small red light spots in green cones could be even reduced following red light stimulation of the far periphery of their receptive field. These results, therefore, indicate that the cells involved in the generation of the feedback depolarization of the green cones are probably of the L2-HC type and support the hypothesis advanced by Leeper.

A simplified schema of the connections between cones and L-HCs, as suggested by our study, is presented in Figure 10. Both the L1- and the L2-HC are supposed to receive input only from red cones. The input from the central cones would be more weighted in the L2-HC than the input from the peripheral cones, whereas the opposite is supposed for the L1-HC. The feedback effect on the red cone is considered to be the result of the action of the L1-HC, whereas the L2-HC would be responsible for the feedback on green cones. The pathway central red cones—L2-HC—green cones would account for the feedback depolarization of the green cones induced by small red light spots. The pathway peripheral red cones—L1-HC—central red cones—L2-HC would be the basis of the peripheral

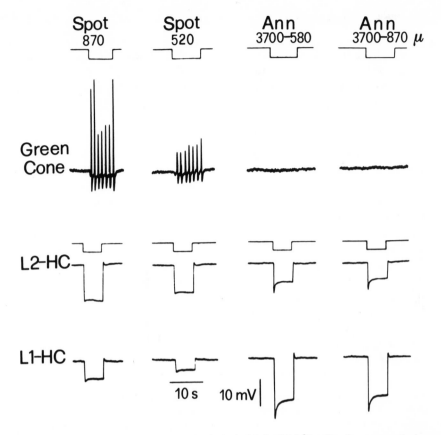

Fig.9. Light responses obtained in a retina bathed with 5 mM Sr^{2+} saline from, respectively, a green cone, an L2-, and an L1-HC. The light stimuli were either spots or annuli of monochromatic red light (700 nm.). The numbers near the stimulus trace give the OD of the light spots, and the OD and ID of the light annuli. The photon flux was 1.2×10^5 quanta μ^{-2} sec^{-1}. Notice that the only the spots elicit the spike discharge in the green cone, whereas the annuli are ineffective. A correlation is evident between the spikes occurrence in the cone and the amplitude of the response of the L2-HC, whereas no correlation exists with the amplitude of the response of the L2-HC.

antagonism acting on the L2-HC. It would account, therefore, for the reduction of the feedback responses of the green cones induced by the illumination of the far periphery of their receptive field. The direct pathway peripheral red cones—L2-HC—would account for the peripheral enhancement of the response of L2-HC which is observed when the effectiveness of the feedback action on central red cones is reduced due to bright central illuminations.

CONCLUDING REMARKS

The results discussed in this paper support the idea that the feedback intervenes in the elaboration of the visual message in the distal retina. Additional studies

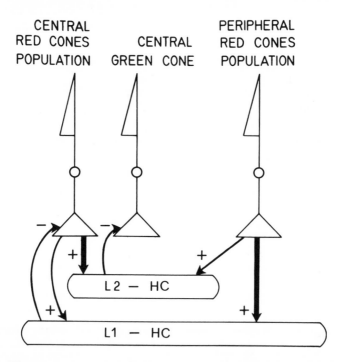

Fig.10. Diagram of the synaptic relations between cones and L-HCs in the turtle retina. Symbols (+) and (−) indicate sign-preserving and sign-inverting synapses, respectively. In the forward pathway the thickness of the line represents the relative weight of the input to the different L-HC types. "Central or peripheral red cone population" refers, respectively, to the pool of cone inside or outside a circular central region of the receptive field of approximately 1000 μm in diameter. (Modified from Neyton et al Proc Nat Acad Sci USA 79:4616, 1981.)

are necessary for a better understanding of the mechanism of cellular interaction at this level. Though it seems rather well established that the final effect of the feedback on the cone membrane is a calcium conductance increase, the mechanism of this effect remains obscure. It has been suggested that L-HCs could influence cones either through a chemical synapse [7] or by means of an electrical effect [41]. The available evidence, however, is not conclusive in this respect. The output of R/G-HCs is not fully indentified. There is anatomical evidence that these cells could be responsible for the feedback on blue cones [23]. Unfortunately, these cones are only occasionally impaled in electrophysiological studies. The notion that HCs have an output on cones does not exclude that they could influence second order neurons also through direct synaptic connections [37,42]. An answer to this problem could be given by selectively blocking the feedback loop. A study of the pharmacology of the feedback synapse might provide an useful experimental tool.

The feedback has been studied almost exclusively in the retina of the turtle. There is also evidence of a similar mechanism in the retina of the fish [43]. Additional studies on other vertebrates would be necessary to know how general this mechanism is.

Finally, it must be considered that the final common pathway for the neural message elaborated in the distal retina is constituted by bipolar cells. The possibility that the response of these cells is modified by the feedback has been already discussed [44]. This problem, however, must be reconsidered in view of most recent results. It would be necessary to distinguish the component of the bipolar cells response due to the direct input from cones, from the components resulting from the feedback loop or from possible direct contacts with HCs or other retinal neurons.

ACKNOWLEDGMENTS

This work would not have been possible without the help and advice of Dr. H. M. Gerschenfeld, to whom we express out profound gratitude. We are also deeply indebted to Mr. Bernard Lacaisse and to Mr. Piero Taccini for technical assistance. The work was supported by grants from the Centre National de la Recherche Scientifique (CNRS), France, Délégational a la Recherche Scientifique et Technique, and Institut National de la Santé et de la Recherche Medicale, France. Marco Piccolino was supported by the Consiglio Nazionale delle Richerche (CNR), Italy, and the CNRS.

REFERENCES

1. Svaetichin G: The cone action potential. Acta Physiol Scand 29 (Suppl 106):565, 1953.
2. Cervetto L, Fuortes MGF: Excitation and interaction in the retina. Ann Rev Biophys Bioeng 7:229, 1978.
3. Maksimova Ye M: Effect of intracellular polarization of horizontal cells on the activity of the ganglionic cells of the retina of fish. Biophysics 14:570, 1969.
4. Naka K-I, Nye PW: Role of horizontal cells in organization of the catfish retinal receptive field. J Neurophysiol 34:785, 1971.
5. Schwartz EA: Organization of on-off cells in the retina of turtle. 230:1, 1973.
6. Lasansky A: Synaptic organization of the cone cells in the turtle retina. Phil Trans R Soc B 262:365, 1971.
7. Baylor DA, Fuortes MGF, O'Bryan PM: Receptive field of cones in the retina of the turtle. J Physiol 214:265, 1971.
8. Naka K-I, Rushton WAH: S-Potentials from colour units in the retina of fish (Cyprinidae). J Physiol 185:536, 1966.
9. Fuortes MGF, Schwartz EA, Simon EJ: Colour dependence of cone responses in the turtle retina. J Physiol 234:199, 1973.
10. O'Bryan PM: Properties of the depolarizing synaptic potential evoked by peripheral illumination in cones of the turtle retina. J Physiol 235:207, 1973.
11. Piccolino M, Gerschenfeld HM: Activation of a regenerative calcium conductance in turtle cones by peripheral stimulation. Proc R Soc B 201:309, 1978.
12. Piccolino M, Gerschenfeld HM: Characteristics and ionic processes involved in feedback spikes of turtle cones. Proc R Soc B 206:439, 1980.

13. Gerschenfeld HM, Piccolino M: Sustained feedback effect of L-horizontal cells on turtle cones. Proc R Soc B 206:465, 1980.
14. Gerschenfeld HM, Piccolino M, Neyton J: Feedback modulation of cone synapses by L-horizontal cells. J Exp Biol 89:177, 1980.
15. Cervetto L, MacNichol EF Jr: Inactivation of horizontal cells in the turtle retina by glutamate and aspartate. Science 178:767, 1972.
16. Dowling JE, Ripps JH: Effect of magnesium on horizontal cell activity in the skate retina. Nature (London) 262:101, 1973.
17. Cervetto L, Piccolino M: Synaptic transmission between photoreceptors and horizontal cells in the turtle retina. Science 191:963, 1974.
18. Kaneko A, Shimazaki H: Effect of external ions in the synaptic transmission from photoreceptors to horizontal cells in the carp retina. J Physiol 252:509, 1975.
19. Trifonov Yu A: Study of synaptic transmission between photoreceptors and horizontal cells by means of electrical stimulation of the retina. Biophisika 13:809, 1968.
20. Katz B, Miledi R: Tetrodotoxin resistant electrical activity in presynaptic terminals. J Physiol 203:559, 1966.
21. Fuortes MGF, Simon EJ: Interactions leading to horizontal cell responses in the turtle. J Physiol 24:177, 1974.
22. Svaetichin G, MacNichol EF: Retinal mechanism for chromatic and achromatic vision. Ann Nat Acad Sci 74:385, 1958.
23. Stell WK, Lightfoot DO, Wheeler TG, Leeper HF: Goldfish retina: Functional polarization of cone horizontal cell dendrites and synapses. Science 190:989, 1975.
24. Leeper HF: Horizontal cells of the turtle retina. II: Analysis of interconnections between photoreceptor cells and horizontal cells by light microscopy. J Comp Neurol 182:795, 1978.
25. Piccolino M, Neyton J, Gerschenfeld HM: Synaptic mechanism involved in the responses of chromaticity horizontal cells of turtle retina. Nature (London) 284:58, 1980.
26. Piccolino M, Neyton J, Gerschenfeld HM: Center surround antagonistic organization in the small field L-horizontal cells of turtle retina. J Neurophysiol 45:363, 1981.
27. Simon EJ: Two types of luminosity horizontal cells in the retina of the turtle. J Physiol (London) 230:199, 1973.
28. Baylor DA, Hodgkin AL: Changes in time scale and sensitivity in turtle photoreceptors. J Physiol 242:729, 1974.
29. Marchiafava PL, Pasino E: The spatial dependent characteristics of the fish S-potentials evoked by brief flashes. Vision Res 13:1355, 1973.
30. Chan RY, Naka K-I: Spatial organization of catfish retinal neurons. II: Circular stimulus. J Neurophysiol 43:832, 1980.
31. Lamb TD: Spatial properties of horizontal cell responses in the turtle retina. J Physiol 263:239, 1976.
32. Ratliff F, Knight BW, Toyoda J-I, Hartline HK: Enhancement of flicker by lateral inhibition. Science 158:392, 1967.
33. Ratliff F, Knight BW, Graham N: On tuning and amplification by lateral inhibition. Proc Nat Acad Sci NY 62:733, 1969.
34. Maffei L, Cervetto L, Fiorentini A: Transfer characteristics of excitation and inhibition in cat retinal ganglion cells. J Neurophysiol 33:267, 1970.
35. Maksimova M Ye, Maksimov VV, Orlov O Yu: Amplified interaction between the signal from cell receptors and sources of S-potentials. Biophysics 11:535, 1966.
36. Negishi K: Reduction and enhancement of S-potential observed with two simultaneous light stimuli in the isolated fish retina. Vision Res 11 (Suppl 3):65, 1971.
37. Lasansky A, Vallerga S: Horizontal cell responses in the retina of the larval tiger salamander. J Physiol 251:147, 1975.

38. Laufer M, Negishi K: Enhancement of hyperpolarizing S-potentials by surround illumination in a teleost retina. Vision Res 18:1005, 1978.
39. Leeper HF: Horizontal cells of the turtle retina. I. Light microscopy of Golgi preparations. J Comp Neurol 182:77, 1978.
40. Neyton J, Piccolino M, Gerschenfeld HM: Involvment of small field L-horizontal cells in the feedback on green cones. Proc Nat Acad Sci USA 78:4616, 1981.
41. Byzov A, Golubtzov KV, Trifonov Yu A: The model of mechanism of feedback between horizontal cells and photoreceptors in vertebrate retina. In Barlow HB, Fatt P (eds): "Vertebrate Photoreception." New York: Academic Press, 1978, p 265.
42. Werblin FS, Dowling JE: Organization of the retina of the mudpuppy, Necturus maculosus. II. Intracellular recording. J Neurophysiol 32:339, 1969.
43. Burkhardt DA: Responses and receptive-field properties of cones in perch retinas. J Neurophysiol 40:53, 1977.
44. Richter A, Simon EJ: Properties of centre hyperpolarizing red sensitive bipolar cells in the turtle retina. J Physiol 248:317, 1975.

The S-Potential, pages 181–192
© 1982 Alan R. Liss, Inc., 150 Fifth Avenue, New York, NY 10011

Formation of Receptive Fields and Synaptic Inputs to Horizontal Cells

Frank S. Werblin and Josef Skrzypek

Our present understanding of vertebrate retinal function is based upon studies that were initiated with the pioneering intracellular recordings of Svaetichin [1] and Svaetichin and MacNichol [2]. These studies showed for the first time that the distal retinal cells, in response to a continuous stimulus, display spikeless, sustained, graded hyperpolarizations. Such forms of response, at first considered heretical, have now been confirmed in a variety of vertebrate preparations, and the original work forms the cornerstone for retinal studies at the intracellular level.

Following the lead of these earlier experiments, horizontal cells have been extensively examined in many laboratories. A great deal has been learned about the response properties of these cells, including spectral qualities, time course, and sensitivity. However, the receptive field structure, the nature of the synaptic inputs, and the electrical changes associated with the horizontal cell response have not yet been adequately defined. This paper addresses some of these issues, and describes some new developments in the evaluation of functional properties of the horizontal cells. First, the role of the horizontal cells in forming the antagonistic surround at the outer plexiform layer is reviewed.

FUNCTIONAL SIGNIFICANCE OF THE HORIZONTAL CELL NETWORK

It is now generally agreed that the visual messages proceed from the photoreceptors to ganglion cells by way of the bipolars, and that this pathway is intersected at two levels by systems of lateral interneurons. Horizontal cells or some of their processes are thought to modulate transmission from the photoreceptors to the bipolars; amacrine cells modulate transmission from the bipolars to the ganglion cells. The horizontal and amacrine cell processes spread laterally across the retina and make synaptic contact with adjacent processes. In this way they form a pathway for relating activity at one part of the visual field to adjacent areas. The role of the lateral interneurons could be inferred from the work of Cajal [3] nearly a century ago. The physiological behavior of the lateral interneurons in modulating bipolar and ganglion cell activity was first described nearly a decade ago [4–6].

The early physiological studies showed that bipolar cells had concentric, antagonistic receptive fields, such that illumination at the receptive field center elicited a response of opposite polarity from that elicited by surround illumination. It was inferred that the horizontal cells provided the pathway for the antagonistic surround. Baylor et al [6] then showed that turtle cones themselves had concentric fields, as was later confirmed by Burkhardt [7]. This study provided evidence that some part of the horizontal cell system formed the antagonistic surround at the outer plexiform layer by feeding back to the receptors through a sign-inverting synapse. A schematic outline of the forms of response at the outer plexiform layer is presented in Figure 1.

It was later shown that the effects of the lateral antagonistic surround measured at the bipolar cells persisted at all levels of center illumination [8]. The graded response of the bipolar cells was affected by lateral antagonism: When the graded bipolar response was plotted against log center stimulus intensity, an S-shaped-intensity-response relation, obeying $R = I^N/(c + I^N)$ was obtained, where N had the value 1.4 [9]. When the intensity of the surround illumination was changed, the bipolar graded response curve was shifted bodily to the right along the log intensity axis as shown in Figure 2 [8,9]. This was interpreted to mean that the surround simply sets the sensitivity or "gain" for the central response. For example, the same bodily shift of the graded response curve would be obtained if a neutral density filter were imposed between the stimulus and the receptive field center of the bipolar cell (the quantal flux would thereby be reduced by a multiplicative factor at all intensities of the stimulator). Thus the effect of increasing surround intensity is similar to the effect of interposing a neutral density filter: Bipolar cell sensitivity is reduced.

How can synaptic interactions between horizontal cells and the receptor–bipolar pathway mediate a change in sensitivity in the bipolar cells? The mechanism for sensitivity control is not yet resolved, but one possibility is clear. The entire graded response in the bipolar cells spans an intensity domain that is only a fraction of that spanned by the photoreceptors: The bipolar domain is about 1 log unit, whereas that of the receptors is about 3 log units as shown in Figure 2. This means that bipolar cells respond only over a narrow range of receptor potentials. We know that lateral interactions mediated by horizontal cells serve to depolarize the cones. This depolarization can act to reset the relationship between stimulus intensity and absolute membrane potential in the receptors. Thus, the potentials in receptors over which the bipolar cells can respond will be shifted to a different intensity domain. This mechanism is discussed in more detail in an earlier paper [8].

To summarize, the horizontal cells perform the essential function of forming the concentric, antagonistic surround for the bipolar cells. The antagonistic surround serves to control the sensitivity of the receptive field center of the bipolar

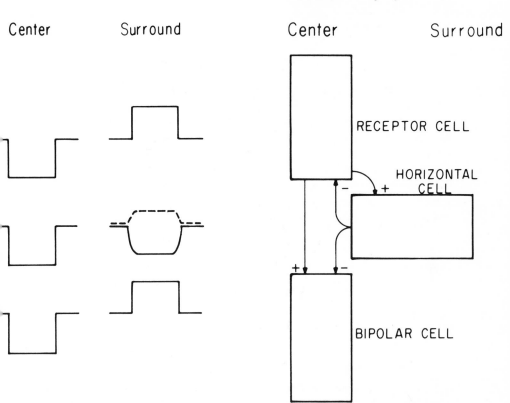

Fig. 1. Schematic relationship between activity and pathways of cones, horizontal cells, and bipolar cells. The response of the cones, horizontal cells, and bipolars is hyperpolarizing for illumination at the center of the receptive fields. Surround illumination elicits an antagonistic response in the cones and bipolar cells. This is presumably mediated by a sign-inverting synapse between horizontal cell processes and the cones and bipolars. Such a scheme requires a hyperpolarizing surround response in the horizontal cell system. In fact, horizontal cell bodies depolarize, precluding their role as lateral antagonistic interneurons. However, the horizontal cell axon terminals always hyperpolarize, making the terminals candidates for lateral interneurons.

cells over their entire response range. Since the higher levels of the visual system must "view" the world through the photoreceptors and bipolar cells, this first stage of lateral interactions could provide a primary and essential sensitivity control for the visual system. The following sections review some of the synaptic mechanisms which control the horizontal cell response.

SYNAPTIC INPUTS TO THE HORIZONTAL CELLS

One of the striking properties of distal retinal neurons is the hyperpolarizing response to light. In most neural systems, including other sensory systems, the

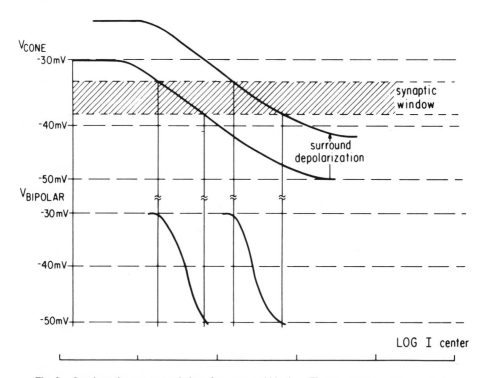

Fig. 2. Log-intensity response relations for cones and bipolars. The cone response spans a greater intensity domain than that of the bipolars. Therefore, only a small portion of the cone potential corresponds to the full bipolar potential range. This small portion of the cone potential range is called the "synaptic window": the potentials that are effective in modulating bipolar activity. Surround illumination acts to depolarize the cones, thus shifting the relationship between the synaptic window and intensity. Therefore, the relationship between bipolar cell response and intensity is shifted.

excitatory stimulus elicits a depolarizing response. This immediately raised the question as to when the synaptic transmitter is liberated: By analogy with other systems, the transmitter would be liberated at the highest rate in the dark, when the retinal neurons were most depolarized. That synaptic transmitter is, in fact, liberated at high rate in the dark has been verified by the experiments of Dowling and Ripps [10], Cervetto and Piccolino [11], Kaneko and Shimazaki [12] and Marshall and Werblin [13]. In all cases, divalent cations, known in other preparations to interrupt release of synaptic transmitter, were applied to the retina. As shown in Figure 3, application of cobalt ions caused the horizontal cells to hyperpolarize to the level of maximum light response. The conclusion is that the synaptic transmitter normally liberated by the photoreceptors depolarizes the horizontal cells in the dark, and that this depolarization is reduced during illu-

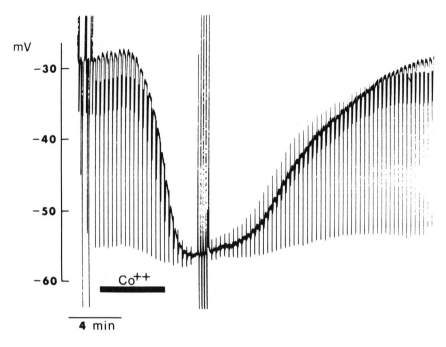

Fig. 3. Effects of light and cobalt ions on the horizontal cell response. The membrane potential in the dark is near -30 mV. The narrow vertical lines show maximal light responses on a very slow time scale. After about 4 min of Co^{2+} application, the membrane is hyperpolarized to the level of the maximum light response. These results suggest that both cobalt and light act to interrupt release of transmitter which normally depolarizes the membrane.

mination when the photoreceptors hyperpolarize, confirming the hypothesis of Trifonov [14]. Interestingly, it appears that saturating test flashes hyperpolarize the photoreceptors sufficiently to turn off transmitter release from the photoreceptors.

The next question of physiological importance is: How can the synaptic transmitter liberated by the photoreceptors act at the postsynaptic membrane to depolarize the horizontal cells? Traditionally, one would look for a conductance change associated with the horizontal cell response. This should be particularly easy to measure since the horizontal cell response can be as great as 50 mV, from a dark level near -20 mV to about -70 mV.

Surprisingly, the conductance change associated with the horizontal cell response has not been easy to measure. Some early studies reported a conductance decrease [15,16], and others, a conductance increase [13,17–19]. Explanations for these inconsistent and negative results invoked two arguments: First, horizontal cells are electrically coupled, so changes in membrane resistance are obscured by the geometry [20,21]; and second, the horizontal cell membrane is strongly inward rectifying, which tends to obscure excitatory conductance changes [22]. Hanani and Valerga [23] have shown both rod and cone inputs to the horizontal cells in tiger salamander. Recently, however, it has been shown that rods and cones may elicit opposing conductance changes in the horizontal cells, at least in fish, presenting yet another factor to obscure the measurement.

The possibility that rods and cones could elicit opposing conductance changes in postsynaptic cells was first suggested by Saito et al [24,25]. They showed that the rod transmitter decreases, whereas the cone transmitter increases membrane conductance in the depolarizing bipolar cells of the carp.

A similar dichotomy has been found by Skrzypek and Werblin (in preparation) for horizontal cells in the retina of the tiger salamander. When rod and cone activity are separated spectrally, it is found in some cases that the cone transmitter appears to decrease conductance, whereas the rod transmitter increases conductance.

Interestingly, it also appears that the cone component of the response can be eliminated in the presence of acetylcholine (ACh). Figure 4 shows the response spectrum of a horizontal cell before and during the application of ACh. The spectrum normally shows a major peak near 600 nm, the response peak for the cones, and a minor peak near 500 nm, the response peak for the rods. In the presence of ACh, the cone peak is lost, and the response spectrum is maximal near 450 nm.

Using the results of Figure 4, it is now possible to interpret an earlier result of Marshall and Werblin [13]. They found that the light response in most horizontal cells was normally not associated with a measurable conductance change, as shown in Figure 5. Acetylcholine itself caused a conductance decrease, and then in the presence of ACh, the light response was associated with a transmitter that increased conductance. (Remember that the transmitter is turned *off* during illumination, as shown in Fig. 3.)

These results suggest that the cone transmitter is cholinergic and acts to decrease membrane conductance. Gerschenfeld and Piccolino [26] have also suggested that the cone transmitter in the turtle retina might be cholinergic, based upon blocking activity with atropine. It is interesting to note that there are numerous examples of muscarinic synapses in vertebrates where ACh acts by decreasing conductance. These results also suggest the rod transmitter is *not* cholinergic, since rod activity persists even in the presence of ACh or atropine.

RECEPTIVE FIELDS FOR HORIZONTAL CELL BODIES AND AXON TERMINALS

In the tiger salamander, two distinct classes of horizontal cell receptive fields can be found, measured in the cell bodies or the axon terminals. The physiology

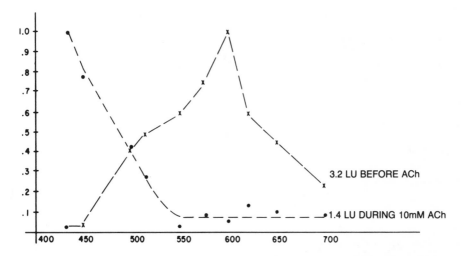

Fig. 4. Spectral response of the horizontal cell under normal conditions and bathed in 10 mM ACh. The spectral response under normal conditions has a peak near 600 nm, the spectral response of the cones. In the presence of ACh, the response peak is shifted far to the left, near the response maximum for the rods. These results suggest that ACh interrupts cone, but not rod, transmission to the horizontal cells.

and morphology of each type, originally shown by Lasansky and Valerga [27], is discussed separately below.

A drawing of a horizontal cell body, derived from a Lucifer Yellow fill obtained after recording is shown in Figure 6B. Cell bodies have clusters of fine processes extending over a limited radius, usually about 100 μm. The processes radiate from the soma with typical diameter near 20 μm. Often the injected dye could be found in neighboring cell bodies, so that the entire stained constellation spanned close to 0.4 mm across the retina.

The physiology for horizontal cell bodies is consistent with the morphology. Receptive fields spanned a range of diameters from about 400 to 1200 μm, when measured as the smallest test disk to elicit the maximal response. In addition, all horizontal cell bodies appear to have a concentric, antagonistic surround response. The strength of the surround response varied with the intensity of the center stimulus. When the center was dark, the surround response was small; at intermediate intensities, the surround response was maximal; and for bright center illumination the surround response inverted and became hyperpolarizing.

The variation of the surround response in horizontal cells with center intensity is similar to that for the cones themselves, except that cones never show a hyperpolarizing surround response. The surround response for cones and hori-

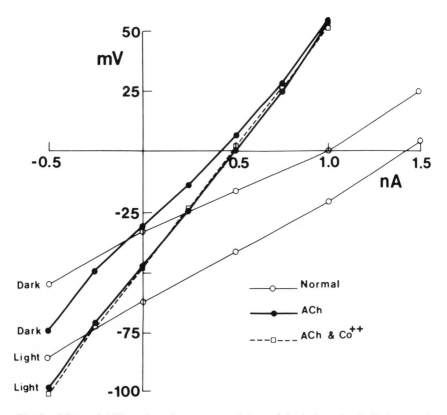

Fig. 5. Effects of ACh on the voltage–current relations of the horizontal cell. Under normal conditions (thin lines), there is little conductance change between light and dark (lines are nearly parallel). ACh itself causes a conductance decrease with negative reversal potential (compare thick and thin lines). Also, in the presence of ACh, the light response shows a clear conductance change: Conductance increases in darkness (when transmitter is released). The results suggest that ACh blocks a conductance-decreasing mechanism, but leaves intact a conductance-increasing system.

zontal cell bodies are compared in Figure 7. The horizontal cell response can be constructed from the cone response by simply shifting the cone surround response downward along the potential axis. This is analogous to introducing a constant hyperpolarization along with the surround response at all center intensities. Coupling between horizontal cell bodies, as described earlier by Kaneko [28], Simon [29], and Skrzypek [30] could generate the additional hyperpolarization needed to convert the antagonistic surround response, probably initiated at the cones themselves, into the complex surround response measured in the horizontal cell bodies.

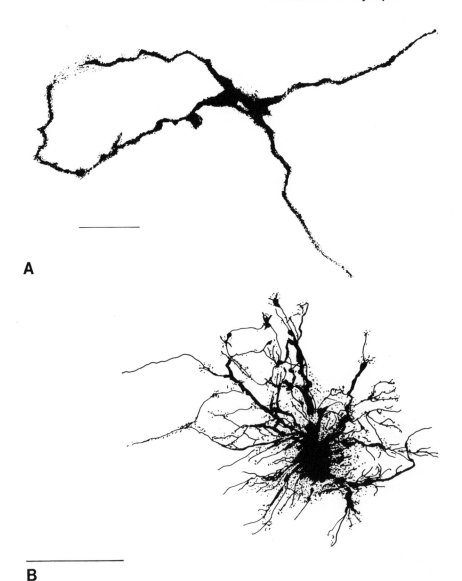

A

B

Fig. 6.   Camera Lucida drawings of the Lucifer Yellow-injected axon terminal (A) and the horizontal cell body (B). Marker for both cells is 50μm.

Horizontal cell axon terminals differ in morphology dramatically from the cell bodies. The axon terminals consist of a few tubular processes, with diameter between 2 and 6 μm, that could be traced over distances up to 0.8 mm, attached

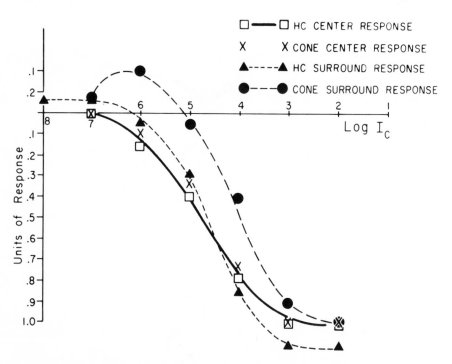

Fig. 7. Relationship between surround responses in cones and horizontal cell bodies. The heavy, solid curve shows the response of a horizontal cell as a function of center intensity. The triangles show the response of the horizontal cell to an annular flash added to the center intensity. At low center intensities, the surround response is depolarizing, whereas at high center intensities, the surround response is hyperpolarizing. The heavy, solid curve and the large dots represent the response of a cone illuminated with a center flash, and the addition of a surround flash, respectively. The surround response in the cone is depolarizing and large for dim center intensities, but progressively smaller for brighter center intensities. The surround response in the horizontal cells seems to follow that in the cones, except that the horizontal cell response is shifted in the hyperpolarizing direction to some constant hyperpolarizing influence coupled to the center of the field from the surround.

to a central portion that was 50 μm in length and about 15 μm in diameter. A sketch of an axon terminal is shown in Figure 6A.

Physiologically, the axon terminals have very broad receptive fields, up to 2 mm in diameter. The axon terminals never show a clear antagonistic surround response, and this is probably because the direct coupling between the axon terminals which extends the dimension of the receptive field, is sufficient to override the antagonistic response initiated in the cones.

Which type of horizontal cell, the axon terminal or cell body, provides the synaptic input to cones mediating the antagonistic surround and controlling sensitivity? If we accept that the synapse from horizontal cells to cones is sign inverting [6], then the horizontal cell bodies are ruled out as the feedback elements. The cell bodies themselves depolarize in response to the annulus, and, therefore, cannot act to depolarize the cones. The axon terminals remain the probable candidates for the feedback elements: They always hyperpolarize, and they have broad receptive fields. To our knowledge, there is no anatomical evidence for a functional polarity between the processes of horizontal cell bodies and axon terminals that make synaptic contact with the cones. Our analysis suggests that such a functional polarity exists: Axon terminals feed back, but cell bodies do not. What, then, is the functional role of the horizontal cell bodies?

ACKNOWLEDGEMENT

This research was sponsored by the National Institutes of Health, Grant EY00561-10.

REFERENCES

1. Svaetichin G: The cone action potential. Acta Physiol Scand 29 Supp 106:565–601, 1953.
2. Svaetichin G, MacNichol EF: Retinal mechanisms for chromatic and achromatic visions. Ann NY Acad Sci 74, 2:385, 1958.
3. Cajal SR: La Cellule 9:119–253, 1822.
4. Werblin FS, Dowling JE: Organization of the retina of mudpuppy, Necturus maculosus. II. Intracellular recording. J Neurophysiol 32:339–355, 1969.
5. Kaneko A: Physiological and morphological identification of horizontal bipolar, and amacrine cells in goldfish retina. J Physiol (London) 207:623–633, 1970.
6. Baylor DA, Fuortes MGF, O'Bryan PM: Receptive fields of cones in the retina of the turtle. J Physiol 214:265–294, 1971.
7. Burkhardt DA: Responses and receptive-field organization of cones in perch retina. J Neurophysiol 40:53–62, 1977.
8. Werblin FS: Control of retinal sensitivity. II. Lateral interactions at the outer plexiform layer. J Gen Physiol 63:62–87, 1974.
9. Thibos LN, Werblin FS: The response properties of the steady antagonistic surround in the mudpuppy retina. J Physiol 278:79–99, 1978.
10. Dowling JE, Ripps H: Effect of magnesium on horizontal cell activity in the skate retina. Nature (London) 242:101–103, 1973.
11. Cervetto L, Piccolino M: Synaptic transmission between photoreceptors and horizontal cells in the turtle retina. Science 183:417–419, 1974.
12. Kaneko A, Shimazaki H: Effects of external ions on the synaptic transmission from photoreceptors to horizontal cells in the carp retina. J Physiol (London) 252:509–522, 1975.
13. Marshall LM, Werblin FS: Synaptic transmission to the horizontal cells in the retina of the tiger salamander. J Physiol 279:321–346, 1978.
14. Trifonov YA: Study of synaptic transmission between photoreceptors and horizontal cells by means of electrical stimulation of the retina. Biofizika 13:809–817, 1968.
15. Tomita T: Electrophysiological study of the mechanism subserving colour coding in the fish retina. Cold Spring Hard Symp Quant Biol 30:559–566, 1965.
16. Tomita T, Kaneko A: An intracellular coaxial microelectrode, its construction and application. Med Electron Biol Engng 3:367–376, 1965.
17. Tasaki K: Some observations on the retinal potentials of the fish. Italian Biol 98:81–91, 1960.

18. Trifonov YA, Utina IA: Investigation of the mechanism of current action on the L-type cells of the retina. Biophysica 11:646–652, 1966.
19. Nelson R: A comparison of electrical properties of neurons in *Necturus* retina. J Neurophysiol 36:519–535, 1973.
20. Lamb TC, Simon EJ: The relation between intercellular coupling and electrical noise in turtle photoreceptors. J Physiol (London) 263:257–286, 1976.
21. Jack JJB, Noble D, Tsien RW: "Electric Current Flow in Excitable Cells." Oxford: Clarendon Press, 1975.
22. Werblin FS: Anomalous rectification in horizontal cells. J Physiol (London) 244:639–657, 1975.
23. Hanani M, Vallerga S: Rod and cone signals in the horizontal cells of the tiger salamander. J Physiol (London) 298:397–405, 1980.
24. Saito T, Kondo H, Toyoda JI: Rod and cone signals in the on-center bipolar cells: Their different ionic mechanisms. Vision Res 18:591–595, 1978.
25. Saito T, Kondo H, Toyoda JI: Ionic mechanisms of two types of on-center bipolar cells in the carp retina. I. The responses to central illumination. J Gen Physiol 73:73–90, 1979.
26. Gerschenfeld HM, Piccolino M: Muscarinic antagonistic blocks cone to horizontal cell transmission in turtle retina. Nature (London) 286:257–259, 1977.
27. Lasansky, A, Vallerga S: Horizontal cell responses in the retina of the larval tiger salamander. J Physiol (London) 251:145–166, 1975.
28. Kaneko A: Electrical connexions between horizontal cells in the dogfish retina. J Physiol (London) 213:95–105, 1971.
29. Simon EJ: Two types of luminosity horizontal cells in the retina of the turtle. J Physiol (London) 230:199–211, 1973.
30. Skrzypek J: "Synaptic Mechanism of the Light Response in Horizontal Cells of the Tiger Salamander Retina." Berkeley: PhD Thesis, University of California at Berkeley, 1979.

The S-Potential, pages 193–205

Quantitative Analysis of Horizontal Cell Response

Ken-ichi Naka and Masanori Sakuranaga

Twenty years ago, a paper was published which was to affect the career of one of us (KIN). The paper was entitled "The Cone Action Potential," a title which precipitated an immediate controversy as well as did much to lessen the paper's apparent historical impact [1]. Not that the paper lacked anything, but it had too much, particularly, of imagination. To be imaginative should be commendable for scientists but the lack of it seems to be a virtue now. Gunnar Svaetichin, to whose honor this volumn is dedicated, authored the paper. One of us (KIN) had the fortune to follow Svaetichin's footsteps and also to be able to associate with many analytical minds in doing so. They showed us beyond any doubt that it was not only possible to analyze potentials from the retina, but it was imperative to do so, if we were to understand, in a quantitative fashion, how the retina works. The popularity of the Michaelis–Menten equation and also of the concept of lamima formed by a layer of cells testifies in favor of this view (cf [2,3]).

HISTORICAL BACKGROUND

In 1953 Svaetichin [1] discovered in a fish retina a large hyperpolarizing potential which was maintained as long as light was kept on. We are now familiar with a maintained hyperpolarizing potential, but 30 years ago, such a potential was quite unbelievable. The potential, unlike the ubiquitous explosive nerve action potential, was graded in its amplitude and it was like the generator potential, a term which was very popular then. Svaetichin believed that the potential he discovered came from the single receptors, as he indicated in the title of the epoc-making paper. Under the circumstances, his belief was not at all unreasonable and a series of papers was published based on that belief.

In 1957 and 1958, Tomita and his collaborators came up with experimental results which were at variance with Svaetichin's idea that the potential came from single cones. The evidence was: (1) When a bar or a dark stripe was swept across the retinal surface, the effects of passing shadow or light were so small that they could hardly be detected; and (2) two electrodes whose tips were separated by more than 100 μm recorded potentials which were essentially similar. This set of evidence showed, argued Tomita [4], that the potential could not come from cones and that the potential had its main source in a layer proximal to the receptors. Tomita and his collaborators [5] argued that the potential must come from the second order neurons which integrated activities of a number of receptors. They suggested that the potential was recorded from a compartment which was isolated electrically from the rest of the neurons in the retina. To circumvent the problem associated with its (morphological) origin, a proposal was made to refer to the potential as the S-potential: it is not at all clear whether S stood for Svaetichin, the discoverer of the potential, or for so-called slow potential [6]. The most direct approach to solve the origin of the potential was to mark, by means of dye, the location of the electrode tip. Attempts were made by a number of authors [6–9]. These earlier results showed that the potential came from the horizontal cell layer which, according to Svaetichin and his associates were glia-like [10]. Elaborate schemes of "control" among the retinal neurons were proposed. Their views, however, did not receive universal recognition and have faded from the memory of those who study the horizontal cells. We had to wait until the arrival of more satisfactory Procion dye to reach a definitive view on the origin of the S-potential. Kaneko [11] used the dye to show that the potential indeed came from the horizontal cell and from its axon, which was known as the internal horizontal cell [12]. More detailed studies have since been conducted using the dye by Saito et al [13] in the turtle retina and by Mitarai et al [14] in the carp retina.

In addition to its origin, there are two more questions about the potential: (1) How such a potential is generated? Or, what are the ionic mechanisms responsible for its generation?; and (2) What is the functional role of the potential? Or, does it have anything to do with vision? We are not qualified to deal with the first question. In what follows, we will present our views on the second question.

EARLIER VIEWS ON THE ROLE OF S-POTENTIAL

The most striking feature of the potential was its "area effect;" the potential's amplitude became larger as the stimulated area on the retina was made larger. Somehow the structure responsible for the generation of the potential behaved as if it gathered signals over a large area, and the early authors referred to it as the "area effect" [5,9,15,16]. Gouras [9] saw that such a summation of potential could occur over an area as large as 8 mm in diameter.

On the other hand, evidence had accumulated in the late 1950s, mainly from psychophysical experiments, to suggest that there was a signal which controlled the sensitivity of a large number of receptors or rods. Rushton [17] coined a phrase "excitation pool" to indicate the source of such a signal. According to the evidence then available, the excitation pool had to be somewhere proximal to the receptor layer, probably in the inner nuclear layer, and it had to integrate signals from a large number of receptors. The notion of excitation pool seemed to have found its physical counterpart in the compartment which generated S-potential. It was common consensus that the potential did not participate in the direct transmission of visual signals, for these large cells would smudge all spatial detail of the images cast on the retina. Rushton [18] suggested that in some way the potential must act to modify transmission of signals from photoreceptors to the optic nerve. The effect of this suggestion is still with us: For example, the bipolar cells could be "sensitized" or "desensitized" by the horizontal cells [19].

The horizontal cells, however, were generally believed to regulate the sensitivity during adaptation, and there were two ways in which this role could be played. The two possibilities were closely related to the two aspects of adaptation, the field and bleaching adaptations [20]. In the field adaptation, the S-potential could be instrumental in raising the incremental threshold according to the steady background light. This could be done, Rushton [20] proposed, in such a manner that signals in the excitation (or summation) pool controlled (through feedback) its own sensitivity to account for the elevation of the threshold. Obviously the excitation pool was the lamina (the S-space) formed by the horizontal cells. In catfish we argued that the incremental sensitivity was simply the local slope of the Michaelis–Menten equation and that there was no need to propose a specialized mechanism such as a parametric feedback to account for the increase in the threshold in field adaptation. The other possibility was the cell's role in bleaching adaptation. In the early 1960s a view was proposed that the increase in sensitivity during bleaching adaptation was due to a decrease in the "dark light" [21] and the S-space, a lamina formed by the horizontal cells, provided a physical realization of the hypothetical screen on which the real and imaginary dark lights were mixed together. If this were the case, the dark potential of the horizontal cell should reflect the progress of dark adaptation. Experiments performed to establish this relationship failed in tench and carp [22]. A similar conclusion was reached in skate [23]. During bleaching adaptation, sensitivity was already scaled before the signals were fed into the horizontal cells. As the receptors were the only cells which were distal to the horizontal cells, the receptors themselves had to be the site of bleaching adaptation.

Werblin and Dowling [24] were the first to suggest that the horizontal cell might provide the surround of bipolar cells' concentric receptive field, possibly by turning off the cells' response to the central illumination. Their view was complicated by their own observation that the presence of the surround illumination, which presumably acted through the horizontal cells, caused a lateral shift of the bipolar cell's V-log I curve. In their view, the horizontal cells either multiplied or divided the bipolar cell's response.

In 1969 Maksimova [25] published her initial results on extrinsic current injected into the horizontal cells to evoke discharges from the ganglion cells. Her observation rejected beyond any doubt the idea that the S-potential was generated by a glia-like element and that the potential did not play a direct role in information transmission in the retina. During the last 10 years we have expanded upon her pioneering effort and we have, in the catfish retina, a fairly good idea about the role played by the horizontal cells.

INPUT–OUTPUT RELATIONSHIP OF S-POTENTIAL

Naka and Rushton [26] noted that the relationship between the intensity of illumination, I, and the amplitude of the resulting response, V, could be expressed by the following equation:

$$V/V_{max} = I/(I + I_{1/2}) \qquad (1)$$

where V_{max} is the amplitude of the response evoked by a very bright light (the greatest possible potential excursion or the potential's ceiling) and $I_{1/2}$ is a constant to give $V = V_{max}/2$ at $I = I_{1/2}$. This relationship was also shown to hold for the responses from single cones by Baylor and Fuortes [27] and was referred to as the Michaelis–Menten relationship by Baylor and Hodgkin [28], who proposed a mechanistic model to produce the relationship. During the last 15 years the relationship has been used to characterize the input–output relation of the responses from the receptors and horizontal cells in numerous retinas and under various conditions. There are, however, two conditions to be met for this relationship to hold:

(1) The response must be generated by signals from a single class of pigments. If a response is generated by signals from more than one class of pigments, the V-log I curve becomes very complex and is no longer represented by Eq. 1. Such a curve could be decomposed into individual Michaelis–Menten curves under some condition [29]. It is possible that the response generated by a multipigment system produced a relationship which is approximated by the following equation:

$$V/V_{max} = I^n/(I^n + I_{1/2}) \qquad (2)$$

This was the relationship which some authors found to give a better fit to their data [30].

(2) The response must be constant-gain low-pass. Equation 1 applies only to a system which produces a step response to a step input. For the equation to hold, a cell must respond to the DC component of the input signal. In the past the equation has often been applied to a response with a large initial transient

peak and has been used to define sensitivity of a system which did not produce a DC response. The absolute (or DC) sensitivity was often confused with the incremental (or AC) sensitivity [31].

If a response is generated by a single class of pigment, the V-log I curves generated by stimuli of various wavelengths are identical in their shapes but are displaced along the log I axis according to the spectral absorption of the pigment. Naka and Rushton [26] referred to such a curve as the template. In Eq. 1, the term $I_{1/2}$ determines the position of the curve on the log I axis. If we observe the positions of templates for each wavelength, the values of positions give the spectral sensitivity curve of the pigment. Conversely, if the templates obtained with lights of various wavelengths could be fitted by Eq. 1, the templates must be generated by signals from a single class of pigments. The template moves laterally along the log-I axis during bleaching adaptation [22], ie, $I_{1/2}$ is also a measure of (absolute) sensitivity. Therefore, a man who monitors only the horizontal cell's potential cannot discriminate whether a lateral shift of a template was due to an increase in the sensitivity or to changes in the spectral composition of light stimulus [23].

AREA EFFECT

In the late 1950s it became apparent that the amplitude of the S-potential was dependent upon the size of the retinal area illuminated, and this was referred to as the area effect [6,9,15]. This area dependency of the potential's amplitude was one of the prime arguments against Svaetichin's original notion that it came from single receptors.

To account for this striking observation, Naka and Rushton [32] advanced a notion of the S-space in which S-potentials propagated freely toward all directions. The S-space was a large flat-cell or a lamina formed by a layer of horizontal cells which were coupled together through a passage of low electrical resistance. In the simplest form, the S-space was a thin, flat layer bounded by two parallel (high resistance) rubber membranes which acted as an insulator. Ten years before we advanced the idea of electrically isolated S-space, Tomita and his collaborators had written, "The recordings (of S-potentials) were made from within some kind of compartments isolated electrically from each other" [5].

It was a relatively simple task to advance a formal model of the S-space. The first version was made by Naka and Rushton [32], and was followed by a more elaborate one by Marmarelis and Naka [33]. Similar ideas of a space formed by electrically coupled cells have been applied to horizontal cells and receptors in other retinas and have become a standard notion in the retinal physiology. Hashimoto et al [34] used a modification of Marmarelis and Naka's equation [33] to describe the spread of potentials in the carp horizontal cells.

Kaneko [35] employed a more direct approach to the problem: He used double electrodes whose tips were separated by a known distance. The electrodes were inserted into the S-space and current was injected through one of them, and the resulting potential changes were recorded from the other. A similar experiment was performed in the catfish retina. In this case two electrodes were inserted into an S-space independently. This was accomplished by putting one of the electrodes into an S-space and injecting current pulses through the electrode. The second electrode was inserted into such a position that the large potential changes due to the current pulses were recorded. As long as the second electrode was not in the same S-space, potential changes were very small, and as soon as it was in the space, large potential changes were registered.

Here we injected white-noise modulated current which had a flat power spectrum from near DC to 100 Hz. We measured the transfer gain and phase shift between the input (injected current) and output (potential change). As shown in Figure 1, the transfer amplitude was flat from near DC to 100 Hz, and there was no phase shift in the frequency range. This was true for current injected from either one of the two electrodes. Two arbitrary points in the S-space were connected by a low resistance passage. As the highest temporal frequency of the S-potential produced by the light stimulus did not go beyond 30 Hz, the S-space was a pure resistive network for any perturbation caused by light stimulus [36].

FUNCTIONAL ROLE OF HORIZONTAL CELLS

In catfish, the horizontal cell soma has threefold functions: (1) to provide the bipolar cells an integrating (or global) signal; (2) to feed its potential back to the receptors to improve their frequency response; and (3) to communicate signals, including the DC components, to the axons. The axons, in turn, communicate with the elements in the inner synaptic layer. In what follows we will advance our arguments for the proposed functions of the horizontal cell soma and axon.

(1) Horizontal cell soma provides the bipolar cells' receptive field surround. There are two sets of direct evidence in favor of this thesis. First, receptive fields of bipolar cells' could be synthesized from those of receptors and horizontal cells. This was shown by Davis and Naka [37] by the use of traveling random grating and cross-correlation technique. They showed that bipolar cells' receptive field could be produced by a simple addition (after proper scaling) of the fields formed by the two distal cells: The polarity of one of the fields was reversed to account for the sign inversion in the transmission. Second, the signal transmission from the horizontal cell soma to the bipolar cells was linear and either sign inverting or noninverting, but was not excitatory or inhibitory. This is shown in Figure 2A. In the experiment, white-noise modulated current was injected into the soma of a horizontal cell and the resulting responses were recorded from a bipolar cell. Input and output signals were cross-correlated to compute the first order kernel (first order correlation). The kernel could predict a bipolar cell's

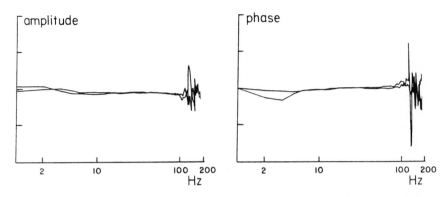

Fig. 1. Transfer function between two points in the S-space. Two electrodes were located in the S-space formed by the horizontal-cell soma. White-noise current which had a flat power spectrum from near DC to 100 Hz was injected into the space through one of the electrodes. Potential changes due to the current spread in the space were monitored by the other electrode. Transfer functions, amplitude and phase, were computed by a Hewlett Packard spectrum anlyzer (Model 3582A). Left plots show the amplitude of the transfer function in 20 dB/div and right plots show the phase of the transfer function of 100°/div. Two curves in each plot were for one of the pairs of the electrodes used for current injection and for monitoring potential changes.

response with a MSE (mean square error) of about 20 to 30%. (If it were 100%, the kernel failed completely to predict a bipolar cell's response; if it were 0%, it predicted the cell's response without any error). The degree of MSE we observed for the neuron chain is expected even for a linear system because of the "noise" in the experiment such as the poor signal-to-noise ratio or the short duration of experiment. It seems reasonable to say that the signal transmission from the soma to bipolar cells was quasi-linear. Results of experiments with step inputs substantiated this conclusion [38].

There are several other indirect evidences to support our thesis that bipolar cells' receptive field surround was formed by signals from horizontal cells. Results from extrinsic current injection into the horizontal cells to evoke ganglion cell discharge were one of them [39].

Taken together, a fairly reasonable case can be advanced in favor of the idea that integrating signals from the horizontal cells were transmitted directly to the bipolar cells.

In other retinas, it is thought that horizontal cells provided the surround of the concentric fields. There are three ways through which the horizontal cell could affect the bipolar čells as pointed out by Rodieck [40]: (a) It could be through the photoreceptors by means of a feedback synapse; (b) the horizontal cell could modulate the signal transmission from receptors to bipolar cells; and (c) the horizontal cell could communicate directly with the bipolar cells. All the evidence from catfish retina favors the case (c).

KERNEL   TIME RECORD

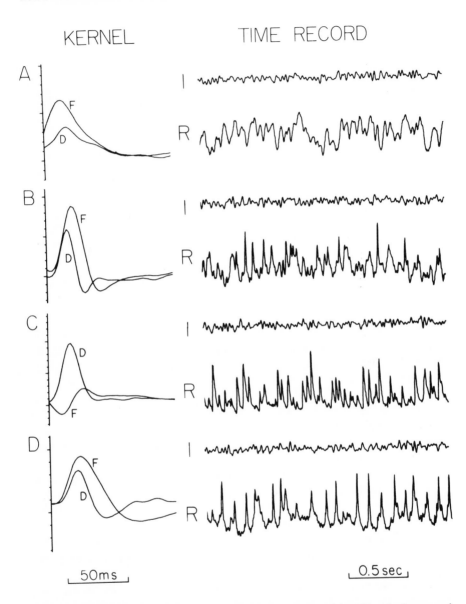

50ms   0.5 sec

Fig. 2. Time records of the responses evoked by white-noise current injected into the S-space and kernels computed from the current injection experiments. In the time record, "I" was the injected current and "R" was the resulting response. Records A, B, C, and D were from the responses recorded from an on-center bipolar cell, type NA cell, type C cell, and an on-center ganglion cell. Records marked "F" were the first order kernels and "D" were the diagonal of the second order kernels.

(2) Horizontal cell soma feeds its potential back to the receptors. A large horizontal cell response (such as the one evoked by a large annulus of light) could follow much faster (temporal) frequency than a small response (such as the one evoked by a small spot of light). The "speeding" up of the response could best be shown by measuring the cell's first order kernel: The peak response time (a measure to indicate how fast a system could follow input signals) of the kernels evoked by a large annulus (or a field) of light were always shorter than that of the kernels evoked by a small spot of light [36]. When the two inputs, a small spot and a large annulus of light, were given simultaneously, the peak response time of the spot-evoked kernels became as short as the one evoked by the annular or field inputs. There are two possible explanations for this observation: Either the soma's response was somehow fed back to the receptors to improve their frequency response characteristics, or the condition which produced larger responses caused some changes in the horizontal cells themselves. The latter possibility was disproved by Lasater's observation to the effect that similar speeding up of the responses was observed in the receptors [41].

Lam et al [42] reported that in the presence of bicuculline, a GABA antagonist, the peak response time of annular-evoked kernels became as long as that of the spot-evoked kernels to suggest that the assumed feedback was blocked by the antagonist. They also showed that, as in other retinas, the horizontal cell soma accumulated GABA in dark. Chemical synapses made by the soma back to the receptors, mostly onto their telodendria, have been observed consistently during the past 10 years (cf. [37]).

These two sets of evidence, one chemical and the other morphological, give credence to the idea of the feedback action. Although experimental evidence is strong, the idea is not so convincing because the synapse's proposed function is very far apart from that of the conventional synapses so far seen in the central nervous system, and the possible mechanism for such a synapse was beyond our comprehension. Our analysis of the feedback synapse by means of modeling showed that such an action was not subtractive because, if it were the case, a concentric receptive field would be seen in the receptors themselves. The feedback must be "zero order" in which the DC level of the horizontal cell controlled it [43].

There are, however, many curious phenomena related to the horizontal cell response. For example, a steep off-response was observed in the tench horizontal cells. The response was a dual function of flash duration and of the state of adaptation. Temporal or spatial contrast of light and darkness was necessary for the appearance of the cut off [44]. In the carp horizontal cells, Usui (personal communication) also noticed a similar complex response pattern. The proposed synapse might provide a mechanism for these curious phenomena.

Extrinsic current injected into the horizontal cells could evoke responses from the cells in the proximal retina, the types C and N and ganglion cells. To identify such signal transmissions, we injected white-noise modulated current into the horizontal cells. We computed the first order kernels and also the diagonal of the second order kernel for the neuron chains. (The latter kernel could be computed in a fraction of time required to compute the whole two-dimensional second order kernel but could still characterize the neuron chains.)

In Figure 2 are shown the kernels ("F" for the first order and "D" for the diagonal cut) and also the time records ("I" for the injected current and "R" for the response) for the on-center bipolar, (Fig. 2A), types NA and C (B and C) and ganglion cells (D). As we have already described, the bipolar cell's time record showed no nonlinear components such as sharp transients or rectification. The cell's second order kernel's diagonal was noisy. Time records from the other three cells had nonlinear features such as depolarizing transients and rectification: These cells produced nonlinear responses. In the type NA and ganglion cells, the amplitude of the second order kernel was comparable, although slightly smaller, to that of the first order kernel, whereas in the type C cell, the first order kernel was much smaller than the second order kernel. In type NA and ganglion cells, their responses had both the linear and nonlinear components and the type C cell's response was dominated by the nonlinear components. Indeed, a step of current injected into the horizontal cells produced an on–off transient depolarization similar to the one evoked by a step of light input [38].

In Figure 3 are shown results from an experiment in which white-noise modulated current was injected into a horizontal cell and the resulting response was recorded from a type NB cell. As in the type NA cell, the type NB cell's time response (RESPONSE in Fig. 3) showed transient depolarizing peaks and rectification. The cell's response was very different from the linear model (LINEAR MODEL in Fig. 3) predicted by the first order kernel alone. The kernel was hyperpolarizing and the second order kernel's diagonal had an initial depolarizing peak as in other proximal cells. We note here that the type NA cell is commonly known as the sustained depolarizing amacrine cell, and the type NB cell as the sustained hyperpolarizing cell. In catfish both cells formed a biphasic receptive field [45]. The polarity of the first order kernel from current injection experiments was that of the center of the cells' biphasic receptive field. In a previous study, we also noted that the type N cell's response to white-noise modulated light stimulus was linear. The light stimulus which was a modulation around a mean intensity had apparently "linearized" the system we studied [46].

Our study has shown that the signal transmission from the horizontal to proximal cells had features characteristic to each (postsynaptic) cell type and the feature was reflected upon the second order kernels. Nonlinear analysis performed on the neuron chains will reveal, in a quantitative fashion, the intricacy of signal processing in the vertebrate retina.

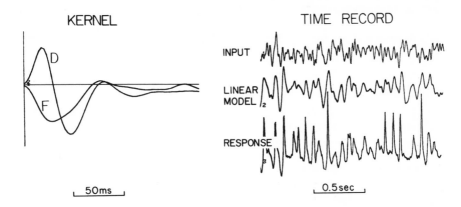

KERNEL

TIME RECORD

INPUT

LINEAR MODEL I_2

RESPONSE

50ms

0.5 sec

Fig. 3.   Time records and kernels from a type NB cell. INPUT was the white-noise current injected into the S-space. LINEAR MODEL was the model response predicted by the first order kernel alone, and RESPONSE was the current evoked response from the type NB cell. Notice the sharp depolarizing transients similar to those seen in the type NA cell of Figure 2. Record "F" was the first order kernel and "D" the diagonal of the second order kernel.

CONCLUSION

In catfish, information processing in the outer retina was essentially linear: receptors, horizontal cells, and bipolar cells formed linear spatiotemporal filters when their responses were evoked by white-noise stimulus [43]. In the distal layer the horizontal cells communicated with both the on- and off-center bipolar cells [38] and, as we have shown in this paper, in the proximal layer horizontal cells communicated with the type C and N cells. Characteristic nonlinearities appeared in the signal transmission from the horizontal cells to the proximal cells.

The function of the S-space which Svaetichin discovered 30 years ago is to provide the integrating or global signal through the S-space: The potential by itself is not excitatory or inhibitory, but is neutral. It is unfortunate that the idea of lateral inhibition is so entrenched in people's mind that the potential is automatically associated with inhibition. This single example illuminates the inherit danger of seeing the neural circuitry in the retina from the conventional point of view which sees the world in the simplistic dichotomy of exitatory and inhibitory synapses. Much more subtle but new approaches have to be taken to appreciate the intricacy of signal processing in catfish retina. Tribute to Gunnar Svaetichin is his willingness to subscribe to bold ideas: They might have been wrong but he stated them clearly.

ACKNOWLEDGMENTS

The authors thank Mr. N. Numata of Rikei Computer Co., and Mr. Y. Ando of the National Institute for Basic Biology for programming assistance.

REFERENCES

1. Svaetichin G: The cone action potential. Acta Physiol Scand 29, Suppl 106:565–600, 1953.
2. Lamb TD, Simon EJ: The relation between intracellular coupling and electrical noise in turtle photoreceptors. J Physiol (London) 263:257–286, 1976.
3. Gold GH: Photoreceptor coupling in retina of the toad, Bufo marinus. II. Physiology. J Neurophysiol 42:311–328, 1979.
4. Tomita T: A study on the origin of intraretinal action potential of the Cyprinid fish by means of pencil-type microelectrode. Japan J Physiol 7:80–85, 1957.
5. Tomita T, Tosaka T, Watanabe K, Sato Y: The fish EIRG in response to different types of illumination. Japan J Physiol 8:41–50, 1958.
6. Tomita T, Murakami M, Sato Y, Hashimoto Y: Further study on the origin of the so-called cone action potential (S-potential): Its histological determination. Japan J Physiol 9:63–68, 1959.
7. MacNichol EF Jr, Macpherson L, Svaetichin G: Studies on spectral response curves from the fish retina. "Symposium on Visual Problems of Color No. 39." Teddington, England, 536–571, 1957.
8. Mitarai G: Determination of ultramicroelectrode tip position in the retina in relation to S-potential. J Gen Physiol 43:95–99, 1960.
9. Gouras P: Graded potentials of bream retina. J Physiol (London) 152:487–505, 1960.
10. Svaetichin G, Laufer M, Mitarai G, Fatechand R, Vallecalle E, Villegas J: Glial control of neuronal networks and receptors. In Jung R, Kornhuber H (eds): "The Visual System: Neurophysiology and Psychophysics." Berlin: Springer–Verlag, pp 445–456, 1961.
11. Kaneko A: Physiological and morphological identification of horizontal, bipolar and amacrine cells in goldfish retina. J Physiol (London) 207:623–633, 1970.
12. Cajal Ramòn y S: "The Structure of the Retina." Translated by Thorpe SA, Glickstein M, Springfield: C. C. Thomas, 1972.
13. Saito T, Miller WH, Tomita T: C- and L-type horizontal cells in the turtle retina. Vision Res 14:119–123, 1974.
14. Mitarai G, Asano T, Miyake Y: Identification of five types of S-potentials and their corresponding generating sites in the horizontal cells of the carp retina. Japan J Ophthal 18:161–176, 1974.
15. Oikawa T, Ogawa T, Motokawa K: Origin of so-called cone action potential. J Neurophysiol 22:102–111, 1959.
16. Tasaki K: Some observations on the retinal potentials of the fish. Arch Ital Biol 98:81–91, 1960.
17. Rushton WAH: The excitation pools in the frog's retina. J Physiol (London) 149:327–345, 1959.
18. Rushton WAH: The retinal organization of vision in vertebrates. Symp Soc Exp Biol 16:12–31, 1962.
19. Werblin FS: Control of retinal sensitivity. II. Lateral interactions at the outer plexiform layer. J Gen Physiol 63:62–87, 1974.
20. Rushton WAH: The Ferrier Lecture, 1962; Visual Adaptation. Proc Roy Soc B 162:20–46, 1965.
21. Barlow HB, Sparrock JMB: The role of afterimages in dark adaptation. Science 120:401–405, 1965.

22. Naka K-I, Rushton WAH: S-potential and dark adaptation. J Physiol (London) 194:259–269, 1968.
23. Dowling JE, Ripps H: S-potentials in the skate retina. Intracellular recordings during light and dark adaptation. J Gen Physiol 58:163–189, 1971.
24. Werblin FS, Dowling JE: Organization of the retina of mudpuppy, Necturus maculosus. II. Intracellular recording. J Neurophysiol 32:339–355, 1969.
25. Maksimova YM: Effect of intracellular polarization of horizontal cells on the activity of the ganglionic cells of the retina of fish. Biofizika 14:537–544, 1969.
26. Naka K-I, Rushton WAH: S-potential from colour units in the retina of fish (Cyprinidae). J Physiol (London) 185:536–555, 1966.
27. Baylor DA, Fuortes MGF: Electrical responses of single cones in the retina of the turtle. J Physiol (London) 207:77–92, 1970.
28. Baylor DA, Hodgkin AL: Changes in time scale and sensitivity in turtle photoreceptors. J Physiol (London) 242:729–758, 1974.
29. Naka K-I, Rushton WAH: S-potential from luminosity units in the retina of fish (Cyprinidae). J Physiol (London) 185:587–599, 1966.
30. Boynton RM, Whitten DN: Visual adaptation in monkey cones: Recording of later receptor potentials. Science 170:1423–1427, 1970.
31. Naka K-I, Chan RY, Yasui S: Adaptation in catfish retina. J Neurophysiol 42:441–454, 1979.
32. Naka K-I, Rushton WAH: The generation and spread of S-potentials in fish (Cyprinidae). J Physiol (London) 192:437–461, 1967.
33. Marmarelis PZ, Naka K-I: Spatial distribution of potential in a flat cell: Application to the catfish horizontal cell layers. Biophys J 12:1515–1532, 1972.
34. Hashimoto Y, Kato A, Inokuchi M, Watanabe K: Re-examination of horizontal cells in the carp retina with procion-yellow electrode. Vision Res 16:25–29, 1976.
35. Kaneko A: Electrical connexions between horizontal cells in the dogfish retina. J Physiol (London) 213:95–105, 1971.
36. Marmarelis PZ, Naka K-I: Nonlinear analysis and synthesis of receptive field responses in the catfish retina. III. Two input white-noise analysis. J Neurophysiol 36:634–648, 1973.
37. Davis GW, Naka K-I: Synaptic communication in the catfish outer plexiform layer: Structure and function. In Pinsker H, Willis WD (eds): "Information Processing in the Nervous System: Communication among Neurons and Neuroscientists." Raven Press, pp 221–240, 1980.
38. Naka K-I: The cells horizontal cells talk to. Vision Res, in press.
39. Naka K-I, Nye PW: Role of horizontal cells in the organization of the catfish retinal receptive field. J Neurophysiol 34:785–801, 1971.
40. Rodieck RW: "The Vertebrate Retina." San Francisco: WH Freeman, 1973.
41. Lasater EM: Physiological and Pharmacological Studies of the Spatiotemporal Receptive Fields of Vertebrate Retinal Neurons." Galveston, Texas: Thesis, University of Texas Medical Branch at Galveston, 1980.
42. Lam DM-K, Lasater EM, Naka K-I: Gamma-aminobutyric acid: A neurotransmitter candidate for cone horizontal cells of the catfish retina. Proc Nat Acad Sci 75:6310–6313, 1978.
43. Krausz HI, Naka K-I: Spatio Temporal testing and modelling of catfish retinal neurons. Biophys J 29:13–36, 1980.
44. Naka K-I: Factors influencing the time course of S-potentials resulting from brief flashes. J Physiol (London) 200:373–385, 1969.
45. Davis GW, Naka K-I: Spatial organization of catfish retinal neurons: I. Single- and random bar stimulation. J Neurophysiol 43:807–831, 1980.
46. Naka K-I, Marmarelis PZ, Chan RY: Morphological and functional identification of catfish retinal neurons. III. Functional identification. J Neurophysiol 38:92–131, 1975.

The S-Potential, pages 207–233
© 1982 Alan R. Liss, Inc., 150 Fifth Avenue, New York, NY 10011

Mammalian Horizontal Cells: Spatial and Temporal Transfer Properties

Otto-Joachim Grüsser

HISTORICAL REMARKS ON THE DISCOVERY OF CAT HORIZONTAL CELL POTENTIALS

The first intracellular microelectrode recordings from horizontal cells in the mammalian retina were performed simultaneously in Motokawa's laboratory in Sendai, by Brown and Wiesel in San Francisco and in our Freiburg laboratory [1–5]. As is frequently the case in science, our discovery was by chance, with systematic studies following. My interpretation of the first data was erroneous, but the data themselves were repeatedly confirmed in later studies. Originally I believed the sources of horizontal cell potentials to be cones and, therefore, called these potentials "Rezeptorpotentiale" or R-potentials [2, 6–8].

After finishing my doctoral thesis on the flicker responses of the cat retina and visual cortex neurons [9], I proceeded with intraretinal recordings of retinal ganglion cell action potentials late in 1956 and 1957, studying the response of on-center and off-center ganglion cells to short flashes of different frequencies or to squarewave flicker stimuli [10–13].

On the advice of J. Lehmann (now at the University of Essen), we had improved our microelectrode pulling technique (by hand) and were able to produce glass micropipettes with a tip diameter far below the resolution limits of the light microscope. These electrodes were filled with 3-M-KCl solution and were thin enough to allow intracellular recordings. Thus, in recording from the ganglion cell layer of the cat retina, we occasionally obtained intracellular recordings from ganglion cells. Due to the pulsation of the retina (open eye preparation, Fig. 1a), however, the membrane potential in most penetrations deteriorated very rapidly. Now and then, I unintentionally moved the microelectrode tip deeper into the retina beyond the ganglion cell layer and recorded large slow "bumps" synchronized with the flashes. Having become curious about these signals, I used two parallel DC amplifiers of different amplifications plus a long-time constant AC amplifier in some experiments. To my surprise, I saw that

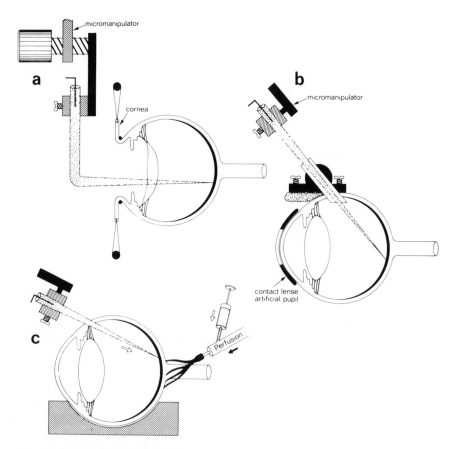

Fig. 1. (a) Schematic drawing of open eye in vivo recording technique with intraretinal microelectrodes applied in the experiments 1956/1957. (b) Schematic drawing of intraretinal recordings with microelectrodes from the cat eye with intact dioptric apparatus and a contact lens with artificial pupil. (c) Schematic drawing of the isolated perfused eye recording technique (from Ref. [45] modified).

these potentials recorded from the inner retinal layers were hyperpolarizing signals superimposed on a rather low membrane potential of −15 to −40 mV. The hyperpolarization varied between −3 and −25 mV and was dependent on the stimulus luminance (Fig. 2). Being interested in flicker phenomena, I applied squarewave flicker stimuli of different frequencies and found that at photopic stimulus intensities—white light from a tungsten filament bulb leading to about 500-Lux stimulus intensity at the retina—the hyperpolarizing potentials showed a pronounced flicker response, continuing up to at least 75 Hz. Relying on the

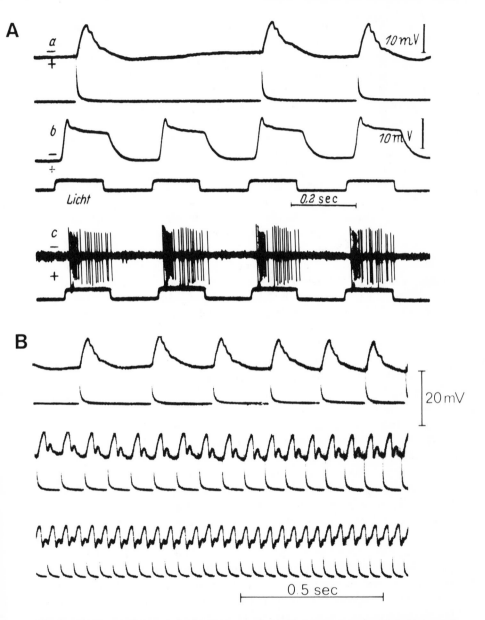

Fig. 2. (A) H-potentials recorded from the cat retina (a,b); responses to short light flashes and to squarewave flicker stimuli of about 500-Lux stimulus intensity; large field stimulation. In comparison to the H-cell potentials (then believed to be "receptor potentials"), the responses of an intraretinally recorded on-center ganglion cell are shown from the same preparation (c). Membrane potential hyperpolarization upwards, opposite to the recordings shown in the other figures (from Ref [2]). (B) Response of H-cell potential to flash series. Note the double peaks in the H-unit responses (from Ref [3]).

results of psychophysical studies and the electroretinographic findings with flicker stimuli [14–16], I concluded that these fast flickering hyperpolarizing potentials must be the result of cone excitation, because rods were (and still are) believed to have a maximum flicker fusion at about 25–28 flashes · sec⁻¹.

On reading the papers of Gunnar Svaetichin [17–21] in which he described the discovery of "cone potentials" in the fish retina, I found that there was a striking parallel between the properties of these cone potentials in the fish and our data from cats: the relatively low membrane potential in darkness, the logarithmic relationship between stimulus intensity and hyperpolarization by light (Fig. 11), the fast initial hyperpolarization, the instantaneous adaptation to a steady state hyperpolarizing plateau, and the difference in the time course of the on- and off-response (Fig. 3). We bought chromatic interference filters and our laboratory engineer H. Kapp built a "Svaetichin wheel" [22] on which the filters were mounted. Being an admirer of Ewald Hering and his "Gegenfarbentheorie," I hoped to find, as Svaetichin (cf also [22a]) had in the fish retina, antagonistic responses of the "cone potentials" to different chromatic stimuli (yellow–blue potentials or green–red potentials). The application of these chromatic stimuli was disappointing, however. All H-potentials responded to light from the whole visible spectrum with a hyperpolarization exhibiting a maximum estimated at around 550–560 nm. This maximum corresponded to that of Granit's dominator curve for the cat retina [16, 23]. During these first chromatic experiments, we had no instruments available to calibrate the stimulus energy. Thus I measured my own flicker fusion frequency for equal area chromatic stimuli to "calibrate" our stimuli. This method only led, of course, to a crude estimate of the spectral sensitivity of the hyperpolarizing R-potentials.

The method to locate the electrode tip position was also not very satisfactory. I measured the distance between the membrana limitans interna, the penetration of which was signaled by a DC shift of −5 to −10 mV and the depths of the H-potential recordings. Comparing these measurements with histological slides of the cat retina, I concluded that the recordings were from the inner part of the receptor layer, in particular, from the synaptic layer between receptors and bipolar cells. Because displacement of the microelectrode tip by 1–3 μm led, as a rule, to the disappearance of the resting membrane potential and a reduction in the "receptor" potential to 3–8% of the intracellular value, I thought that the microelectrode tip might be situated in a very tiny structure, perhaps the synaptic contacts between receptors, bipolars, and horizontal cells. In addition, I tried to locate the hyperpolarizing potentials by another experiment: The central retinal arteries were coagulated at the papilla nervi optici. 15 min later no action potentials from the ganglion cell layer could be recorded, whereas typical "receptor potentials" were still present. Erroneously, I concluded that this finding might be taken as proof that receptors are the source of these potentials, because it was known from the work of Noell [24] that after coagulation of the central retinal

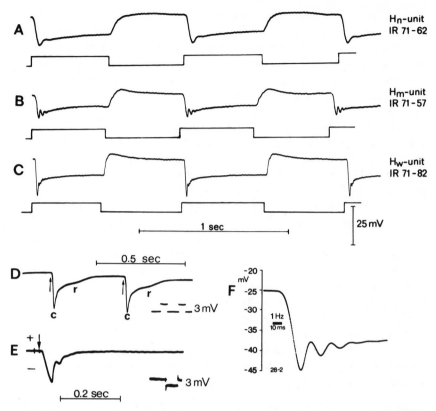

Fig. 3. Response of three different types of H-units in the light-adapted cat retina (A–C). Square-wave modulation of stimulus luminance; 15° × 15° stimulus area. H_n-unit: $L_0 = 200$ cd/m², m = 0.9. H_m-unit: $L_0 = 190$ cd/m², m = 0.72. H_w-unit: $L_0 = 190$ cd/m², m = 0.8. (D) Responses of an H_m-unit to a short (1-msec) light flash. The presumed cone response is marked "c," the presumed rod response "r." (E) Flash response of an H-unit lacking the rod response. (F) Average responses of an H_m-unit to 10 squarewave, 1 per second, photopic light stimuli. Note the oscillatory potentials. A–C from [37], D from [8], E from [72], F from Grehn and Stange unpublished measurements, 1976.

arteries, all retinal cell layers except those of rods, cones, and pigment cells degenerate. Evidently, the horizontal cells in the region around the area centralis still respond to light (at least temporarily) when the blood flow in the central retinal arteries is interrupted and supply is only provided via the choroidal vessel system. This localization of R-potentials, however, was not in accordance with one curious finding which I did not mention in the publication: Short flashes in a frequency range somewhat below the flicker fusion frequency led now and then to a 1:2 response of the units. The amplitude of every second response was relatively high, that of the responses in between, low. Such a response pattern was difficult to interpret as originating in a single receptor cell and pointed toward an interaction on the part of different receptors. This argument was also supported by the incidental finding that short flashes led in some of the units to a double response after each flash, which could be easily explained by the assumption that two different receptor signals with different latency properties interact (Fig. 2b).

Within a few years it became evident that the "cone potentials" or "S-potentials" of the fish are horizontal cell responses [25]. The careful study by Steinberg and Schmidt [26], applying intracellular staining techniques, proved that the "R-potentials" of the cat retina also originated in horizontal cells. We call these potentials therefore "H-potentials." Steinberg [27–30] performed extensive studies on the chromatic response properties of H-potentials and the rod/cone interaction in horizontal cells. His work was extended by Nelson and co-workers [31–33], who demonstrated that the morphologically different types of cat horizontal cells are the source of different H-potentials, which have in part different chromatic response properties.

Toward the end of 1957 I discontinued the intraretinal recordings, and it was not until 10 years later in our Berlin laboratory that we began to study the responses of H-potentials evoked by sinewave flicker stimuli (1967 together with H.-U. Lunkenheimer and 1970/1971 with M. Foerster and W.A. van de Grind). The latter work extended our knowledge of the spatial and temporal frequency response properties of cat H-potentials. These more recent data will be the main subject of the present report.

THREE METHODS TO RECORD HORIZONTAL CELL POTENTIALS FROM THE CAT RETINA

In our early Freiburg experiments (1956/1957) the head of the anesthetized and immobilized cat was fixed in a simple stereotaxic instrument in a horizontal position. Only one eye was used, its cornea being cut horizontally and along the limbus and fixed with thin strings to the headholder. The lens was removed and the lens capsule covering the vitreous body was opened with a small vertical slit. A glass micropipette was advanced horizontally under direct visual control through the vitreous body (Fig. 1a). The mechanical contact of the microelectrode tip with the inner surface of the retinal layer could be seen on the oscilloscope by the appearance of oscillatory potentials followed by a DC shift of -5 to -10 mV; the depth of the microelectrode tip was read off from this "landmark." An Eccles-micromanipulator built by H. Kapp was used. It allowed a movement precision of about 2 μm. Light was projected onto the central retina parallel to the microelectrode. Pulsation of the retina was a hindrance for stable intracellular recordings, which lasted at best about 20 min. Reliable measurements of the receptive field sizes were not possible with this technique.

In the Berlin experiments [34–38] we applied a recording technique which preserved the optics of the eye [5] (Fig. 1b). The head of the anesthetized and immobilized cat was fixed in a stereotaxic apparatus. The upper eyelid, conjunctiva, orbital fascia, and osseous part of the upper orbita were removed on the left side to expose the upper quarter of the left bulbus oculi. A double plate with a central balljoint socket was fastened to the frontal bone by means of a dental acrylic bridge. The metal balljoint was perforated to hold a trocar; this joint could be fixed by tightening four screws on the corner of the double plate. The entrance angle of the micropipette could thus be altered during the experiments by changing the position of the balljoint (Fig. 1b). With the aid of a metal rod, in the place of the microelectrode initially, the central axis of the micromanipulator system and the trocar were aligned before the microelectrode was moved into the eye through the trocar. The position of the microelectrode within the eye was controlled by an ophthalmoscope. The microelectrodes were advanced via the trocar by a stepmotor-driven hydraulic microdrive. Molenaar and van de Grind [39] have further developed this method into a sophisticated technique by which intraretinal recordings and precise stereotaxic adjustment of the microelectrode for recordings from a large range of the cat retina are possible.

As with the "open eye method," all our recordings were obtained in the region of the area centralis and about 15° around it. The optics of the eye (dilated pupil) were improved by a corneal contact lens with a vertical artificial oval pupil of 3 × 6 mm in size. The tangent screen onto which the stimuli were projected, placed at a distance of 180 cm from the eye, was brought into focus with spectacle lenses. With this improved recording technique, area functions and the extension of the receptive field (RF) of individual H-units were measurable.

A further technical improvement in recording from mammalian horizontal cells was the development of the isolated and perfused mammalian eye preparation [32, 40–44]. This preparation has the advantage of eliminating pulsation movement artifacts, because the oxygenized plasma flows continuously through the retina. Niemeyer [45] recently demonstrated by light microscopic and electronmicroscopic studies that no morphological signs of serious disturbance in retinal metabolism can be found in such a preparation (Fig. 1c).

THREE DISTINCT TYPES OF CAT HORIZONTAL CELL RESPONSES TO ACHROMATIC FLICKER STIMULI

On the basis of the critical flicker frequency (CFF)—defined as the frequency at which the H-potentials disappear into the noise of the recording—the H-cell responses to large (15° × 15°) high modulation (m = 0.6–0.9), photopic (average stimulus luminance L_0 = 140–200 cd · m^{-2}), sinewave or squarewave flicker stimuli could be grouped unequivocally into three distinct classes:

H_n-units had a CFF of 25–40 Hz; H_m-units 55–70 Hz; H_w-units 95–110Hz. These three classes of H-potentials recorded from cat eyes with an intact optic system (method Fig. 1b) had altogether the following properties:

(a) They were all recorded near the margin between the inner nuclear and outer plexiform layer (depth estimation according to [5]).

(b) They never discharged action potentials.

(c) A stable membrane potential of -25 to -50 mV was found with a background luminance level of approximately 0.1 cd $\cdot$ m^{-2}.

(d) A well-defined receptive field (RF) was found covering an area of at least 2–4° in diameter with no antagonistic surround, as in bipolar cells (Necturus retina [46, 47]; fish retina [48]; cat retina [49]).

(e) In all three classes of H-potentials, the increase in hyperpolarization to a step-up in luminance was considerably faster than the decrease in hyperpolarization by an equal darkening (Fig. 3). Therefore, the responses to high modulation slow sinewave stimuli showed the anticipated nonlinear waveform distortions (Figs. 4, 5).

(f) The "overswing" of the hyperpolarization in the on-response was present in all three classes, but the oscillatory responses during this overswing were faster in H_m and H_w-units than in H_n-units.

(g) H_n-units and H_m-units were recorded throughout the entire central retina, whereas H_w-units were only recorded at or near the center of the area centralis.

THE DYNAMIC RESPONSES OF H-UNITS

(a) The risetime of H_n-potentials was slow and contained few oscillatory components, if at all, in the responses to squarewave light stimuli (Fig. 3). With squarewave or sinewave photopic flicker stimuli, H_n-units reached a response maximum at about 1.5–2 Hz (Fig. 5). The amplitude attenuated slowly with a slope of about -3dB/octave when the flicker frequency f_s increased up to a frequency of about 15 Hz. Above this corner frequency, a maximal attenuation of about -18 dB/octave was found for the sinewave flicker responses. The phase angle φ between the sinewave stimuli and the H_n-unit response depended on stimulus frequency f_s according to the following equation:

$$\varphi = \Delta t \; 2\pi f_s \; \text{[degrees]} \tag{1}$$

Δt is a constant delay and amounts to about 40 msec in H_n-units.

Due to the low CFF and the strong response attenuation above 15 Hz, we presume that H_n-units have a dominant rod input. From the work of Steinberg [27, 28], Niemeyer and Gouras [44], Niemeyer [40], and Nelson [33], it is known that some H-units in the cat retina are dominated by a rod input and have a spectral sensitivity curve with a peak sensitivity at about 505 nm. It is, of course, tempting to correlate these rod-dominant H-potentials with the axonal arborization seen in some of the H-cells of the cat retina (Fig. 6).

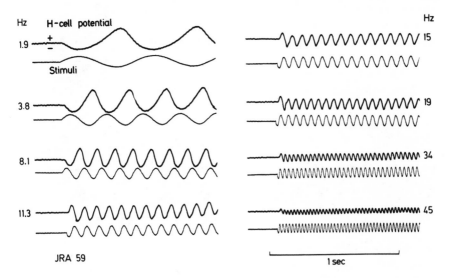

Fig. 4. H_m-unit response to a sinusoidal flicker stimulus. Stimulus parameters as indicated. The upper tracing of each pair is the H_m-potential, the lower tracing is the signal from a photocell monitoring the light stimulus. Note the distortion of the H_m-potential in the low frequency range. Hyperpolarization is recorded in the downward direction (from Ref [38]).

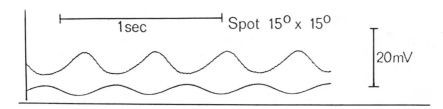

Fig. 5. H_n-unit responses to sinusoidal stimuli of 2.4 Hz. L_0 about 180 cd/m², m = 0.8; stimulus size 14 × 14 degrees centered to the RF-center (from [71]).

(b) A typical flicker response of an H_m-unit is shown in Figure 4: At low stimulus frequencies (< 5 Hz), nonlinear components in the responses are visible. The hyperpolarization phase caused by the increase in stimulus luminance was faster and lasted for a shorter period of time than the depolarizing phase caused by light dimming. This response asymmetry slowly disappeared at stimulus frequencies above 7–10 Hz, but in some responses a kink suggesting the su-

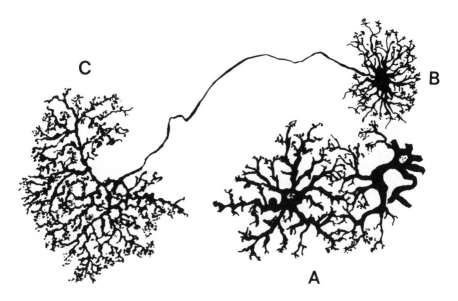

Fig. 6. Two types of horizontal cells found in the cat retina. Schematic drawing after morphological studies [53, 54, 56–59]. (A) two (one incomplete) A-cells without axon, (B) cell soma of B-cell. (C) axonal terminal arborization of B-cell. A possible correlation between histology and physiology is: A = H_m-units, B = H_w-units, C = H_n-units.

perposition of two components with different delays appeared at frequencies between 12 and 20 Hz. The amplitude and phase response characteristics (Bode-plots) of an H_m-unit are shown in Figures 7A and B. At photopic stimulus conditions the response maximum was reached in a frequency range between 1 and 4 Hz. Above this frequency the amplitude was diminished at − 3 dB/octave up to a corner frequency of about 40 Hz. Above this value a strong attenuation with about − 36 dB/octave characterized the Bode-plot. Some H_m-potentials exhibited a second maximum at frequencies between 30 and 45 Hz. The second resonance peak corresponded well to the frequency of the oscillatory potentials seen in the squarewave responses (Fig. 3). For the phase angle φ between stimulus and response, Eq (1) was also valid, but the constant delay Δt was about 25–30 msec.

The amplitude response characteristics expressed by the Bode plots depended on stimulus intensity and size. For very small-field photopic or large-field scotopic sinewave stimuli, the Bode plots of H_m-units were very similar to those described for H_n-units with large fields and high intensity stimulation. The flicker fusion frequency under upper scotopic or mesopic stimulus conditions ($L_0 < 0.1$ cd $\cdot$ m^{-2}) corresponded to that known for mammalian rods [16, 50].

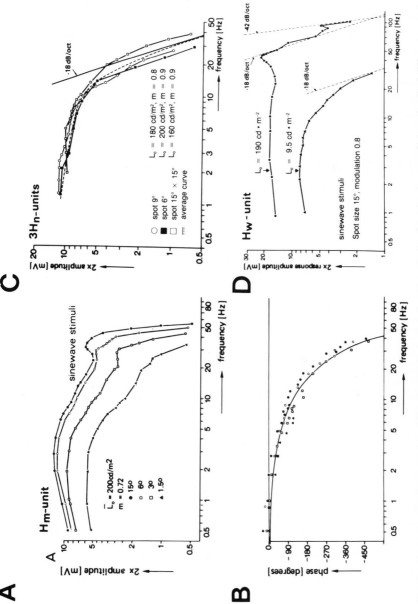

Fig. 7. Frequency transfer properties of H-units. (A) Bode plot of an H_m-unit stimulated by sinewave flicker stimuli of different areas (as indicated). (B) Phase relationship of the responses of the same H_m-unit. The curved line was computed according to eq (7). (C) Bode plots of three H_n-units stimulated with flicker stimuli of two different L_0-values, as indicated (from [37, 38]).

(c) Figure 8 illustrates recording examples of H_w-unit responses to squarewave flicker stimulation. This response was significantly different from the flicker responses obtained in H_m-units. The amplitude response characteristics of H_w-units are shown in Figure 7D. Their Bode-plots exhibited two response peaks obtained in a frequency range in which only cones respond to flicker stimuli. The lower peak was at 40–45 Hz, the higher at 90–95 Hz. These peaks were also visible with a fast frequency sweep (Fig. 9). When the average luminance L_0 of large-area flicker stimuli was reduced to lower mesopic levels, the Bode-plots of H_w-units, as those for H_m-units, again resembled the rod-dominated H_n-response characteristics.

SYSTEM ANALYSIS APPLIED TO H-POTENTIALS

The Fourier description of a periodic function F (x) can be written as

$$F(x) = C_0 + C_1 \sin (x + \psi_1) + C_2 \sin (2x + \psi_2) + \ldots + C_n \sin (nx + \psi_n) \quad (2)$$

where C_i and ψ_i represent the amplitude and phase of the ith harmonic components. In our case x is the stimulus frequency $\omega = 2\pi f_s$. The contribution of a given ith harmonic to the non-linear response of a system described by Eq (2) is usually specified by the distortion coefficient d_i defined as:

$$d_i = \frac{C_i}{C_1}, i \geqslant 2 \quad (3)$$

From this value the harmonic distortion factor h can be computed:

$$h = \sqrt{\sum_{i=2}^{n} d_i^2} \quad (4)$$

Applying Eq (2), one can reconstruct the H-potential when the constants C_i are correctly chosen (Fig. 10) and, using d_i and h of Eqs (3) and (4), the influence of the stimulus parameters on the nonlinear waveform distortion can be estimated. With both techniques we found that harmonics higher than the third order are not necessary for the simulation of the H-potentials evoked by sinewave stimuli, because they contribute very little to the response. It was further evident that the influence of the higher harmonics decreased as the stimulus frequency increased. An increase in stimulus luminance and/or stimulus area, however, led to an increase in the non-linear components of H-potential responses (Fig. 11, [38]).

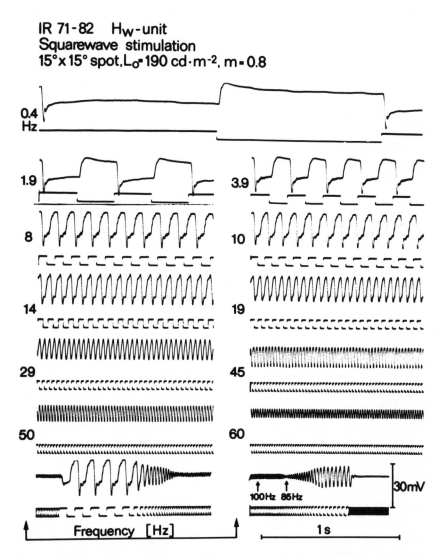

Fig. 8. Flicker responses of cone-dominated H_w-units. (A) H_w-unit response to squarewave flicker stimuli. Note the high-frequency oscillatory response at "light on." Squarewave stimulus frequencies as indicated. The bottom row shows responses to rapid changes in stimulus frequency. A resonance is visible at about 95 Hz (from [37]).

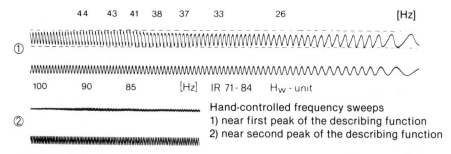

Fig. 9. H_w-unit responses to sinewave flicker stimuli. Rapid changes in stimulus frequency. Photopic flicker stimuli $L_0 = 190$ cd/m², m = 0.8. The two response peaks of the describing function (43 and 95 Hz, Fig. 7) are visible (from [69]).

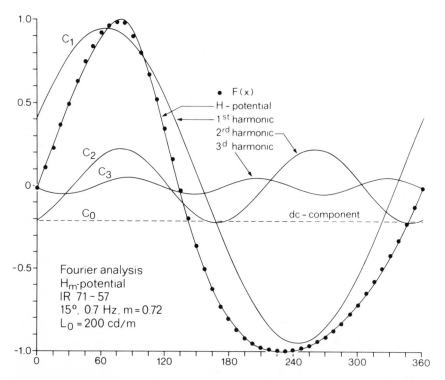

Fig. 10. H_m-potential elicited by 0.7 Hz sinewave stimuli ($L_0 = 200$ cd/m⁻², m = 0.72, 15 × 15 degree stimulus area) plotted in normalized form. It can be approximated very well by the sum of a constant + 3 "harmonics" (dots) according to eq (2) with the parameters: $C_0 = 0.211$, $C_1 = 0.949$, $C_2 = 0.220$, $C_3 = 0.049$, $\psi_1 = 25.4°$, $\psi_2 = 66.5°$, $\psi_3 = 10.6°$. The harmonic components are also drawn separately (from [38]).

A

Distortion as a function
of frequency
15°spot, L = 200 cd/m², m = 0.72

H_m-unit

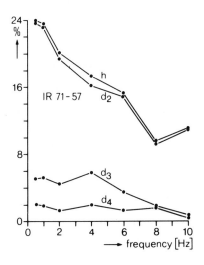

Fig. 11. Harmonic distortion factor h and the
contribution of the second (d_2), third (d_3) and
fourth (d_4) harmonics to horizontal cell responses
are plotted as a function of stimulus frequency (A),
stimulus area (B), and average stimulus luminance
(C). Responses from H_m-unit (A, B) and an H_n-
unit (C) (Dotted lines are model calculations [38]).

B

Distortion as a function
of stimulus area
1 Hz, L = 200 cd/m², m = 0.72

H_m-unit

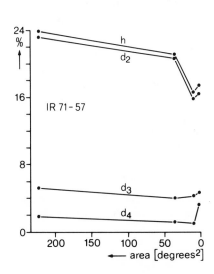

C

Distortion as a function
of luminance
1 Hz, m = 0.9.9°spot

H_n-unit

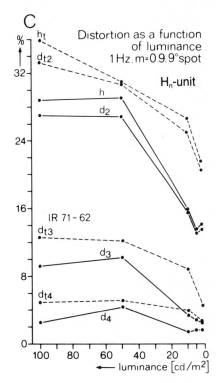

THE EFFECT OF STIMULUS AREA

All H-units had a maximum sensitivity in the center of their receptive fields. From this center the sensitivity decreased approximately symmetrically and exponentially toward the RF-periphery. Recently, however, employing light spots orbiting around the center of the RF at different radii, Molenaar and van de Grind [51] demonstrated that discontinuities in excitability exist within the RF ("troughs and peaks of excitability"). These inhomogeneities in the RF-structure probably correspond to the nonhomogeneous branching of horizontal cell dendrites. The discontinuities, however, are averaged out by circular stimuli increasing symmetrically with respect to the center of the RF. Using the finding that the responses to small light stimuli decreased with the distance from the RF-center toward the RF-periphery according to an exponential function (cf also [33, 49]) we searched for a reliable method to estimate the RF-size. For this purpose we defined a parameter d* [degrees] as the diameter of a round light stimulus centered to the RF giving half the maximum response as compared to a 15° diameter stimulus. The parameter d* was found to be about the same with an increasing and decreasing stimulus area; d* was on the average about 1.4° in H_m-units and 2.2° in H_n-units at 2 Hz sinewave flicker stimuli. In both classes of H-units, however, d* increased with increasing stimulus frequencies. Thus the temporal and spatial nonlinearities of H-unit responses seemed to influence each other.

Comparing morphological data [52–59] with the d*-values and the approximative size of H-unit receptive fields, the latter were always larger than a dendritic spread of a single H-cell [38]. Therefore, one has to assume that signals from more than one H-cell contribute to the responses of an "H-unit." This assumption is in good agreement with the morphological findings of gap-junctions between the dendrites of Cajal-type horizontal cells in the cat retina [60].

We tested whether a linear or nonlinear spatial summation is valid for H-unit responses by computing the expected area response function from the exponential sensitivity distribution across the RF and the stimulus area (linear convolution technique). The results of these computations were compared with the measured area–response relationship of H-units. In H_n-units there was a close correspondence between data and computed responses, whereas a significant deviation in H_m-unit area response functions from the computed values was found. Therefore, nonlinear spatial summation of the membrane potential changes elicited in different regions of the H_n-unit receptive field has to be assumed. The area response relationship of H_w-units was not studied in detail.

THE INTENSITY FUNCTION

We could confirm the experimental results obtained in 1956/1957, that the amplitude R_H of the hyperpolarizing H-potential corresponds within a range of

2–3 $\log_{10}$-units to the so-called Weber–Fechner law:

$$R_H = a \log \frac{L}{L_{Th}} \; [mV] \tag{5}$$

whereby a is a constant and L_{Th} a theoretical luminance threshold value. Above and below this range, however, a deviation from a simple logarithmic function was found. Throughout the entire stimulus range, the S-shaped curves are better described by a hyperbolic relationship first proposed by Ewald Hering [61, 62] and applied by Naka and Rushton [63]:

$$R_H = \frac{k_o L}{1 + k_i L} \; [mV] \tag{6}$$

Naka [64] proposed the modified normalized formula:

$$\frac{R_H}{R_{max}} = \frac{L^b}{L^b + \delta^b} = \left\{ 1 + \left(\frac{L}{\delta}\right)^{-b} \right\}^{-1} mV \tag{7}$$

R_{max} is the saturation response. Figure 12 shows intensity functions of an H_m-unit and an H_n-unit. The curves fitting the experimental data best (dashed lines) are computed according to Eq (7). For the cone-dominated H_m-units the exponent b was 1, whereas in the rod-dominated H_n-units b was 0.5 [38].

Steinberg [27] analyzed the intensity functions of mixed input horizontal cells in the dark-adapted cat retina and computed Eq (7) for an optimal fit to his results. The curves that best fitted his data for orange flashes (cone-dominated responses) were much steeper than those fitting the data for blue flashes (rod-dominated responses). These findings correspond to our assumption that the intensity function of the cone-dominated response isolated by high flicker frequency is represented by a higher exponent b of Eq (7) than the rod components.

INTERACTION BETWEEN RECEPTORS, HORIZONTAL CELLS, AND BIPOLAR CELLS

Horizontal cells form a network regulating the signal flow between receptors and bipolar cells, but they are only one of several mechanisms of lateral signal spread throughout the neuronal network of the retina. Receptors probably transmit information to bipolar cells only by conventional chemical synapses; two types of such synaptic structures were found (Fig. 13). Presumably, horizontal cells contribute mainly to the RF-periphery response of bipolar cells (1 in Fig. 13), but, in addition, interplexiform cells (2 in Fig. 13) have to be considered as a

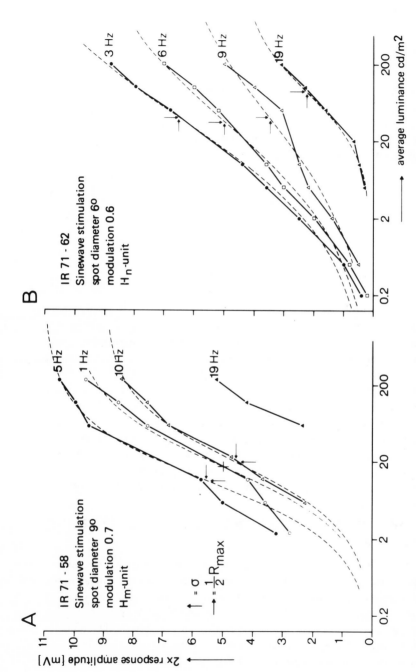

Fig. 12. Peak-through values of an H_m-potential (A) and an H_n-potential (B) obtained at different stimulus frequencies as a function of the average luminance level (abscissa, L_0). The dotted curves in (A) are hyperbolic functions (eq. (7) with b = 1). The half-ceiling response levels are indicated with small horizontal arrows and the corresponding average luminance (eq. 7) with small vertical arrows. The dotted curves in (B) represent square-root hyperbolic curves (eq. 7, with b = 0.5). The small arrows in (B) have the same meaning as those in (A) (from [38]).

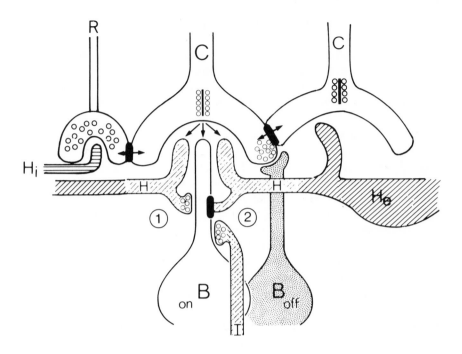

(1) C $\longrightarrow$ H $\longrightarrow$ H   (4) R $\longrightarrow$ H

(2) C $\longrightarrow$ C $\longrightarrow$ H   (5) R $\longrightarrow$ C $\longrightarrow$ H

(3) C $\longrightarrow$ R $\longrightarrow$ H

Fig. 13. Scheme of connections between cat retina photoreceptors (cones C, rods R), Horizontal cells (H) and on-center and off-center bipolar cells (B_{on}, B_{off}). I is an "axon" from an "interplexiform cell." (1) to (5) give schematically five different pathways from receptors to horizontal cells (from [71]). ①: Chemical synapses according to Fisher and Boycott [66]; ②: Chemical synapses according to Kolb [57].

second source providing lateral control of the signal flow through the bipolar cells [65]. The lateral interaction between adjacent receptors and feedback signals from horizontal cells to the receptors is another mean by which lateral signal flow is obtained in the retinal layer distal to the bipolar cells.

One can conceive of different modes by which the horizontal cells could interact with the signal transmission from photoreceptors to bipolar cells.

(a) The depolarization or hyperpolarization of horizontal cells may be fed back to the receptor membrane, especially the cone membrane, whereby a slow chemical process involved in light-dark adaptation could play a role. Through the membrane contacts between adjacent photoreceptor pedicles, such a feedback mechanism will increase the functional receptive field size of a single photoreceptor far beyond the area of its outer segment and also the RF-size of the bipolar cells.

(b) Horizontal cells form perhaps conventional chemical synapses on the bipolar cell dendrites outside the parts invaginating into the receptor pedicles (Fig. 13). According to Fisher and Boycott [66], however, such conventional synapses are formed by the axonless A horizontal cells. Kolb [57] described in her electronmicroscopic studies that the chemical synapses found at bipolar cell dendrites in the outer plexiform layers are endings from interplexiform cells. She assumes that the axonless horizontal cells form nonconventional synapses with the membrane of bipolar cell dendrites (? electrotonic junctions, Fig. 13). By both types of synapses horizontal cells could directly modify the signal flow from receptors through the bipolar cells.

(c) Svaetichin et al [67, 68] proposed a third interaction possibility between horizontal cells and the signal flow from cones to bipolar cells. They considered a chemical interaction between the transmitter released from the receptor synaptic terminals (at the site of the ribbon structure, Fig. 13) and an inactivating enzyme released by horizontal cell dendrites proportional to the polarization state of their membrane. This proposed chemical interaction is thought to take place within the synaptic cleft. It determines the transmitter efficacy at the dendritic surface of the bipolar cells.

(d) A few years ago, I speculated about another mechanism by which the invaginating dendrites of horizontal cells could influence the synaptic interaction between receptor terminals and bipolar cell dendrites [69] (Fig. 13). It is the "interaction by competition for the same transmitter" released within a very restricted part of the presynaptic photoreceptor membrane in the region of the ribbon structure. If the synaptic transmitter is an electrically charged molecule, it does not move only by free diffusion across the synaptic cleft. The movement and distribution of transmitter molecules also depend on the voltage gradient between the site of transmitter release and transmitter action. The local distribution of this voltage gradient is in turn a function of the current flowing through the inner segments of the photoreceptors and the synaptic terminals and also depends on the current flowing through the membrane of bipolar cell and horizontal cell dendrites, invaginating into the receptor pedicles. The fraction of transmitter molecules discharged per unit of time which reaches either the bipolar cell dendrite or the horizontal cell dendrite membrane would then depend on the voltage gradient between the site of release at the receptor synapse and the membrane of bipolar cell and horizontal cell dendrites, respectively. The higher the voltage gradient between the site of transmitter discharge and the invaginating horizontal cell dendritic membrane, the smaller the relative flow of transmitter to the membrane of the invaginating bipolar dendrite. Thus the degree of polarization of the horizontal cell membrane potential controls the relative number of transmitter molecules reaching the molecular receptors in the bipolar cell dendritic membrane, whereby no direct contact between bipolar cells and horizontal cells is necessary.

A similar "control of synaptic efficacy by competition for the same transmitter" is conceivable if one assumes that the rate of the transmitter–molecular receptor interaction (transmitter turnover) in the postsynaptic membrane depends upon the membrane potential. The electrical voltage gradient across the horizontal cell membrane may influence the configuration of large molecules responsible for the transmitter turnover and a change in molecular configuration may in turn change the speed of transmitter–molecular receptor interaction. The concentration gradient between the site of transmitter release at the synaptic terminal and the site of transmitter action at the horizontal cells will then be dependent on the transmitter turnover at the respective postsynaptic membranes competing for the same transmitter.

This interaction by competition for the same transmitter certainly constitutes a rather unorthodox way by which neighboring neurons might interact. I think, however, that whenever neurons involved in a neuronal circuit only generate slow membrane potential changes and no action potentials, one has to consider unorthodox interaction between neighboring neurons. For further details of this problem, the reader is referred to the discussion about "local neuronal circuits" in the book edited by Schmitt and Worden [69].

A PHENOMENOLOGICAL MODEL DESCRIBING THE FREQUENCY TRANSFER PROPERTIES OF HORIZONTAL CELLS

The Bode plots shown in Figure 7 can be derived from a phenomenological H-unit model in which inputs from different types of receptors converge on a single H-cell. The receptor responses are simulated by a nonlinear model consisting of a first order low-pass filter, a fixed time delay, a nonlinear amplitude compression according to Eq (7) and a second order low-pass filter (Fig. 14). Rods and cones have different time constants and different amplitude compressions, as described previously. In addition, the three different cone types of the cat retina are assumed to have different temporal frequency transfer properties [70]. H_n-units receive predominantly rod input signals, H_m-units receive signals from rod and cones in parallel, and in H_w-units the cone input is dominant. In the phenomenological model describing the response of H_m-units [37, 38], the two types of receptors are represented by two different frequency filters with a 3 dB frequency cut-off for rods at 15 Hz and for cones at 40 Hz. The H-unit

A General phenomenological receptor model

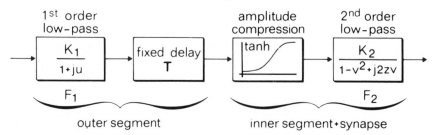

B Phenomenological H-units model
(steady state, constant input amplitude)

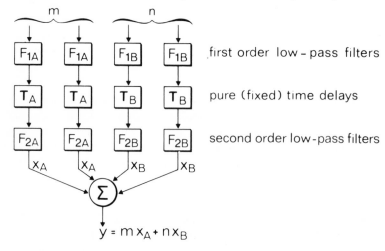

Fig. 14. (A) Block diagram of the receptor model, including an amplitude compression mechanism first proposed by E. Hering, 1874; slightly modified. Response of the amplitude compression: $R_H = -cL^b/(a + L^b)$ mV, where a, b, and c are constants, and L = stimulus luminance. (B) H_m-unit model with inputs from cones (m) and rods (n) (from [37]).

model consists of a first order low-pass filter, a fixed time delay, and a second order low-pass filter. As Figure 15 indicates, the Bode plots of H_m-units are well described by such a model. In simulating the experimental data, the coupling parameters, ie, the ratio of cone influence and rod influence, were varied to approximate the model responses to the experimental data. Similarly, the responses of H_n-units can be simulated by assuming a rod-dominant receptor input. For the H_w-units, however, a dominant input from two or three different cone

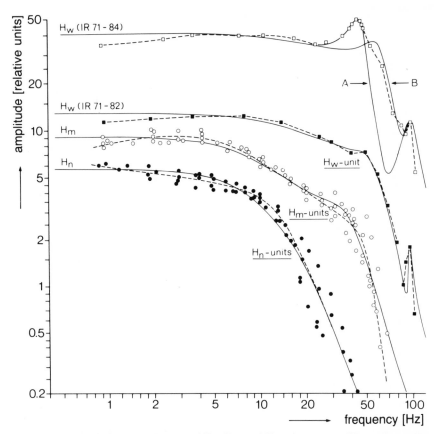

Fig. 15. Amplitude frequency diagrams of H_n-, H_m-, and H_w-unit responses. The continuous lines are model predictions (Fig. 14). Calibration of ordinate units: H_n: 10 = 20 mV, H_m: 10 = 11.5 mV, H_w(IR71–82): 10 = 10 mV, H_w(IR71–84): 10 = 4.5 mV. A and B are results from two different model calculations (from [38]).

types was necessary to simulate the experimental data (Fig. 15; for details see [37,71]).

In the model it is assumed that the horizontal cell membrane itself does not affect the dynamic response properties in the frequency range investigated (< 120 Hz); however we cannot exclude the possibility that the input synapses to the horizontal cells and the very small terminal dendrites may modify the frequency response contents of the signals. A combination of intracellularly applied electrical AC signals and flicker stimulation might lead to an answer to this question.

SUMMARY

(a) A short review of the history of intracellular recordings from horizontal cells of the cat retina is presented. Three different methods to record from cat horizontal cells are described.

(b) The responses of horizontal cells in the cat retina to sinewave and square-wave flicker stimuli of a different temporal frequency, stimulus luminance, and stimulus area are discussed. With large-field, high modulation, white-light stimuli, three distinct classes of H-units were found. The critical flicker frequency to large-field photopic (200 cd $\cdot$ m^{-2}) flicker stimuli was one unequivocal criterium for classification: H_n-units had a CFF of 25–40 Hz, H_m-units of 55–70 Hz, and H_w-units of 95–110 Hz. When low frequency photopic squarewave stimuli were applied, characteristic differences between the three different H-unit types were also obtained.

(c) The responses to squarewave and sinewave light stimuli were in all H-units clearly nonlinear. The nonlinear distortion was mainly due to the contribution of the second and third harmonics and increased with the stimulus luminance, the area of the light stimuli, and the depth of modulation of the sinewave flicker stimuli. An increase in the sinewave flicker frequency, however, led to a decrease in nonlinear components.

(d) The responses of H_n-units at photopic luminance levels were dominated by rod inputs, whereas, under the same stimulus conditions, the responses of H_m-units and H_w-units were dominated by cone inputs. In H_w-units two or three different cone types contribute to the responses.

(e) The area function indicates some nonlinear properties in spatial summation within the receptive field of H_m-units which is certainly larger than the dendritic arborization of a single horizontal cell. This finding indicates an efficient distribution of signals within the horizontal cell layer beyond the single cell.

(f) Possible interactions between horizontal cells and the signal transmission between receptors and bipolar cells are discussed.

(g) A phenomenological model simulating the frequency transfer properties of the three different classes of horizontal cells is described.

ACKNOWLEDGMENTS

The work was supported by a grant from the Deutsche Forschungsgemeinschaft (Grant 161) and an ETP Twinning Grant of the European Science Foundation, Strassburg.

REFERENCES

1. Motokawa KT, Oikawa T, Tasaki K: Receptor potential of vertebrate retina. J Neurophysiol 20:186, 1957.
2. Grüsser O-J: Rezeptorpotentiale einzelner retinaler Zapfen der Katze. Naturwissenschaften 44:522, 1957.

3. Jung R, Creutzfeldt O, Grüsser O-J: The microphysiology of cortical neurones. Germ med Mth 3:269, 1958.
4. Brown KT, Wiesel T: Intraretinal recording in the unopened cat eye. Amer J Ophthal 46:91, 1958.
5. Brown KT, Wiesel TN: Intraretinal recording with micropipette electrodes in the intact cat eye. J Physiol 149:537, 1959.
6. Grüsser O-J: Rezeptorpotentiale einzelner retinaler Zapfen der Katze. Pflügers Arch 268:47, 1958.
7. Grüsser O-J: Rezeptorabhängige Potentiale der Katzenretina und ihre Reaktionen auf Flimmer-licht. Pflügers Arch 271:511, 1960.
8. Grüsser O-J: Rezeptorabhängige R-Potentiale der Katzenretina. In Jung R, Kornhuber H (eds): "Neurophysiologie und Psychophysik des visuellen Systems." Berlin: Springer–Verlag, 1961, p 56.
9. Grüsser O-J: Reaktionen einzelner corticaler und retinaler Neurone der Katze auf Flimmerlicht und ihre Beziehungen zur subjektiven Sinnesphysiologie. Doctoral dissertation, Freiburg i Br, 1956.
10. Grüsser O-J, Grützner A: Neurophysiologische Grundlagen der periodischen Nachbildphasen nach kurzen Lichtblitzen. Graefes Arch Ophthalmol 160:65, 1958.
11. Grüsser O-J, Rabelo C: Reaktionen retinaler Neurone nach Lichtblitzen. I. Einzelblitze und Blitzreize wechselnder Frequenz. Pflügers Arch 265:501, 1958.
12. Grüsser O-J, Reidemeister C: Flimmerlichtuntersuchungen an der Katzenretina. II. Off-Neurone und Besprechung der Ergebnisse. Z Biol 111:254, 1959.
13. Reidemeister C, Grüsser O-J: Flimmerlichtuntersuchungen an der Katzenretina. I. On-Neurone und On-Off-Neurone. Z Biol 111:241, 1959.
14. Schatternikoff M: Über den Einfluß der Adaptation auf die Erscheinung des Flimmerns. Z Sinnesphysiol 29:241, 1902.
15. Kries J von: Über die Wahrnehmung des Flimmerns durch normale und durch total farbblinde Personen. Z Sinnesphysiol 32:113, 1903.
16. Granit R: "Sensory Mechanisms of the Retina." London: Oxford University Press, 1947.
17. Svaetichin G: Spectral response curves from single cones. Acta Physiol Scand 39:17, 1956a.
18. Svaetichin G: Receptor mechanisms for flicker and fusion. Acta Physiol Scand 39:47, 1956b.
19. Svaetichin G: Notes on the ERG analysis. Acta Physiol Scand 39:55, 1956c.
20. Svaetichin G: The cone function related to the activity of retinal neurons. Acta Physiol Scand 39:67, 1956d.
21. Svaetichin G: Aspects on human photoreceptor mechanisms. Acta Physiol Scand 39:93, 1956e.
22. Svaetichin G, Jonasson R: A technique for oscillographic recordings of response curves. Acta Physiol Scand 39:3, 1956.
22a. Laufer M, Millan EE, Vanegas H: Spectral sensitivity of L-type S-potentials in a teleost retina. Vision Res 11:77, 1971.
23. Dodt E, Walther JB: Der photopische Dominator im Flimmer-ERG der Katze. Pflügers Arch 266:175, 1958.
24. Noell WK: The origin of the electroretinogram. Amer J Ophthal 38:78, 1954.
25. MacNichol EJ, Svaetichin G: Electric responses from the isolated retinas of fishes. Amer J Ophthal 46:26, 1958.
26. Steinberg RH, Schmidt R: The evidence that horizontal cells generate S-potentials in the cat retina. Vision Res 11:1029, 1971.
27. Steinberg RH: Rod and cone contributions to S-potentials from the cat retina. Vision Res 9:1319, 1969a.
28. Steinberg RH: Rod–cone interaction in S-potentials from the cat retina. Vision Res 9:1331, 1969b.
29. Steinberg RH: The rod after-effect in S-potentials from the cat retina. Vision Res 9:1345, 1969c.

30. Steinberg, RH: Incremental responses to light recorded from pigment epithelial cells and horizontal cells of the cat retina. J Physiol 217:93, 1971.
31. Nelson R, Kolb H, Famiglietti EV, Gouras P: Neural responses in the rod and cone systems of the cat retina: Intracellular records and procion stains. Invest Ophthal 15:946, 1976.
32. Nelson R, Lützow A, Kolb H, Gouras P: Horizontal cells in cat retina with independent dendritic systems. Science 189:137, 1975.
33. Nelson R: Cat cones have rod input: A comparison of the response properties of cones and horizontal cell bodies in the retina of the cat. J Comp Neurol 172:109, 1977.
34. Grüsser O-J, Lunkenheimer HU: Responses of cat horizontal cells to sinewave light shimuth: unpublished, 1967.
35. Grind WA van de, Grüsser O-J, Lunkenheimer HU: Temporal transfer properties of the afferent visual system. Psychophysical, neurophysiological and theoretical investigations. In Jung R (ed): "Handbook of Sensory Physiology, VII/3." Berlin, Heidelberg, New York: Springer–Verlag, 1973, p 431.
36. Foerster MH, Grind WA van de, Grüsser O-J: Intracellular recordings from different layers of the cat retina. Eur J Physiol 343:90, 1973.
37. Foerster MH, Grind WA van de, Grüsser O-J: Frequency transfer properties of three distinct types of cat horizontal cells. Exp Brain Res 30:347, 1977a.
38. Foerster MH, Grind WA van de, Grüsser O-J: The response of cat horizontal cells to flicker stimuli of different area, intensity and frequency. Exp Brain Res 30:367, 1977b.
39. Molenaar J, Grind WA van de: A stereotaxic method of recording from single neurons in the intact in vivo eye of the cat. J Neurosci Meth 2:135, 1980.
40. Niemeyer G: Intracellular recording from the isolated perfused mammalian eye. Vision Res 13:1613, 1973.
41. Niemeyer G: ERG dependence on flow rate in the isolated and perfused mammalian eye. Brain Res 57:203, 1973.
42. Niemeyer G: Some properties of the isolated, perfused mammalian eye. Experientia 30:682, 1974.
43. Niemeyer G: The function of the retina in the perfused eye. Doc Ophthal 39:53, 1975.
44. Niemeyer G, Gouras P: Rod and cone signals in S-potentials of the isolated perfused cat eye. Vision Res 13:1603, 1973.
45. Niemeyer G: The perfused cat eye: A model in neurobiologic research. Albrecht v Graefes Arch klin exp Ophthal 203:209, 1977.
46. Dowling JE, Werblin FS: Synaptic organization of the vertebrate retina. Vision Res 11:1, 1971.
47. Werblin FS, Dowling JE: Organization of the retina of the mudpuppy, Necturus maculosus. II. Intracellular recording. J Neurophysiol 32:339, 1969.
48. Kaneko A: Receptive field organization of bipolar and amacrine cells in the goldfish retina. J Physiol 235:133, 1973.
49. Nelson R, Kolb H, Robinson MM, Mariani P: Neural circuitry of the cat retina: cone pathways to ganglion cells. Vision Res (in press), 1981.
50. Granit R: The organization of the vertebrate retinal elements. Ergeb Physiol 46:31, 1950.
51. Molenaar J, Grind WA van de: Anisotropic receptive field structure of cat horizontal cells. Exp Brain Res 37:253, 1979.
52. Ramon y Cajal A: Die Retina der Wirbeltiere, translated by Graeff A, Wiesbaden: Bergmann, 1894.
53. Boycott BB, Kolb H: The connections between the bipolar cells and photoreceptors in the retina of the domestic cat. J Comp Neurol 148:92, 1973.
54. Boycott BB, Peichl L, Wässle H: Morphological types of horizontal cell in the retina of the domestic cat. Proc R Soc London B 203:229, 1978.
55. Gallego A: Horizontal and amacrine cells in the mammal's retina. Vision Res 11:33, 1971.

56. Kolb H: The connections between horizontal cells and photoreceptors in the retina of the cat: Electron microscopy of Golgi preparations. J Comp Neurol 155:1, 1974.

57. Kolb H: The organization of the outer plexiform layer in the retina of the cat: Electron microscopic observations. J Neurocytol 6:131, 1977.

57a. Kolb H, Famiglietti EV: Rod and cone pathways in the retina of the cat. Invest Ophthal 15:935, 1976.

58. Wässle H, Boycott BB, Peichl L: Receptor contacts of horizontal cells in the retina of the domestic cat. Proc R Soc London B 203:247, 1978a.

59. Wässle H, Peichl L, Boycott BB: Topography of horizontal cells in the retina of the domestic cat. Proc R Soc London B 203:269, 1978b.

60. Sobrino JA, Gallego A: Células amacrinas de la capa plexiforme de la retina. Actas Soc Esp Cienc Fysiol 12:373, 1970.

61. Hering E: Zur Lehre vom Lichtsinne. V. Grundzüge einer Theorie des Lichtsinnes. Sitzungsber Kais Akad Wiss Wein (Math-Nat Classe, Abth III) 69:179, 1874.

62. Hering E: "Zur Lehre vom Lichtsinn." Berlin: Springer, 1920.

63. Naka KI: Computer assisted analysis of S-potentials. Biophys J 9:845, 1969.

64. Naka KI, Rushton WAH: S-potentials from luminosity units in the retina of fish (Cyprinidae). J Physiol (London) 185:587, 1966c.

65. Kolb H, West RW: Synaptic connections of the interplexiform cell in the retina of the cat. J Neurocytol 6:155, 1977.

66. Fisher SK, Boycott BB: Synaptic connections made by horizontal cells within the outer plexiform layer of the cat and the rabbit. Proc R Soc London B 186:317, 1974.

67. Svaetichin G, Negishi K, Drujan B, Muriel C: S-potentials and retinal automatic control systems. In Broda E, Locker A, Springer-Lederer, H (eds): "Proceedings of the First European Biophysics Congress." Vienna: Verlag der Wiener Medizinischen Akademie, Vol 5, 1971, p 77.

68. Svaetichin G, Negishi K, Fatehchand R, Drujan BD, Testa AS de: Nervous function based on interactions between neuronal and non-neuronal elements. Prog Brain Res 15:243, 1965.

69. Grüsser O-J: Cat ganglion-cell receptive fields and the role of horizontal cells in their generation. In Schmitt FW, Worden FG (eds): "The Neurosciences IV." Cambridge Mass: MIT Press, 1979, p 247.

70. Saunders R McD: The spectral responsiveness and the temporal frequency response (TFR) of cat optic tract and lateral geniculate neurons: Sinusoidal stimulation studies. Vision Res 17:285, 1977.

71. Grind WA van de, Grüsser O-J: Frequency transfer properties of cat retina horizontal cells. Vision Res, in press, 1981.

72. Grüsser O-J, Kapp H: Reaktionen retinaler Neurone nach Lichtblitzen. II. Doppelblitze mit wechselndem Blitzintervall. Pflügers Arch 266:111, 1958.

The S-Potential, pages 235–256
© 1982 Alan R. Liss, Inc., 150 Fifth Avenue, New York, NY 10011

Studies on S-Potential Control Mechanisms in the Fish Retina

Mustafa B.A. Djamgoz, Sonia H. Reynolds, and Keith H. Ruddock

The first recording of intracellular potentials from the vertebrate (fish) retina by Svaetichin [1,2] constituted a major advance in the electrophysiological study of the visual pathways. Previous studies had used only extracellular recording methods, either on the whole optic nerve [3], on dissected single optic nerve fibres [4], or, with metal tipped microelectrodes, on single neurones in intact retinae [5]. The introduction of intracellular methods made possible the investigation both of slow potential response mechanisms and of the effects of pharmacological agents on membrane potentials, neither of which can be adequately studied by extracellular methods. The potentials recorded by Svaetichin and further characterized by MacNichol and Svaetichin [6] and Svaetichin and MacNichol [7] are called S-potentials and are the subject of the work to be reported here. There are two principal classes of S-potential, the L-type which hyperpolarize in response to all stimulus wavelengths, and the C-type, which depolarize in response to some stimulus wavelengths and hyperpolarize in response to others. C-type responses can be diphasic, for which there is only one spectral region where response polarity reverses, or triphasic [8], for which there are two such spectral regions. Depolarizing components of biphasic C-unit responses and the long-wavelength hyperpolarization of triphasic responses are characterized by a lag in response to light stimulation relative to L-unit responses. In fish, there is considerable species variation in the spectral characteristics of both L- and C-units (see, for example, [9–11]), although there is broad correlation between environment and complexity of the chromatic organization [7]. S-potentials were at first recorded only from neurones receiving input from cones, but rod-dominated S-potentials were subsequently reported [8]. The relationship between S-potential voltage amplitude (V) and illumination level (I) is given by V equals $K_\lambda I (I + I_{1/2})^{-1/2}$, where $I_{1/2}$ and K_λ are constants [10] with the value of K_λ dependent upon the stimulus wavelength (λ). By recording the V-I function for different λ values, Naka and Rushton were able to obtain spectral sensitivity functions for the different classes of S-potential responses in cyprinid fish retinae.

They were particularly concerned with the correlation between absorption spectra of single cone photopigments and the spectral sensitivities of the S-potential responses. The absorption spectra of single fish cones are well characterized [12] and Naka and Rushton successfully identified the contributions of different spectral classes of cones to the various S-potential units, with the exception of the red-sensitive depolarizing C-type responses. These gave peak sensitivity at about 680 nm, quite unlike any known cyprinid photopigment absorption spectrum and a similar problem has been noted in later S-potential spectral analyses [13,14]. We have applied Naka and Rushton's method of spectral analysis in our work and the accurate identification of the spectral input to different S-potential units plays a significant role in the analysis of the retinal microcircuits (see eg, Fig. 6). The receptive fields of S-potential units are considerably larger than the dendritic extensions of any single horizontal cell and can extend over virtually the whole retina (eg,[15]). It was proposed that S-potentials spread laterally by electrotonic coupling between horizontal cells [16] and such coupling between neighboring and functionally similar S-potential units in dogfish was established by intracellular current injection and recording [17]. It should be noted, however, that the influence of pharmacological agents on S-potential spread, which is reviewed below, has yet to be related to the electronic model of horizontal cell coupling. We present observations on the spread of L-type S-potentials which support the view that this coupling is electrotonic in nature.

The neuronal origin of retinal S-potentials has been elucidated by intracellular staining methods. Early observations with crystal violet [6] and lithium carmine [18] indicated that in fish they arise at the level of the horizontal cells, and the horizontal cell origin of the potentials was confirmed by staining with Niagara Sky Blue [19] and procion yellow [20]. The horizontal cells are particularly well developed in the teleost fish retina, with up to four layers of cells extending laterally across the retina [21–23]. In the cyprinid fish (roach and rudd) used for the present investigation, there are three layers of horizontal cells of which the central is connected to rods and the inner forms the layer of axonal extensions arising in the outer layer of cone horizontal cell bodies. These species are, therefore, similar to the goldfish [24] in the arrangement of retinal horizontal cell layers.

The mode of excitation of horizontal cells and the neurotransmitters which control this excitation have been subject to considerable investigation, particularly since the successful recording of intracellular receptor potentials [25,26]. The primary effect of light absorption appears to be receptor hyperpolarization, and Trifonov [27] proposed that in darkness, photoreceptors release excitatory neurotransmitter which depolarizes the horizontal cells. The hyperpolarization of photoreceptors by light suppresses transmitter release, causing the horizontal cells to hyperpolarize. The hypothesis was formulated from observed changes in S-potential levels produced by radially directed, transretinal electrical currents.

A solution to the problem of depolarizing S-potentials was suggested by Fuortes and Simon [28] who attribute them to inhibitory interactions between different spectral classes of cone. Light-evoked depolarization in one spectral class of cone resulting from absorption in another spectral class is observed in the turtle retina [29,30]. Fuortes and Simon, therefore, proposed that negative feedback from red-sensitive cones via horizontal cells causes depolarization in the green-sensitive cones, and these provide the input signals to red-depolarizing, green-hyperpolarizing C-units. Although the amplitudes of the feedback-depolarizing signals in turtle cones are much smaller than the amplitudes of C-type-depolarizing responses, Fuortes and Simon's suggestion has received support from anatomical and pharmacological studies on goldfish retina [24,31]. The interpretation of depolarizing C-type potentials is one of the problems examined in this chapter.

The susceptibility of S-potentials to physiologically active chemical agents has been widely investigated, with particular attention paid to the neurotransmitter release by photoreceptors. Structures associated with chemical synapses have been observed at the contact points between horizontal cells and photoreceptors [22,32,33], and identification of the transmitter activity at these putative synapses is of obvious importance. Furukawa and Hanawa [34] showed that the b-wave of the retinal ERG is suppressed by amino-acid salts (glutamate and aspartate) and with the development of intracellular recording methods, the effects of amino acids on retinal S-potentials could be readily examined. There is general agreement that the membrane potentials of all S-potential units are reversibly depolarized by aspartate and glutamate and hyperpolarized by GABA, with suppression of light-evoked potentials [35,36]. Effective concentrations are of the order of 5–10 mM, about 100 times greater than those at which glutamate is effective at the neuromuscular junction of crayfish [37], thus reservations have been expressed regarding the mode of amino acid action on horizontal cells. GABA uptake in external horizontal cells of the goldfish retina has been demonstrated by autoradiographic methods [31] and the functional implications of such uptake were discussed by them.

Acetylcholine was reported to have no effect on S-potentials in carp [36] but in larval tiger salamander, it causes contraction of S-potential receptive fields [38]. Since the discovery that retinal interplexiform cells [39] accumulate dopamine [40], there has been considerable interest in the retinal action of catecholamines, in particular dopamine. The interplexiform cells make both pre- and postsynaptic contacts in the inner plexiform layer, mostly with amacrine cells, but only presynaptic contacts in the outer plexiform layer, with external horizontal cell bodies, horizontal cell processes, and bipolar cell dendrites [40]. Binding studies with radioactive agonists and antagonists of dopamine have shown that the dopamine receptor sites in guinea pig and carp retina are of the D_1-type, which are associated with adenylate cyclase activity, rather than D_2-type, which are not [41]. The anatomy suggests, therefore, that interplexiform cells exert control over cone horizontal cells by release of dopamine (DA). Application of DA to the goldfish retina produces depolarization of cone L-type S-potential units, sometimes depolarizes C-type units but does not affect rod S-potential units [42]. In contrast, Negishi and Drujan [43] found that in Eugerres plumieri, a marine teleost, all L-type S-potential units depolarize under application of DA and other catecholamines such as noradrenaline and adrenaline, whereas C-units sometimes depolarize and sometimes hyperpolarize. They also noted that reduction in lateral spread of the S-potential occurs with higher concentrations of catecholamines. We show that retinal stimulation with bright lights elicits responses from some classes of S-potential units which are similar to those induced by application to the retina of catecholamines.

EXPERIMENTAL METHODS

We have studied S-potentials recorded from the retinae of cyprinid fish, roach (Rutilus rutilus), and rudd (Scardinius erythrophthalmus). The retina was isolated in dim red light from the dark-adapted eye of a freshly killed fish by severing the optic nerve, and was placed receptor side up in an open chamber (RC; Fig. 1a) supplied with moist oxygen. Special care was taken to maintain the retina in a dark-adapted state when studying rod responses. The retina was stimulated from below by light beams provided by a three-channel optical system and was irradiated from above by a laser beam, reflected into the chamber by a prism (P_2) and focused by a $\times 10$ microscope objective (MO) onto the retina. In the experiments to be described, the laser beam was focused into a 1-mm spot, which covered the area stimulated by the 1.0-mm diameter (or smaller) light beams from the stimulator, thus light-evoked responses could be recorded both before and after bleaching with the laser beam. Such local laser bleaching has advantages over general retinal bleaching; for example, the bleaching spot can be moved systematically across the retina, enabling us to carry out a number of independent bleaching experiments on each retina. Again, the bleaching area can

Fig. 1. (a) Schematic diagram of the equipment used for recording electrical signals from the isolated fish retina (R) placed receptor side up in a recording chamber (RC). The retina was stimulated from below by light from the optical system (O) and from above by a laser beam (L) reflected by the prism (P_2) and imaged by a $\times 10$ microscope objective (MO). The recording electrode (E) is connected via an impedance matching Xl amplifier to an oscilloscope (CRT). (b) Stimulus and electrode arrangement for local perfusion of cobalt chloride. S_1 and S_2 were circular light spots with center-to-center separation of 1 mm, of wavelength 635 nm and diameter 0.5 mm. S_1 was concentric with the recording electrode and S_2 provided peripheral stimulation. E_1 and E_2, the recording and injection electrodes, were filled with 2.5 M KCl and 20 mM $CoCl_2$ respectively. Compressed air (CA) provided pressure injection for electrode E_2. The different retinal layers are illustrated schematically: (RCL) receptor cell layer; (OPL) outer plexiform layer; (INL) inner nuclear layer; (IPL) inner plexiform layer; (GCL) ganglion cell layer.

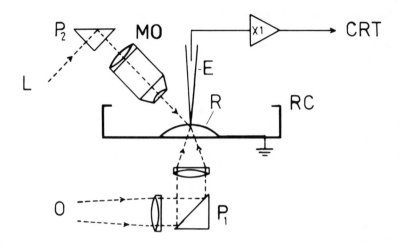

a

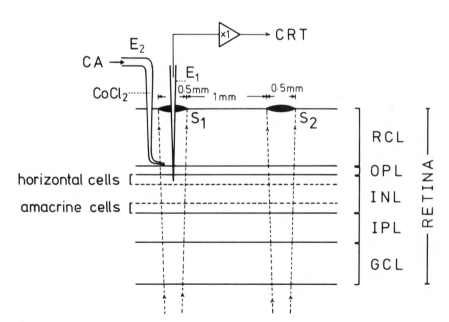

b

be easily restricted to the central region of center-surround antagonistic receptive fields, thus permitting us to suppress selectively the central response component. In the experiments to be described, we used two lasers, in somewhat different ways. An Ar^+-Kr^+ laser provided a number of spectral lines, including those of wavelength 647.1 nm and 488 nm, giving peak flux levels of 0.13 W/mm^2 and 0.03 W/mm^2, respectively, corresponding to some 10^{17} photons/mm^2/sec. An 0.1-sec duration flash of either beam produced spectrally selective retinal bleaching, but we could usually record S-potentials, albeit of reduced amplitude, after such a flash and could, therefore, determine whether the S-potential spectral characteristics were modified by chromatic adaptation. We also used a He–Ne laser, giving a 632.8-nm beam of peak flux 1 mW/mm^2. The flux level of this beam could be readily controlled by neutral density filters and it was used for sustained retinal stimulation in order, for example, to examine the time course of S-potentials under continuous illumination. The illumination levels of the stimulator light beams were controlled, stepwise, with neutral density filters, which could be inserted manually or by motor drive. In the latter case, filters with decreasing optical density in steps of 0.4 over a total density range of 4.0 were introduced successively into the beam. Thus response voltages (V) elicited by light flashes could be readily determined as a function of the logarithm of stimulus illumination level, log I. The spectral composition of the stimulator light beams were controlled by Balzers B.40 interference filters (half-width 5 nm) and the duration of light flashes was controlled by electromagnetic shutters (Ledex) driven by electronic timers (Grass; Digitimer). Spectral response data were obtained by recording V-log I curves for a number of stimulus wavelengths, and in all cases to be described these curves were well fitted by the template $KI(I + I_{1/2})^{-1/2}$ (see introductory section). The relative position of the templates for different wavelengths along the I axis defines the spectral sensitivity function of the response [10]. Spectral sensitivity curves have been expressed in relative quantum sensitivity for comparison with the absorption spectra of the red-sensitive (R-), green-sensitive (G-), and blue-sensitive (B-) cones of the cyprinid retina. The cone absorption spectra plotted in our figures were derived from the published data of Marks [12]. When required, pharmacological agents could be sprayed from above, through an atomizer, onto the retina and the effective concentration at retinal level was estimated by spraying dye onto small disks of acetate sheet and measuring the resulting optical density after collecting the dye in standard solution [44].

Electrodes were manipulated into position under visual control with a stereomicroscope placed above the retina. This provided ready alignment of the different light beams, including the laser beam. Recording electrodes were filled with 2.5 mM KCl and were of DC resistance in the range of 40 to 150 MΩ, whereas procion injection electrodes were of much greater resistance, between 200 and 800 MΩ. Recording electrodes were connected through preamplifiers

(WPI 701) to an oscilloscope (Tektronix 5103N) and traces photographed from the screen. Procion yellow was injected iontophoretically with 2-nA current and standard fixation and sectioning methods were used to locate the stained neurones.

Local perfusion experiments were performed by pressure injection of the perfusate from the tip of a course microelectrode (Fig. 1b) and the tip of the injection electrode was turned so that it lay tangentially across the retina. In this way, the tendency of the recording electrode to dislodge during injection was minimized.

EXPERIMENTAL OBSERVATIONS

We have observed five spectral classes of S-potential response in the roach and rudd retina, four driven by cone and one by rod input. Of the four cone S-potential response classes, two are L-type and two C-type, one of the latter being diphasic and the other triphasic. This last class, which depolarizes to green and hyperpolarizes to red and blue lights, accounts for fewer than 1% of the observed S-potential responses in roach, but was more commonly observed in the Rudd (Scardinius erythrophthalmus). As the recording electrode was driven vertically through the retina, cone-driven S-potential units were found at two separate levels, whereas rod S-potentials occurred at a level intermediate between the two. The horizontal cell generators of the different S-potential response classes were identified by iontophoretic injection of procion yellow dye, and it was established that the horizontal cells which generate rod S-potentials form a layer intermediate between the two layers in which the cone S-potentials are generated. The stains also, on occasion, revealed the extension connecting the outer layer of cell bodies to the inner layer which has been shown to consist of axonal extensions of the external horizontal cell bodies [45]. We noted greater diffusion of procion dye along the horizontal cell layer when we injected C-type neurones, which may indicate tighter coupling between neurones of this particular class.

The electrophysiological properties of the different classes of S-potential unit are briefly reviewed below.

Rod-type

The spectral response curve of the hyperpolarizing S-potentials arising in the rod horizontal cells peaks at about 530 nm (Fig. 2a) and follows the expected spectral absorption curve for a retinene$_2$-based rod photopigment [46]. The S-potentials appear to saturate with increased light adaptation without significant shift in spectral sensitivity, as has also been reported for goldfish [47] and a marine teleost, Eugerres plumieri [48]. After 0.1-sec bleaching with a 488-nm laser beam, the rod S-potential units hyperpolarize from the dark resting potential of some -30 mV to a level of some -50 mV to -60 mV and are insensitive to further light stimulation. Neither relaxation of this hyperpolarization level nor recovery of sensitivity to light flashes was observed over a period of at least 15

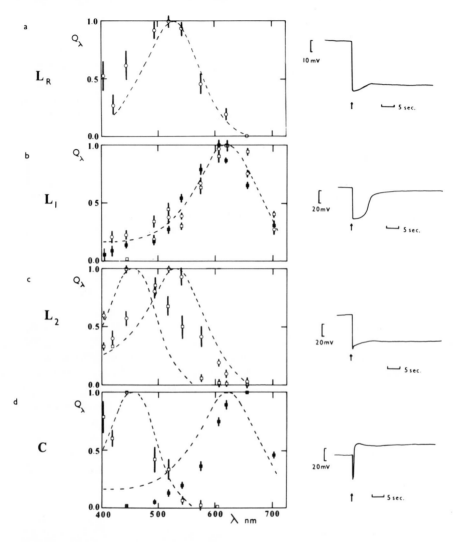

Fig. 2. Response characteristics of four classes of S-potential units observed in roach and rudd retinae. Each row refers to a different S-potential class; (a) rod-type L_R, (b) L_1-type cone, (c) L_2-type cone, and (d) biphasic C-type cone. The left hand column shows data points for the quantum spectral sensitivity (Q_λ) plotted against wavelength, λ; open circles show data for the dark-adapted retina, full squares were determined after 0.1 sec bleaching with a 647.1 nm, 0.13 W/mm^2 laser beam and open squares after 0.1 sec bleaching with a 488 nm, 0.02 W/mm^2 laser beam. The broken lines denote spectral absorption of cyprinid photoreceptors as follows: (a) rods (530-nm peak); (b) red-sensitive (625-nm peak) cone; (c) green- (535-nm peak) and blue-sensitive (455-nm peak) cones; (d) red- (625-nm peak) and blue-sensitive (455-nm peak) cones. The right hand column shows the membrane potentials for the different response units following 0.1-sec irradiation with either a 488-nm, 0.02-W/mm^2 (a and c), or a 647.1-nm, 0.13-W/mm^2 laser beam (b and d).

min following bleaching, and indeed, the hyperpolarization level sometimes tended to fall over the first 30 sec or so of this period (Fig. 2a). Thus, bleaching induces long-term hyperpolarization of rod S-potential units, which behave as if they were subject to continuous light stimulation, ie, they are clamped in a state of light adaptation. Expressed in terms of Trifonov's hypothesis, there is long-term suppression of neurotransmitter release from the rod photoreceptors.

L_1 Cone Type

Of the cone S-potential responses, that designated L_1-type, yields a spectral response which follows closely the absorption spectrum of R-cones, with peak sensitivity at about 620 nm. The spectral response is essentially the same for dark adapted retinae and after 0.1-sec bleaching with either red (647.1-nm) or blue–green (488-nm) laser beams, (Fig. 2b). We conclude that this response class receives input signals exclusively from the R-cones. Psychophysical experiments suggest that pigment bleaching may produce narrowing of the photopigment spectral absorption curves [49] which in turn implies that peak optical density of the pigments must be greater than 0.2 [50]. There is some indication, in our data that after 647.1-nm bleaching, the L_1-type spectral response curve is somewhat narrower than that obtained before bleaching, but the signal amplitudes in the former case are so small that it would be difficult to detect the effect. Like all other S-potential classes in roach, the L_1-type possesses extensive spatial summation properties, with linear summation (Ricco's law) extending to diameters of some 2.5 mm for circular stimuli.

We examined the nature of lateral signal spread in the L_1-type units by means of local injection, under pressure, of cobalt chloride into the region of the recording electrode, whereas the S-potentials were elicited by light flashes located alternately at the point of recording (beam 1) and 1.5 mm peripherally (beam 2) (see Fig. 1b). Following injection, the amplitude of the S-potential elicited by the central flash falls steadily, whereas the response to the peripheral stimulus remains unchanged (Fig. 3a). In view of the fact that cobalt chloride inhibits activity at chemical synapses, we interpret this result in the following way. The response to the central beam represents direct synaptic input from photoreceptors located in the central beam, and injection of cobalt chloride suppresses synaptic activity in this region, thereby reducing the response to light. The peripheral beam stimulates the impaled unit by lateral transmission of signals from the point of light excitation along the coupled horizontal cell layer and the experimental data show that this is not influenced by the injection of cobalt chloride at the recording site. This result is consistent with the view that the signal spread occurs by electrotonic coupling, which is not affected by cobalt chloride, rather than by chemical synaptic coupling, which would be interrupted by the cobalt chloride injection in the region of the impaled neurone.

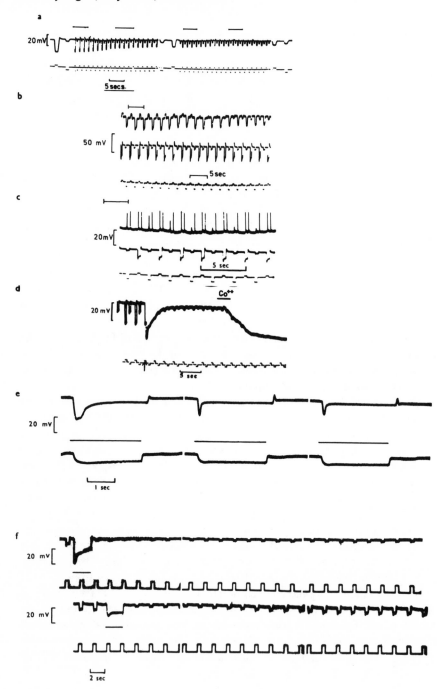

In contrast, lateral spread of signals between transient amacrine cells is blocked by cobalt chloride [51]. Membrane potentials and light-evoked potentials of L_1-type response units are influenced neither by 10^{-5} M picrotoxin, which suppresses depolarizing C-type S-potentials (Fig. 3b), nor by 10^{-5} M strychnine, which suppresses components of transient amacrine cell responses [52] (Fig. 3c). In contrast, Murakami et al [53] report that both L- and C-type S-potential units in the carp retina hyperpolarize after application of 5mM GABA and depolarize by some 10 mV in response to its antagonist, picrotoxin. Our experimental results [52] establish, however, that C-type S-potentials are more sensitive to the action of picrotoxin than are L-type S-potentials. Perhaps the most interesting feature of L_1-type S-potentials is their behavior following bleaching with a 0.1-sec red (647.1-nm) laser beam. As is illustrated in Figure 2b, the membrane potential repolarizes within some 8 to 10 sec after bleaching to a level close to the prebleaching dark resting potential. At the same time, the light-evoked S-potentials are almost completely suppressed, so that the units are effectively clamped in a dark adapted state. We have observed that this postirradiation depolarization is maintained for at least 10 min following bleaching,

---

Fig. 3. Single neuronal responses. The membrane voltage is displayed against time, with hyperpolarization denoted by downward displacement of the trace. The lowest trace of each record denotes the stimulus monitor. (a) Effect of localized $CoCl_2$ perfusion on L_1-type S-potentials. Presentation of beam S_1 (seen in Fig. 1b) located concentrically around the recording elctrode, is denoted by upward displacement of the stimulus monitor and presentation of the peripheral beam, S_2, by downward displacement of the stimulus monitor. The scan speed was periodically increased to display the response waveform. $CoCl_2$ was injected in 0.5-sec bursts for the periods denoted by the horizontal bars above the trace. Note the selective reduction of the S-potentials elicited by the central beam. (b) Effects of spraying 4 mM picrotoxin on to the retina during the period indicated by the horizontal bar above the response traces. The S-potentials were elicited by alternative 1-μW/mm^2, 636-nm and 0.5-μW/mm^2, 493-nm light flashes, denoted, respectively, by upward and downward displacement of the stimulus monitor. Upper trace: biphasic C-type unit; lower trace: L_1-type unit. Note that picrotoxin selectively depolarizes the C-type unit and reverses the polarity of its depolarizing signal. (c) Effects of spraying 4 mM strychnine on to the retina, during the period indicated by the horizontal bar above the trace. Upper trace, transient amacrine cell; lower trace, L_1-type unit. Other parameters as in Fig. 3b. Note the selective suppression of the amacrine cell "on" spike elicited by the 493-nm light flash. (d) The effect on L_1-type responses of 0.1-sec irradiation with a 647.1-nm, 0.13-W/mm^2 laser beam at the time denoted by the arrow below the time base. The 30 mM $CoCl_2$ was sprayed onto the retina during the period denoted by the horizontal bar above the response trace. Other parameters as in Figure 3b. Note that the maintained depolarization which follows laser irradiation is abolished by $CoCl_2$. (e) L_1-type S-potentials elicited by 2.5-sec exposure, denoted by the horizontal bars, to a 2-mW/mm^2, 632.8-nm laser beam, with successive exposures taken every 10 sec. The upper trace refers to a normal retina and the lower to a retina perfused for 2 min with Ringer's solution containing 2.5 mM phentolamine. Note the relaxation of membrane potential following the onset of the laser beam in the upper trace, and its absence from the lower trace. (f) As (e), but with the addition of continuous stimulation of the retina with diffuse, 650-nm light flashes, denoted by upward displacement of the time base. Note the recovery of sensitivity to the diffuse light flashes in the phentolamine perfused retina.

but it is rapidly abolished following application by spraying of cobalt chloride (Fig 3d), which suggests that it is associated with chemical synaptic activity. The postirradiation response was further characterized by recording L_1-type S-potentials under a 2.5-sec exposure to a 632.8-nm laser beam with flux level 1 mW/mm. At this illumination level, the beam was about 1.0 log units greater than the level which produced saturation of the S-potential hyperpolarization and some 0.5 log units greater than the minimum level required to produce rapid relaxation of the membrane potential after the initial hyperpolarization. The time course of membrane potential change during a single exposure to the laser beam varied considerably from unit to unit, but with repeated exposure, the membrane potential always returns rapidly toward the dark adaptation level (Fig 3e, upper trace). When the retina is perfused for 2 min with 2.5 mM phentolamine, however, the L_1-type S-potentials are sustained during laser exposure ([54]; Fig 3e, lower trace). Phentolamine reduces the response amplitude at the onset of laser exposure, but the response to a 5-mm diameter light spot (effectively diffuse illumination) is essentially the same in the normal and phentolamine treated retina (Fig. 3f), thus the reduced response to laser irradiation does not indicate general loss of sensitivity. The records of Figure 3f also show that there is rapid recovery of sensitivity to flashes of diffuse light in the phentolamine perfused, but not in the normal retina. The significance of these observations is disscussed below, in relation to retinal circuits involving horizontal cells.

L_2 - Cone Type

The second class of cone L-type S-potentials, designated L_2-, are sensitive primarily to green and blue lights (Fig. 2c). After 0.1 sec bleaching with a red (647.1-nm) laser beam, the spectral response curve changes, and becomes similar to the absorption spectrum of B-cones, but after 0.1 sec bleaching with a blue–green (488-nm) beam, the amplitudes to light-evoked potentials were too small for accurate spectral analysis. We conclude that this response class receives a mixed input from both G- and B-cones, and in addition, about 50% of such units exhibit a small amplitude (<5 mV) depolarization response for stimulus wavelengths greater than 670 nm. We classify these units as L-type because this depolarizing response is present in only half the units and is of such small amplitude. These depolarizing responses may reflect inhibitory feedback signals, of the kind observed in turtle cones (see introduction section) and in the perch [55]. After 0.1 sec bleaching by either red (647.1-nm) or, particularly, blue–green (488-nm) laser beams, L_2-units display extended hyperpolarization with reduction of light-evoked responses (Fig. 2c). Thus, like rod S-potential units, but in sharp contrast to L_1-type units, they are clamped in a light-adapted state by bleaching lights.

Biphasic C-type

The biphasic C-type units depolarize under long wavelength and hyperpolarize under short wavelength light stimulation, but the "neutral" wavelength at which the response polarity reverses varies between 540 and 650 nm from one dark-adapted retina to another. After 0.1 sec bleaching by a red (647.1-nm) laser beam, C-units depolarize to a level approximately equal to the saturation level of depolarizing responses elicited by flashes of red light (Fig. 2d). Light-evoked responses are then essentially hyperpolarizing for all stimulus wavelengths, with a spectral response which follows closely that of B-cones (Fig. 2d). After 0.1-sec bleaching with a blue–green (488-nm) laser beam, the C-units display membrane potential changes similar to those observed in L_1-type units, and their subsequent light-evoked responses are entirely depolarizing for all stimulus wavelengths. The spectral characteristics of these depolarization responses, with peak sensitivity at about 650 nm, is shifted to the long wavelength side of the R-cone absorption spectrum, in a manner similar to that found in other studies (see introduction section). We consider that this shift in spectral sensitivity reflects hyperpolarizing activity arising in the G-cones, which is not completely eliminated by the bleaching light. The fact that the "neutral" wavelength sometimes occurs at 650 nm in the dark-adapted retina indicates that the G-cones exert hyperpolarizing influence which opposes the long wavelength-sensitive depolarizing response. (As B-cones have insignificant absorption for wavelengths greater than 560 mn, they cannot be responsible for this hyperpolarizing activity). We have been unsuccessful, however, in our efforts to isolate the G-cone contribution to C-type responses. As was previously discussed, 10^{-5} M picrotoxin depolarizes C-type units and causes reversal of depolarizing responses to light (Fig. 3b). The responses thus become entirely hyperpolarizing, with spectral sensitivity similar to the B-cone absorption spectrum, but with a bulge in the range 500 to 560 nm. We can use the effects of bleaching lights to test the feedback hypothesis of depolarizing C-type S-potential generation (see introduction section.) We recorded simultaneously L_1- and C-type S-potentials, and initially we determined V-log I characteristics for a series of 0.3-sec, 656-nm light flashes (Fig. 4a). A 0.1 sec 647.1-nm laser bleach was then applied, and the time course of subsequent membrane potential changes was recorded. The V-log I characteristics define the relationship between hyperpolarizing L_1-responses and depolarizing C-responses, thus if there were direct inhibitory coupling between L_1- and C-units, we could predict the C-unit potential level corresponding to a given L_1-potential level. The time course of C-unit membrane potential following bleaching has been calculated in this way from the L_1-unit potential values, and is plotted together with the experimental values (Fig. 4b,c). It is apparent that the two sets of values deviate considerably from each other, particularly when equilibrium is reached, at which point the C-units maintain

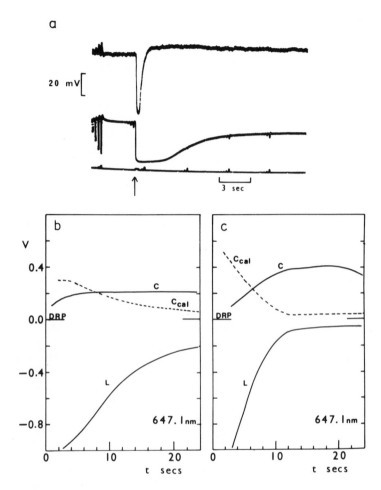

Fig. 4. (a) C-type (upper trace) and L_1-type (lower trace) S-potential responses. Calibration responses for a series of 0.3-sec light flashes (wavelength 656 nm), with illumination level increased by 0.4 log units between successive flashes, are shown at the beginning of the trace. These flashes were repeated at regular intervals, as indicated by the stimulus monitor trace. The retina was irradiated for 0.1 sec by a 647.1-nm, 0.13-W/mm² laser beam, applied at the time indicated by the arrow below the stimulus monitor trace. (b,c) Normalized membrane potentials for two pairs of C- and L-type response units, taken from records such as those of Figure 4a, plotted against time after exposure to the laser beam. The voltage scale is normalized such that the maximum amplitude of L_1-type hyperpolarization is -1.0, and the pre-irradiation dark-resting potentials of all units are adjusted to $V = 0$ (DRP). Experimental values are denoted by full lines and the broken lines, C_{cal}, represent the values of C-unit membrane potentials derived from the calibration responses of the kind shown in Figure 4a.

steady depolarization, whereas the calculation shows that they should repolarize to their dark resting potential. These results establish that simple inhibitory feedback between L_1- and C-units cannot, by itself, describe the effects of bleaching, and we examine this conclusion below in relation to the retinal circuitory.

Other Neuronal Classes

We have recorded data for bipolar, amacrine, and ganglion cells under conditions similar to those applied in the study of horizontal cells. In particular, we have examined the effects of bleaching lights on resting potentials and on light evoked responses, as is illustrated in Figure 5. In general, spike potentials exhibit greater recovery following bleaching than do slow potentials. This is especially so in the case of amacrine cells, where units which give sustained responses to light in the dark-adapted retina generate spike potentials after bleaching (Fig. 5c) and the slow components which in dark adaptation accompany "on" and "off" transient amacrine cell responses are selectively suppressed by bleaching (Fig. 5d). The time course of cell membrane changes induced by bleaching has proved an essential factor in the analysis of horizontal cell function given in the following section, thus we consider it important that intracellular responses are characterized even for those units, such as ganglion cells, from which extracellular spike potentials may be readily recorded.

Retinal Circuits Involving Horizontal Cells

We have summarized the experimental observations presented above in the network diagrams of Figure 6. In these diagrams, Trifonov's [27] hypothesis is assumed, thus excitatory synapses between photoreceptors and horizontal cells, denoted by plus signs, release neurotransmitter in darkness and the neurotransmitter flow rate at these synapses is reduced by light. Spectral classes of cone which give maximum light absorption at 625, 535, and 455 nm [12] are denoted respectively by R-, G-, and B- cones. The characteristics of the local networks can be summarized with reference to each class of S-potential unit.

Rod-type response units (Fig. 6a).   We have detected no cone input to to the rod-type S-potential units, nor do they display relaxation of membrane potential during or following excitation with strong lights such as laser beams 2a). We therefore show only rod input to these units, which correspond to the to the intermediate layer of horizontal cells. Coupling between these cells is implied by the large receptive field area associated with each response unit.

L_2-type cone-driven units (Fig. 6b).   Spectral analysis shows that L_2-type S-potential units receive excitatory synaptic input from G- and B- cones

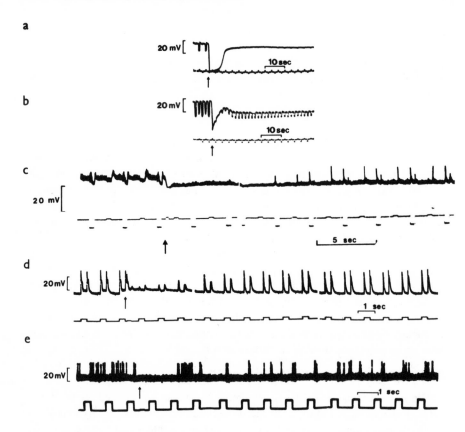

Fig. 5. Traces showing the responses of different retinal response units before and after 0.1-sec irradiation with a 647.1-nm, 0.13-mW/mm² laser beam, presented at the points denoted by the arrows. Responses were elicited by repeated, alternate presentation of two light flashes, one of wavelength 636 nm and flux 1.0 μW/mm², and the other of wavelength 493 nm and flux 0.5 μW/mm² (denoted by upward and downward displacement of the stimulus monitor trace, respectively). All stimuli were circular spots of 1.0 mm in diameter. (a) L$_1$-type S-potential, (b) L$_2$-type S-potential, (c) sustained amacrine cell, (d) transient amacrine cell, and (e) ganglion cell. Note the suppression of sustained response components in records (c and d).

(Fig. 2c) and in addition, about 50% receive a weak inhibitory input from R-cones, which results in depolarization responses for λ ≥ 670 nm. This input is represented in Figure 6b by a broken line, but we have no evidence on whether or not it involves feedback from the R- onto G- and B-type cones. Superficially, the spectral responses of L$_2$-units are similar to those of the biphasic C-type units (Fig. 6c) but the two can be readily differentiated, because in the presence of a maintained green background field, C-units always depolarize in response to superimposed light flashes of wavelength 620 nm, whereas L$_2$-units always

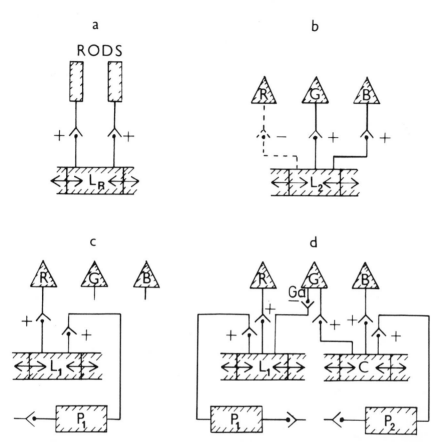

Fig. 6. Network diagrams showing synaptic connections involving the horizontal cells which generate the different classes of S-potential (a) Rod horizontal cells, L_R, receiving excitatory input from rods (b) L_2-type horizontal cells receiving excitatory input from B-and G-cones, and, in some 50% of cases, inhibitory input from R-cones. (c) L_1-type horizontal cells receiving excitatory input from R-cones and P_1-units. (d) Biphasic C-type horizontal cells receiving excitatory input from G-and B-cones and inhibitory input from R-cones via the Gabanergic synapse Ga. They also receive excitatory input from P_2-units.

hyperpolarize. Procion yellow injection shows that L_2-units have significantly larger cell bodies and thicker axons than C-units and, most importantly, L_2-type units give sustained hyperpolarization during stimulation by the red or blue–green laser beams whereas C-type units exhibit rapid relaxation of membrane potential to the dark resting potential.

L_1-type cone-driven response units (Fig. 6c). Spectral analysis shows that these units receive excitatory input only from R-cones (Fig. 2b) but in addition, their membrane potential depolarizes rapidly from the initial hyper-polarization induced by the laser beams (Fig. 2b). This depolarization is blocked by cobalt chloride (Fig. 3d) and by the α-adrenergic blocker phentolamine (Fig. 3e), which implies that it depends on the activity of a synapse sensitive to phentolamine. Spatially localized stimulation by the laser beam not only produces sustained depolarization of L_1-type S-potential units, but also depresses their response to subsequent stimulation by diffuse illumination (Fig. 3f). In the phentolamine perfused state, however, the response to diffuse illumination re-covers rapidly after laser stimulation (Fig. 3f). As the bleaching effects of the laser beam should be the same in both normal and phentolamine-treated retinae, the loss of sensitivity to diffuse light which occurs only in normal retinas cannot be attributed to desensitization of bleached photoreceptors, and in order to in-terpret our observations we have invoked the activity of a second synaptic mech-anism, driven by a neurone designated P_1 (Fig. 6c). We propose that in response to bright lights, retinal neurone P_1, which is presynaptic to the L_1-type horizontal cells, depolarizes and releases an excitatory neurotransmitter to which phento-lamine acts as antagonist. This transmitter both depolarizes the L_1-class response units and decouples them from each other, thereby preventing lateral transmission of signals along the horizontal cell layer. Following stimulation with bright lights, these effects are long lasting, eg, after 0.1-sec irradiation with a 0.13-W/mm^2, 647.1-nm laser beam, no significant recovery in sensitivity to subsequent light flashes was observed over 15 min of recording from the same unit. Phen-tolamine blocks the action of the P_1-cell transmitter and consequently bright light stimuli yield maintained hyperpolarization of L_1-units (Fig. 3e) and there is rapid recovery of response to diffuse light after the bright light stimulus is extinguished (Fig. 3f). We recall that the dopaminergic interplexiform cell makes presynaptic contact with the cone-driven external horizontal cells, but not with the rod-driven medial horizontal cells, and the application of dopamine causes depolarization and decoupling of S-potential units [42,43]. It seems probable therefore, that the P_1-cells of Fig. 6c represent interplexiform cells, but phentolamine is not a specific dopamine blocker and application of the dopamine specific antagonists haloperidial (in the form Serenace) and chlorpromazine gave only marginal blocking of the laser induced S-potential response characteristics. This may reflect the inability of the drugs to penetrate adequately the retinal tissue and we are currently examining the effects of other agents. The data of Figure 3e show that phentolamine reduces the amplitude of the initial hyperpolarization response of L_1-units to the laser beam, thus it appears to change the response properties of the dark-adapted retina. We conclude, therefore, that the transmitter to which phentolamine acts as antagonist is active in darkness. Local perfusion of cobalt chloride does not influence the coupling between horizontal cells, (Fig. 3a) which is consistent with the view that this coupling is mediated by electrotonic rather than chemical synapses. Thus, in order to influence the horizontal cell coupling, dopamine must act on the electrotonically coupled horizontal cell membranes. As the retinal dopamine receptors are all associated with adenylate cyclase [41], we are currently examining the action of cyclic AMP and related agents on the response characteristics of L_1-type horizontal cells.

Biphasic C-type cone-driven response units. C-type units receive excitatory input from B-cones and inhibitory input from R-cones, both of which can be revealed by spectral analysis following spectrally selective retinal bleaching [14]. The spectral sensitivity of the depolarizing responses is displaced to the long-wavelength side of the R-cone absorption spectrum and we interpreted this as evidence that G-cones also make excitatory synaptic contact with C-units, although we were unable to isolate this spectral response component. The red-sensitive depolarizing component of C-type S-potentials is selectively abolished by the GABA antagonist picrotoxin [52,53]. The network diagram of Figure 6d contains a feedback loop between R- and G-cones, operating through L_1-type horizontal cells, as suggested by Fuortes and Simon [28] and supported by the anatomical observations of Stell and Lightfoot [24] and Marc et al [31]. Thus in darkness, L_1-units are depolarized by excitatory transmitter released by R-cones, and as a result, the inhibitory transmitter GABA is released at synapse Ga (Fig. 6d), which hyperpolarizes G-cones and reduces release of excitatory neurotransmitter to C-units. Long-wavelength lights hyperpolarize R-cones, thereby reducing the release of GABA at synapse Ga and depolarizing G-cones, which, in turn, depolarize C-units. Picrotoxin blocks the GABAergic synapse, and thus abolishes the depolarizing component of C-type responses (Fig. 3b). We note that the networks of Figures 6b and 6d imply that only those G-cones which drive C-units receive significant feedback from L_1-units. Biphasic C-type units also exhibit rapid changes in membrane potential during or following laser beam stimulation (Fig. 2d), and thus like the L_1-type units, they appear to receive more than one synaptic input. We have, therefore, shown biphasic C-type units in post-synaptic contact with P_2-cells (Fig. 6d), which are analogous to the P_1-cells of Figure 6c. We have not characterized the properties of the P_2-cell synaptic input to C-units as fully as those of the P_1-cell input to L_1-units, but the two may differ at least in their spectral characteristics, with the former being blue sensitive and the latter red sensitive. We showed previously, under the results section (Fig. 4), that after 0.1-sec exposure to the 647.1-nm laser beam, the experimental values of the C-unit membrane potential differ significantly from those predicted by the feedback model. We attribute this to the sustained activity elicited by the laser of the P_2-cell driven synapse onto the C-units.

SUMMARY

The principal conclusions of our work may be summarized as follows.
(1) Rod and cone-driven horizontal cells can be classified according to their

spectral response characteristics, as was originally demonstrated by Svaetichin [1,2]. The feedback model of C-unit depolarization requires that those G-cones which drive C-units receive significant inhibitory input from R-cones (Fig. 6d). In contrast, such feedback must be virtually absent from G-cones which drive L_2-units (Fig. 6b) as about half the L_2-units exhibit no depolarization at any wavelength and the remainder only weak depolarization for wavelengths greater than 670 nm.

(2) Cone-driven horizontal cells can also be differentiated on the basis of their responses to strong lights. We propose that L_1- and C-type S-potential units, which give rapid relaxation of membrane potential from the initial hyperpolarization level, are postsynaptic to both photoreceptors and P_1-(or P_2-) cells.

(3) The P-cell input to horizontal cells can be blocked by phentolamine and although dopamine-specific antagonists are less effective in this respect than is phentolamine, the P_1-cells probably correspond to the dopaminergic interplexiform cells.

(4) The lateral electrotonic coupling between horizontal cells is modified, through a mechanism which has yet to be elucidated, by P_1-cell synaptic activity.

(5) The effect of phentolamine is to increase the time constant of the S-potentials (Fig. 3e) and correspondingly to maintain coupling between horizontal cells (Fig. 3f). P1-cell synaptic input, which is blocked by phentolamine, therefore, provides a mechanism for control of the horizontal cell receptive field sizes.

(6) An essential problem in the interpretation of retinal circuitry is the identification of the associated neurotransmitters; horizontal cell depolarization appears to be mediated through sites sensitive to the excitatory neurotransmitter agonists kainic and quisqualic acids, but not to N-methyl-D-aspartate [56].

ACKNOWLEDGMENTS

Our studies on S-potential and associated retinal responses were stimulated by a visit made by K.H. Ruddock to the laboratory of the late Dr. G. Svaetichin at IVIC Caracas, and we have subsequently benefited greatly from his advice and encouragement. K.H. Ruddock acknowledges with thanks the receipt of a grant from the Nuffield Foundation which supported the experimental work reported here; M.B.A. Djamgoz thanks the Worshipful Company of Spectacle Makers for the award of a 350th Anniversary Fellowship for retinal research and S.H. Reynolds thanks the Science Research Council for the award of a postgraduate research studentship. We wish to thank Dr. R.W. Smith of the Physics Department, Imperial College, for his generous loan of some of the laser equipment used in these experiments and our colleague, Dr. J.S. Rowe, who collaborated in some of the experiments for helpful discussion.

REFERENCES

1. Svaetichin G: The cone action potential. Acta Physiol Scand 29 Suppl 106:565, 1953.
2. Svaetichin G: Spectral responses of single cones. Acta Physiol Scand 39 Suppl 134:18, 1956.
3. Adian Ed, Matthews R: The action of light on the eye. Part 1. The discharge of impulses in the optic nerve and its relation to the electric charge in the retina. J Physiol (London) 63:378, 1927.

4. Hartline HK: The response of single optic nerve fibers of the vertebrate eye to the illumination of the retina. Amer J Physiol 121:400, 1938.

5. Granit R, Svaetichin G: Principles and techniques of the electrophysiological analysis of colour reception with the aid of micro-electrodes. Upsala Läkareför, Förh 65:161, 1939.

6. Macnichol E,F Jr, Svaetichin G: Electrical responses from the isolated retinas of fishes. Amer J Ophthal 46 No. 3 Pt II:26, 1958.

7. Svaetichin G, MacNichol EF Jr: Retinal mechanisms for chromatic and achromatic vision. Ann NY Acad Sci 74:385, 1958

8. Mitarai G, Svaetichin G, Vallecalle E, Fatehchand R, Villegas J, Laufer M: Glia-neuron interactions and adaptational mechanisms of the retina. In Jung R, Kornhuber H (eds): "The Visual System: Neurophysiology and Psychophysics." Berlin: Springer–Verlag, 1961, pp463–481.

9. Svaetichin G, Negishi K, Fatehchand R: Cellular mechanisms of a Young–Herring visual system. CIBA Symp. on colour vision, physiology and experimental psychology. London: Churchill, 1965, pp 178–203.

10. Naka KI, Rushton WAH: S-potentials from colour units in the retina of fish (Cyprinidae). J Physiol (London) 185:536, 1966.

11. Mitarai G, Asano T, Kijake Y: Identification of five types of S-potential and their corresponding generating sites in the horizontal cells of the carp retina: Japan J Ophthal 18:161, 1974.

12. Marks WB: Visual pigments of single goldfish cones. J Physiol (London) 178:14, 1965.

13. Ruddock KH, Svaetichin G: The effects of maintained light stimulation on S-potentials recorded from the retina of a teleost fish. J Physiol (London) 244:569, 1975.

14. Djamgoz MBA, Ruddock KH: Adaption effects in electrical responses recorded from postreceptoral neurones in the isolated fish (roach) retina. Vision Res 19:413, 1979.

15. Norton AL, Spekreijse M, Wagner HG, Wolhbarsht ML: Receptive field organization of the S-potential. Science 160:1021, 1968.

16. Naka KI, Rushton WAH: The generation and spread of S-potentials in fish (Cyprinidae). J Physiol (London) 192:437, 1967.

17. Kaneko A: Electrical connexions between horizontal cells in the dogfish retina. J Physiol (London) 231:95, 1971.

18. Mitarai G: The origin of the so-called cone potential. Proc Japan Acad 34:299, 1958.

19. Werblin FS, Dowling JE: Organization of the retina of the mudpuppy, Necturus maculosus II. Intracellular recording. J. Neurophysiol 32:339, 1969.

20. Kaneko A: Physiological and morphological identification of horizontal, bipolar and amacrine cells in goldfish retina. J Physiol (London) 207:623, 1970.

21. Ramon y Cajal S: La retine des vertebres. Cellule 9:119, 1893.

22. Stell WK: The structure and relationship of horizontal cell and photoreceptor–bipolar synaptic complexes in goldfish retina. Amer J Anat 121:401, 1967.

23. Parthe V: Horizontal, bipolar and oligopolar Cells in the teleost retina. Vision Res 12:395, 1972.

24. Stell WK, Lightfoot DO: Colour specific interconnections of cones and horizontal cells in the retina of the goldfish. J Comp Neurol 159:473, 1975.

25. Tomita T, Kaneko A, Murakami M, Pautler EL: Spectral response curves of single cones in the carp. Vision Res 7:519, 1967.

26. Baylor DA, Fuortes MGF: Electrical responses of single cones in the retina of the turtle. J Physiol (London) 207:77, 1970.

27. Trifonov YA: Study of synaptic transmission between photoreceptors and horizontal cells by means of electrical stimulation of the retina. Biofizika 13:809, 1968.

28. Fuortes MGF, Simon EJ: Interaction leading to horizontal cell responses in the turtle retina. J Physiol (London) 240:177, 1974.

29. Baylor DA, Fuortes MGF, O'Bryan PM: Receptive fields of cones in the retina of the turtle. J Physiol (London) 214:265, 1971.

30. O'Bryan PM: Properties of depolarizing synaptic potentials evoked by peripheral illumination in cones of the turtle retina. J Physiol (London) 235:207, 1973.

31. Marc RE, Stell WK, Bok D, Lam DMK: GABAergic pathways in the goldfish retina. J Comp Neurol 182:221, 1978.
32. Dowling JE, Werblin FS: Organization of the retina of the mudpuppy Necturus maculosus 1. Synapsic structure. J Neurophysiol 32:315, 1969.
33. Witkovsky P, Dowling JE: Synaptic relationship in the plexiform layers of carp retina. Z Zellforsch 100:60, 1969.
34. Furukawa T, Hanawa I: Effects of some common cations on electroretinogram of the toad. Japan J Physiol 5:284, 1955.
35. Cervetto L, MacNichol EFJ: Inactivation of horizontal cells in turtle retina by glutamate and aspartate. Science 178:767, 1972.
36. Murakami M, Ohtsu K, Ohtsuka T: Effects of chemicals on receptors and horizontal cells in the retina. J Physiol (London) 227:899, 1972.
37. Takeuchi A, Takeuchi N: The effect on crayfish muscle of iontophoretically applied glutamate. J Physiol (London) 170:296, 1964.
38. Marshall LM, Werblin FS: Synaptic transmission to the horizontal cells in the retina of the larval tiger salamander. J Physiol (London) 279: 321, 1978.
39. Gallego A: Horizontal and amacrine cells in the mammal's retina. Vision Res Suppl 3:1971.
40. Dowling JE, Ehinger B: Synaptic organization of the aminecontaining interplexiform cells of the goldfish and monkey retinas. Science 188:270, 1975.
41. Watling JK, Dowling JE, Iversen LL: Dopamine receptors in the retina may all be linked to adenylate cyclase. Nature (London) 281:578, 1979.
42. Hedden WL, Dowling JE: The interplexiform cell system. II. Effects of dopamine on goldfish retinal neurones. Proc Roy Soc Lond B 201:27, 1978.
43. Negishi K, Drujan BD: Effects of catecholamines and related compounds on horizontal cells in the fish retina. J Neurosci Res 4:311, 1979.
44. Negishi K, Sugawara K, Kato S: Effects of chemicals on light-induced responses in the isolated carp retina. Annais da Academia Brasileira de Ciencias 45 (Suppl):111, 1973.
45. Stell WK: Horizontal cells axons and axon terminals in goldfish retina. J Comp Neurol 159:503, 1975.
46. Crescitelli F, Dartnall HJA: A photosensitive pigment of the carp retina. J Physiol (London) 125:607, 1954.
47. Kaneko A, Yamada M: S-potentials in the dark adapted retina of the carp. J Physiol (London) 227: 261, 1972.
48. Ruddock KH, Svaetichin G: Fast and slow components of intracellulary recorded responses from retinal units of a teleost fish (Eugerres plumieri). Vision Res 13:1785, 1973.
49. Brindley GS: Effects on colour vision of adaptation to very bright lights. J Physiol (London) 122:1332, 1953.
50. Dartnall HJA: "The Visual Pigments" London: Methuen, 1957.
51. Djamgoz MBA, Ruddock KH: Effects of local cobalt chloride injection on lateral spread of signals in fish (roach) retina. Neurosci Lett 10:23, 1978.
52. Djamgoz MBA, Ruddock KH: Effects of picrotoxin and strychnine on fish retinal S-potentials: Evidence for inhibitory control of depolarizing responses. Neurosci Lett 12:329, 1979.
53. Murakami M, Shimoda Y, Nakatani K: Effects of GABA on neuronal activities in the distal retina of the carp. Sens Proc 2:334, 1978.
54. Djamgoz MBA, Reynolds SH, Rowe JS, Ruddock KH: Control of retinal S-potentials in dark adapted and bleached retinae. Vision Res 21:1581, 1981.
55. Burkhardt DA: Responses and receptive-field organization of cones in perch retinas. J. Neurophysiol 40: 1977.
56. Rowe JS, Ruddock KM: Identification of neurotransmitter binding sites on retinal horizontal cells. J. Physiol (London) 318:20P, 1981.

The S-Potential, pages 257–279
© 1982 Alan R. Liss, Inc., 150 Fifth Avenue, New York, NY 10011

Electrophysiological Studies of Drug Actions on Horizontal Cells

Miguel Laufer

INTRODUCTION

The rare potentials that Svaetichin described in 1953 [1], recorded by means of glass microelectrodes upon illumination of the isolated retina, were unheard of and indeed strange to neurophysiologists. The maintained hyperpolarization of up to 30 mV induced by light was interpreted by many as an experimental artifact. Unsuspected as those potentials were, they generated great suspicion from colleagues. The original interpretation of a cone origin gave way to a more internal generation site [2, 3], although doubts were cast upon their actual origin as they did not seem to be intracellular [4, 5]. In recognition to the discoverer this peculiar form of neuronal activity was termed S-potential after 1959 [6], and the horizontal cell (HC) was definitively established as its cellular origin by means of intracellular fluorescent dye injections [7]. The large size of HCs in the retinas of various lower vertebrates has permitted the stable recording of their membrane potentials during periods of time long enough to characterize their properties and to essay the actions of exogenous agents. Furthermore, the possibility to isolate the tissue from the rest of the animal, and yet be able to stimulate it with its physiological stimuli and to apply foreign substances to it while it remains in apparent good, testable functional conditions, has made the retina of cold-blooded animals an extensively probed preparation. A large number of reports exist that deal with the actions of ions, of probable neurotransmitters, and of very diverse chemicals on the electrical potentials generated by HCs—the S-potentials. To review them comprehensively is not our aim; only some significant recent findings and their implications will be examined. First, some of the ideas developed by Svaetichin during the 1960s will be presented and discussed, as they are based to a very large extent on observations of the effects of chemicals on HCs.

OVERVIEWS OF SVAETICHIN'S VIEWS

The series of papers published by Svaetichin and his colleagues during the 1960s [8–15] postulated an important role for HCs, thought initially to be glial elements, in the control of retinal excitability. The basic supports for their conclusions were morphology and the effects of diverse agents. The cells that generate S-potentials were considered to be axonless glial cells, a notion that was soon overridden by the present concept of HCs as neuronal elements. HCs were found to be particularly sensitive to many agents and conditions applied to the isolated retina, such as temperature variations, CO_2, NH_3, and anoxia [9]. The effects produced were always opposite to those observed on typical neuronal structures, such as spinal ganglion cells or peripheral nerves. Cooling the retina, for instance, resulted in depolarization of the HC membrane with an increase in the amplitude of S-potentials, whereas heating it led to hyperpolarization with S-potential reduction. On typical neurons, conversely, hyperpolarization or depolarization of the membrane potential were observed after cooling or heating. Similar complementary effects were found after the application of CO_2 and NH_3. The membrane potentials of HCs were also found to be very sensitive to anoxia, which resulted in a transient depolarization followed by hyperpolarization and S-potential reduction. The effects were found to be irreversible if anoxia was maintained for about 10 minutes or more, and the high temperature sensitivity was then lost.

The initial observations were confirmed repeatedly [12–15] and the idea of a complementary function of neurons and "controller cells" was developed. The term "controller cell" was coined by Svaetichin [12] to denote cells that, although they were no longer considered to be glia, had a characteristic nonspiking electrical behavior and a particular sensitivity to the agents tested, which was clearly different from and in many cases opposite to that of typical neurones. Such cells could, in Svaetichin's view, exert control over neuronal excitability through two mechanisms: metabolic interrelation and feedback. His vision of a metabolic interrelation was based on an energy-supplying machinery in the controller cell, and energy transfer mechanisms through respiratory chains located at the cell membranes. The membrane of the neurons was considered to be a rather passive element, concerned mainly with ionic movements for which the energy was supplied by the controller cell. These ideas served him to explain the changes observed in the firing patterns of retinal ganglion cells, and he further extended his views to the control of neural activity in general. Acceleration and deceleration of cellular respiration by CO_2 and NH_3, for example, led to an indirect modulation of excitability, resulting in depression or augmentation of neuronal activity.

The understanding of the complex effects produced by agents that interfere with cellular metabolism is extremely difficult, and much more so in an intricate and heterogeneous neuronal circuitry such as the retina. A major flaw in the interpretation given by Svaetichin and his colleages to their observations was that the effects of the agents applied to the retina were considered to be exerted directly on the HCs. Photoreceptors were considered as simple light detectors and transducers, and the interposed synapse was practically ignored. Many of the effects reported, indeed, could have been explained as being due to changes in the photoreceptors or in the transmission of signals between them and HCs. Large transreceptoral extracellular voltages, observed upon illumination after application of NH_3 vapors, were considered to be the result of an action of this agent on HC metabolism [12, 16]. It is now known that the blockade of the activity in second order neurons, as seen after aspartate application [17] results in a large distal P III. This could explain the findings with NH_3 vapors, although the initial depolarization of the dark potential of HCs remains to be explained. It could be the result of a transient increase in the neurotransmitter liberation from the photoreceptors, or of a secondary ionic imbalance. The effects of anoxia, on the other hand, have been characterized in more detail. While the transreceptoral field potential evoked by light remains unchanged, electrical activity ceases in the proximal retina [18], implying that photoreceptors can still operate as transducers but transmission is blocked. Furthermore, it has been shown that the lateral spread of S-potentials continues to take place in an anoxic area of the retina [19], and that isolated HCs have a very small oxygen consumption while that of photoreceptors is high [20]. Thus, the primary effects of anoxia appear to be exerted on the photoreceptor synapse. Transmission is blocked, leading to HC hyperpolarization, and this happens before the photoreceptors cease to respond to light, as revealed by the transreceptoral potentials. But, contrary to the case of NH_3 vapors, the transreceptoral potentials do not increase in amplitude. The reason could be that photoreceptors themselves are affected by anoxia. The initial dark level depolarization of the HC under anoxia could similarly be due to a transient increase in the liberation of neurotransmitter.

Besides metabolic interactions, Svaetichin postulated a second form of excitability control excerted by HCs. It consisted in a feedback mechanism leading to the control of excitability and resulting in the various activity patterns of retinal neurons. The idea of a feedback control, first hinted at in 1961 [11] and further developed later [21, 22], was based on the observation of oscillatory potentials in HCs, on the correspondence between HC membrane potential and ganglion cell excitability, and on the convenience of the consideration of feedback to explain the wide range of luminosities under which the eye can operate, as well as to explain the genesis of the opponency in the polarity of C-type S-potentials. A nonspecific negative feedback from the HC, which was conceived both as a comparator and as a regulator, onto the photoreceptor-bipolar transmission mechanism was thought to set the gain of the system and explained the changes in sensitivity during neural adaptation to different light levels, despite a linear receptor process [16]. The same principle, but with appropriate, or specific, channeling of the negative feedback effect onto selective bipolar types could determine the opponent firing patterns of ganglion cells [21]. In Svaetichin's example [22] a given HC connected to cones containing 610-nm absorbing photopigment would be hyperpolarized by its direct cone input. Through feedback, it would change the input into itself, and would also, through "crossed" feedback, elicit a response of opposite polarity (ie, depolarizing) in the horizontal and bipolar cells connected to the cone containing 465-nm absorbing pigment.

It is now accepted that negative feedback indeed exists and is responsible for spectral opponency, although it is exerted on photoreceptors. Even though speculative and in many aspects erroneous, Svaetichin's views were conceptually so close to the ideas put forward by Fuortes and Simon [23] and extensively discussed in other chapters of this book!

MANIPULATION OF THE IONIC ENVIRONMENT

In both eyecup and isolated retina preparations the effects of changes in the ionic composition of the bathing solution can be tested. The most conclusive evidence obtained with such manipulation has supported a depolarizing transmitter liberated by photoreceptors in darkness. The original hypothesis of Trifonov [24] was supported by his experiments with extrinsic current application. Substitution of Ca^{2+} by other divalent ions in order to block synaptic transmitter liberation has provided direct evidence for the validity of Trifonov's theory. In the turtle [25] and mudpuppy [26] 2 mM Co^{2+} hyperpolarizes HCs, eliminating their responses to light while cones remain relatively unaffected. We have observed the same effect in HCs of the teleost Eugerres plumieri. In the skate [27] 50 mM Mg^{2+} has a similar effect, which is also obtained with 20 mM Mg^{2+} in the carp [28]. Experiments performed on the eugerres retina show that above 1 mM Co^{2+} the transmission block is complete after 1 or 2 minutes of perfusion, and that during the beginning of the effect, and particularly during Co^{2+} washing, submaximal HC responses show an increased amplitude. Lower Co^{2+} concentrations reveal more clearly this phenomenon (Fig. 1A). The progressive transmission block leads to hyperpolarization due to diminished Na^+ permeability of the HC membrane (see below). In this condition the membrane potential is dominated by K^+ permeability, which is not affected by Co^{2+}. The light-induced arrest of remaining transmitter liberation is then able to bring the membrane closer than before to the K^+ equilibrium. This increase of submaximal light responses is not merely a consequence of the potential level attained by the HC membrane, since a similar hyperpolarization produced by an equivalent light background leads to reduction of the responses. However, when different receptor populations are illuminated, mutual enhancement of HC responses takes place [29]. Another common observation is that the ratio between the response elicited by a local spot illumination and that elicited by a concentric light annulus decreases. The relative dominance of the response elicited at a distance implies that direct transmission is more affected than is lateral spread, through intercellular coupling, in HCs.

A comparable result to that obtained with Co^{2+} or Mg^{2+} should be accom-

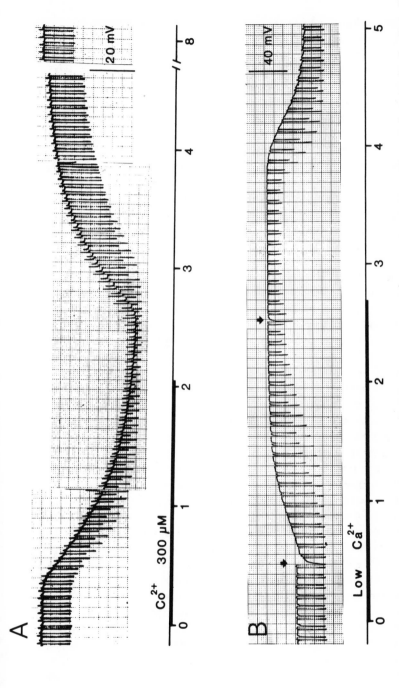

Fig. 1. A. Recording from a cone-connected horizontal cell in the isolated perfused Eugerres plumieri retina. During the period indicated by the thick lower tracing, a Ringer solution containing 300 μM Co^{2+} was applied. Pairs of alternating concentric light spots and annuli were used to stimulate the retina, with intensities eliciting responses less than half-maximal in normal Ringer. During the Co^{2+}-produced hyperpolarization, responses to spots are smaller than those to annuli. Time is in minutes. B. Similar recording, showing the effect of low Ca^{2+} (about 5 μM). Pairs of stimuli in this case elicited maximal responses. The ceiling potential of the cell was ascertained by applying supramaximal stimuli (arrows). During the induced depolarization, responses to light spots are larger than those to annuli. Time is in minutes.

plished by Ca^{2+} withdrawal from the bathing solution, as the former cations are considered to block transmission by interfering with Ca^{2+} entry at the synaptic terminal. Carp [28] and turtle [25] cones, as well as frog rods [30], depolarize slightly and generate larger responses to light in Ca^{2+}-free medium, while HCs hyperpolarize and their responses dissappear, as expected. In eugerres, however, Ca^{2+} withdrawal depolarizes, instead of hyperpolarizing, cone-connected HCs [31, 32] (Fig. 1B). Such HC depolarization is maintained in the presence of low Ca^{2+} for more than 10 minutes. Responses to low-level illumination usually decrease from the beginning of low Ca^{2+} effects. On the other hand, maximal responses show a marked increase in amplitude during the initial phase of depolarization and decrease thereafter, disappearing completely if Ca^{2+} falls below 10^{-6} M. During recovery, a similar response increase ensues. The depolarization appears to be the result of an increased Na^+ permeability of the HC membrane (see below) as well as of photoreceptors. The transient increase of maximal responses results from the larger potential gradient to the unchanged K^+ equilibrium, while there is enough transmitter release from photoreceptors, whose light responses also increase [28]. Eventually, release is impaired and the HC responses are reduced or abolished. A similar HC depolarization with response reduction by low Ca^{2+} has been reported in the axolotl retina [33]. The ratio of locally and distantly evoked HC response amplitudes is generally in favor of the local one under low Ca^{2+}, and implies that lateral spread through HC coupling is reduced.

The experimental variation of the extracellular ionic composition has promoted understanding of some of the mechanisms responsible for the generation of HC potentials. After synaptic blockade with high Mg^{2+} in the carp, the HC membrane behaves very closely to a K^+ electrode [28]. In normal solution the K^+ dependence of both the eugerres and turtle HC membranes, relatively low in the dark, increases and approximates a K^+ electrode under strong illumination [31, 32] (Fig. 2A), which also blocks transmitter release from photoreceptors. Under low Ca^{2+} the HC membrane becomes even less dependent on extracellular K^+ concentration. This is due to its high dependence upon Na^+ under these conditions, and not to a low K^+ permeability.

The membrane potential of the HC is thus dependent upon K^+ gradients in its "resting" condition, ie, without synaptic input from photoreceptors, in the light or after Co^{2+} or high Mg^{2+} application. In the dark, on the other hand, the membrane potential is dominated by the Na^+ gradient. The reversal potential of the HC response, slightly above zero [34], points to this fact. Reduction of Na^+ content in the bathing fluid reveals a very strong dependence of HC membrane potential in the dark, and of responses to light, upon Na^+ in both photoreceptors and HCs of axolotl retina [33]. In eugerres, the HC membrane potential in the dark is markedly dependent upon external Na^+ [31, 32] (Fig. 2B) as a result of the Na^+ dependence of the presynaptic cell (the photoreceptor),

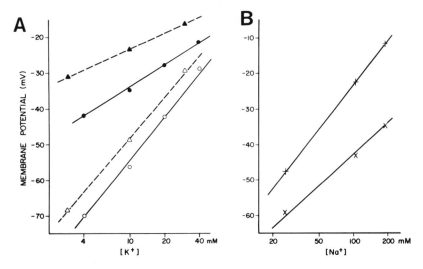

Fig. 2. A. Dependence of horizontal cell membrane potentials upon K^+ concentration of the perfusion solution in the Eugerres isolated retina (circles) and in the Pseudemys scripta elegans eyecup preparation (triangles). Filled symbols, membrane potential in the dark; open symbols, maximal membrane potential under strong illumination. Hand-drawn lines represent approximate relationship in each case. B. Dependence of the horizontal cell membrane potential in the dark upon Na^+ concentration of the perfusion solution in the Eugerres isolated retina. Normal Ca^{2+} (2.5 mM, X) or low Ca^{2+} (5 μM, +).

added to the Na^+ dependence of the HC (probably the subsynaptic membrane) under the action of a depolarizing neurotransmitter. This Na^+ dependence in the dark is further increased by perfusion with low Ca^{2+}, despite an impaired transmitter liberation. Under low Ca^{2+} conditions the HC membrane is very close to a Na^+ electrode (Fig. 2B).

Variations of gradients and movements of Cl^-, alone or accompanying other ions, must also be of importance to HCs, but the situation is less clear. Cl^--free solutions have been reported to hyperpolarize the HC in the mudpuppy retina [35], but this happens after more than 5 minutes of perfusion with such solutions. We have observed a similar effect, after a short transient period of depolarization, in the eugerres isolated retina. In the eyecup of the turtle, substitution of Cl^- by either methylsulfate or isethionate does not markedly alter the membrane potential of the HC for 10 to 15 minutes, after which it shows a slow oscillatory behavior (Fig. 3).

The existence of different ionic permeabilities in different regions of the HC membrane [36] does not permit a simple comprehensive explanation of the ionic dependence of its potentials. The depolarizing photoreceptor neurotransmitter

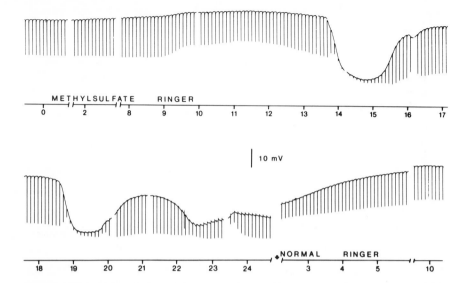

Fig. 3. Recording from a horizontal cell in the Pseudemys eyecup. At time 0 methylsulfate was substituted for chloride. No changes took place in the membrane potentials during the initial 9 minutes. Thereafter the cell membrane depolarizes and hyperpolarizes alternately. Normal solution was restituted at arrow, after 28 minutes of Cl⁻-free perfusion. Recovery is almost complete after 5 or 6 minutes. Similar results were obtained substituting Cl⁻ with isethionate.

appears to modulate HC membrane potential by its ability to increase Na^+ permeability at the subsynaptic sites. This ion dominates HC membrane potencial in the dark, but the existence of a not negligible and voltage-dependent K^+ permeability of the membrane results in a potential of about -30 mV. The reduction of Na^+ permeability when photoreceptors are hyperpolarized by light or their synapse is blocked leads to a potential dominated by the K^+ permeability of the nonsynaptic membrane, and tends to a value of -70 mV. A further complexity results from the electrical coupling between HCs of a given layer [37], which is variable (see below). The synaptic modulation of a given HC will influence the membrane potential of its neighbors, and the whole layer acts as a coupled network, which minimizes the changes taking place in one or a few cells. This results in the large receptive field of the HC.

EFFECTS OF PUTATIVE NEUROTRANSMITTERS ON THE HC

As stated by Gerschenfeld and Piccolino in their review of the pharmacology of photoreceptor transmission, "few problems in neurobiology are as difficult as that of establishing beyond doubt that a substance is a transmitter at a specific synapse," including the vertebrate retina as well [38]. Extensive reviews on this problem have been published [38–40]; and we will only remark upon some recent findings that, rather than clarifying the issue of the chemical nature of HC synaptic activation, illustrate the complexity of the experimental identification of the pertinent transmitters.

Amino Acids

Excitatory, or depolarizing, amino acids have been extensively tested. Both L-glutamate (Glu) and L-aspartate (Asp) depolarize turtle and fish HCs [41, 42], but the effects reported require concentrations of at least several millimoles, a fact that casts doubt on their actual physiological role. The depolarizations are due to postsynaptic effects since they occur after synaptic transmission has been arrested by saturating lights or Co^{2+} application. In the carp, contrary to early reports [43], it has been found that low doses of around 0.1 to 0.3 mM of L-Asp are sufficient to exert a half-maximum effect, which is blocked by αDL-aminodipic acid [44]. In contrast, 5 mM of L-Glu and L-lysine were needed for a comparable result and were not blocked by GDEE and GDME. The method of application used in these experiments [44]—atomization of a solution on the isolated retina—does not permit an accurate knowledge of the actual concentration, but comparatively L-Asp appeared to be 10 times more potent than the other amino acids tested. Thus L-Asp was considered as a good candidate for the cone transmitter in the carp. A recent report [45] concludes that in goldfish cones the possible neurotransmitter is glutamate, not aspartate. Both L-isomers depolarize the HC at several mM, but L-Glu can do it at 15 times less concentration if applied together with D-Asp, which blocks Glu uptake.

In the isolated retina of eugerres millimolar concentrations of either L-Glu or L-Asp depolarize the HC membrane and abolish light responses. Their effects persist after Co^{2+} application and are not blocked by GDEE or αDL aminoadipic acid [46, 47]. However, at 500 μM or less they have a hyperpolarizing effect. Such hyperpolarization in the case of L-Glu is blocked by picrotoxin but not by GDEE, and has been tentatively interpreted as resulting from a metabolic conversion of L-Glu into GABA, which similarly hyperpolarizes the cone-connected HCs when applied exogenously (Fig. 4). The results obtained so far in this species do not point to L-Glu or L-Asp as likely photoreceptor neurotransmitters. Synthesis, accumulation, and liberation studies have not been performed, but the identity in the actions of both amino acids suggests a lack of specificity, further indicated by the high concentration needed to observe depolarizing effects on the HC. Finally, whatever the mechanism of the observed hyperpolarization with low doses, which are likely to be closer to physiological concentrations, the effect is opposite that of depolarization of the HC expected from the photoreceptor transmitter.

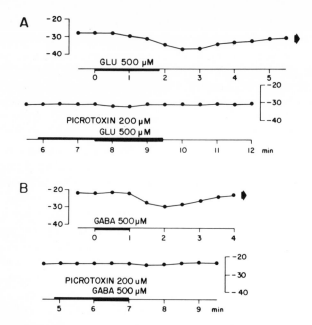

Fig. 4. A. Hyperpolarization of the membrane potential in the dark by perfusion with low L-glutamate concentration in a cone horizontal cell of the isolated Eugerres retina. Without interruption the drug was again applied during perfusion with picrotoxin, which blocks the effect. B. Similar experiment in another preparation, perfused with low GABA concentration. Scales in millivolts.

Besides the search for a depolarizing and effective neurotransmitter, inhibitory amino acids have been extensively probed on HCs. In goldfish, the HC connected to red pigment cones contains GAD [48] and accumulates GABA [49], and its light-induced hyperpolarization leads to an increase of GABA content [49], thought to occur as the result of liberation arrest. Furthermore, GABA, which hyperpolarizes the HC membrane in carp [50] is a likely transmitter for the feedback synapse from HC to photoreceptor. Indeed, in carp [50] and rudd [51] it has been shown that excess GABA, or picrotoxin, eliminates the depolarizing responses to long wavelength lights in C-type HC. In the retina of eugerres, GABA similarly hyperpolarizes cone-connected HCs and blocks depolarizing responses to red light in C-type cells (which are also blocked by picrotoxin), but does not affect the membrane potential of rod-connected HCs, even at 10 mM (Fig. 5). In the superfused turtle eyecup, on the other hand, GABA at millimolar concentrations depolarizes the HCs, an effect that persists after Co^{2+} application because of its postsynaptic nature (Fig. 6). The observed effects on the HC membrane potential, which are opposite in teleosts and turtle, need not

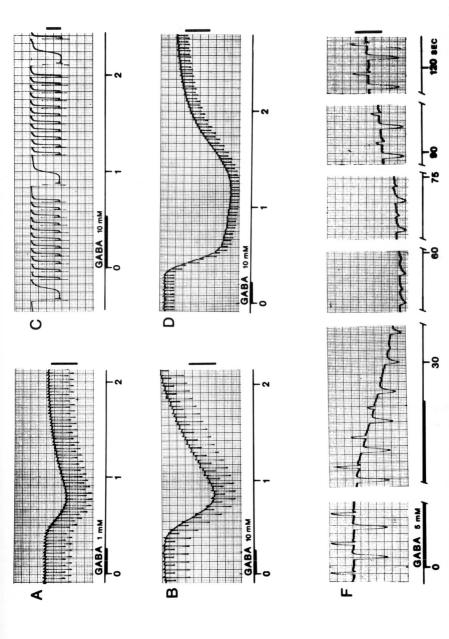

Fig. 5. Recordings from horizontal cells in the perfused isolated Eugerres retina. Effects of GABA applications in cone horizontal cells (A,B,D), in red horizontal cell (C), and in G/R⁺ color horizontal cell (F). Note absence of hyperpolarization in red horizontal cell (C) and inversion of depolarizing responses to red flashes in cell in F. In A to D, time is in minutes. Vertical calibration bars: 10 mV.

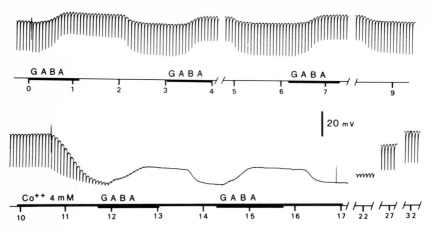

Fig. 6. Recording from a horizontal cell in the perfused eyecup of Pseudemys. Three successive applications of 20-mM GABA result in similar depolarizing effects. During membrane hyperpolarization resulting from synaptic blockade produced by Co^{2+}, reapplication of GABA results in depolarization similar to that observed previously in the maximal potential attained under illumination. This was observed also in other instances, irrespective of the magnitude of the GABA-induced depolarization. Time is in minutes.

be related to a functional role of GABA. Specific GABA receptors have not yet been reported in HCs and the effects could be due to changes in different ionic conductances in different species, or to the same conductances but in opposite directions. It is interesting that glycine, which hyperpolarizes the HC membrane as GABA does in carp [50] as well in eugerres, has an effect opposite to that of GABA in the HC of the turtle. In this retina glycine hyperpolarizes whereas GABA depolarizes the HC membrane (Fig. 7).

Cholinergic Agents

The search for a depolarizing neurotransmitter from photoreceptors has steered studies on the effect of cholinergic agents on HC membrane potentials. The machinery for acetylcholine (ACh) biosynthesis has been reported to exist in turtle photoreceptors [52]; and nicotinic binding sites have been found in the outer plexiform layer of turtle, goldfish, and chick retinas [53, 54]. Electrophysiological probing, on the other hand, has not rendered a clear picture. In an early study no effect on the HC was found when ACh was sprayed on the isolated carp retina [43]. In another study [55] on the same preparation it was reported that ACh, perfused at 10^{-5} M, produced a depolarization of the HC with disappearance of light responses, but the effect was deemed presynaptic, as it was absent after synaptic blockade. In an extensive study of the effects of

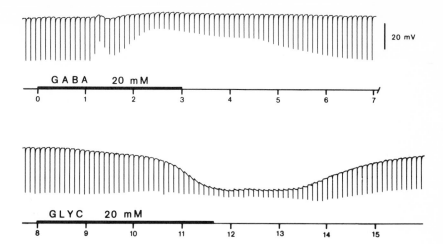

Fig. 7.   Recording from a horizontal cell in the perfused eyecup of Pseudemys. Effects of successive applications of 20-mM GABA and glycine. Time is in minutes.

cholinergic agents on HCs of the perfused turtle eyecup [38], no changes of membrane potential or responses were observed with Ach, and carbachol was reported to have a variable and discrete effect. Whereas nicotine depolarized the cone connected HC, the nicotinic agonist decamethonium and several nicotinic antagonists were ineffective. Of muscarinic agents, only pilocarpine produced a marked depolarization, whereas various antagonists, particularly atropine, hyperpolarized the HC. We have confirmed most of these results on the turtle retina, and compared the effects with those obtained in the isolated carp retina.

In the carp, ACh was found not to modify the membrane potentials of the HCs. Both carbachol and betanechol produce very small and variable effects. Application of 5 mM of either drug resulted in membrane potential changes of only up to about 5 mV, in either direction. Small depolarizations reduced the dark membrane level or the response maximum in an irregular fashion, whereas small hyperpolarizations were more noticeable in the dark membrane level. Pilocarpine and nicotine had more powerful effects at 5 mM, but were practically ineffective at 1 mM. Pilocarpine reduced and abolished light responses, while the dark level changed very little and irregularly. Nicotine, on the other hand, produced a marked depolarization of the dark level and also abolished the light responses (Fig. 8). These observations do not fit the picture of a specific cholinergic effect: high concentrations of carbachol do not produce clear effects. Some muscarinic and nicotinic agonists are active, but only at very high doses in both turtle and fish, while other agonists are not. It is tempting to conclude

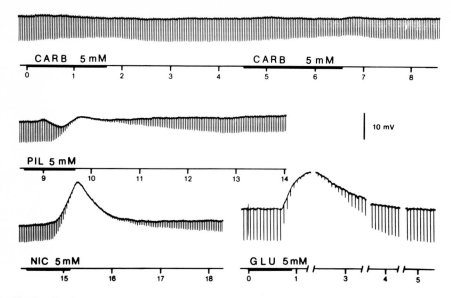

Fig. 8. Continuous recording from a cone horizontal cell in the perfused isolated retina of Cyprinus carpio. Successive applications of 5-mM carbachol (twice), pilocarpine, and nicotine as indicated. The effect of L-glutamate, at the same concentration in a cell from another carp retina, is shown for comparison. Time is in minutes.

that the observed changes are nonspecific effects at concentrations so high that little expectation remains for a physiological role of the substances tested. The effects of atropine on HCs of the turtle retina [56] are of particular interest. At 5 mM atropine hyperpolarizes the L-type HC and completely blocks S-potentials after some 20 minutes of perfusion but does not affect the center hyperpolarizing bipolars. It leads to the disappearance of feedback onto photoreceptors, due to HC block, as revealed in recordings from both HCs and cones. The high dose of atropine needed and the prolonged application required do not favor the blockade of a specific synaptic effect. In the isolated carp retina, we have observed a similar effect of atropine on HCs, in less time and with 10 times lower concentrations than in the turtle eyecup, but this does not afford an argument for specificity.

Another observation pertaining to the actions of cholinergic agents on the HC is that of a contraction of the receptive field in both the salamander [57] and the eugerres [58, 59] retina upon application of millimolar concentrations of ACh. Also in the turtle eyecup preparation, 5 mM carbachol leads to an increase in the HC responses to small centered light spots and a reduction of the responses

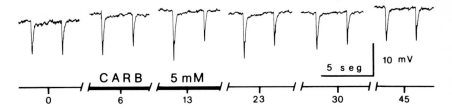

Fig. 9. Effect of carbachol application on a horizontal cell in the perfused Pseudemys eyecup. Perfusion time in minutes. Fast recordings are shown of pairs of responses to a local light spot and a concentric light annulus. Note relative predominance of the response to the light spot during carbachol perfusion.

evoked by a light annulus indicating a marked contraction of the receptive field (Fig. 9). These effects will be discussed in the next section.

Catecholamines

Several aspects of the morphology of catecholamine-containing cells, and of the effects of various catecholamines on the HC membrane potential and its responses to retinal illumination, are treated in the chapter by Drujan. We will only discuss the mechanisms by which dopamine could modulate the extent of the receptive field of HCs in the fish retina. As stated above, ACh was found to produce a contraction of the size of the receptive field, together with a membrane resistance increase, in the tiger salamander retina [57]. We have observed a similar contraction by carbachol (Fig. 9) and dopamine in the turtle retina. In the fish, ACh and various catecholamines have also been shown to contract the HC receptive field [58]. Several experimental manipulations point to dopamine as the immediate agent responsible for the effect. The effect of ACh is blocked by hexamethonium, which does not interfere with that of dopamine [58]. On the other hand, the effects of both substances disappear when the dopamine antagonists phentolamine [58] or haloperidol [59] are used. These antagonists also impede the HC receptive field contraction produced by substance P [59]. A possible interpretation is that both ACh or carbachol and substance P are able to depolarize dopaminergic cells and thus induce the liberation of dopamine. Since these agents do not produce a marked direct effect on the HC membrane potentials, the effect of dopamine liberation can be observed [59]. This hypothesis is supported by the finding that carbachol and substance P, which produce only small contractions of the HC receptive field, become very active after the retina has been perfused with dopamine [59] (Fig. 10). Dopaminergic cells would be capable of dopamine uptake, and after they have been loaded with dopamine the depolarizing agents

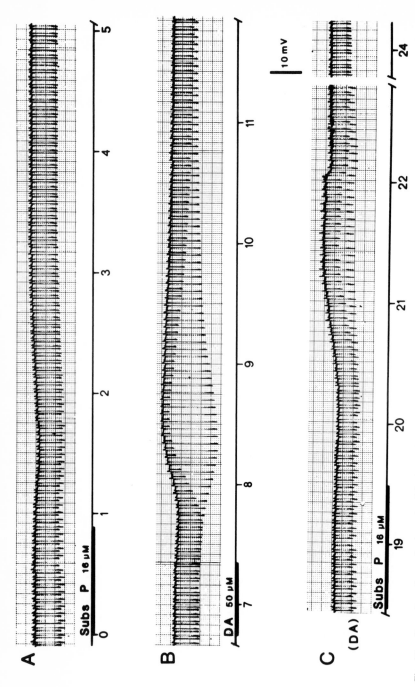

Fig. 10. Recordings from a horizontal cell in the perfused isolated retina of Eugerres, stimulated by pairs of light spots and concentric light annuli. Substance P, which had no obvious effect in the relation between the two responses when applied in A, became effective in C, after two dopamine applications, one of which is shown in B. Time is in minutes. From [59].

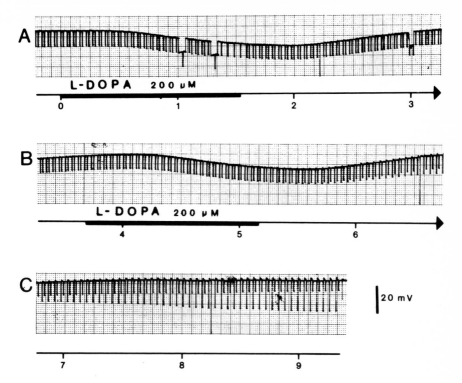

Fig. 11. Continuous recordings from a horizontal cell in the perfused isolated retina of Eugerres. Pairs of responses were elicited by spots and concentric annuli of light. Two equal L-DOPA applications preceding A were also ineffective, but after the fourth application, in B (accumulated DOPA administration of 6 minutes), a pronounced contraction of the receptive field is observed (C). Time is in minutes.

could liberate it in significant amounts. Indeed, histofluorescence studies [60] reveal that dopamine is taken up by dopaminergic cells, and that carbachol, ACh, and substance P reduce their dopamine content. L-dopa also enhances fluorescence, because of dopamine, in dopaminergic cells [60]. L-dopa was reported to be ineffective in producing contraction of the receptive field in HCs [61]. However, when perfusion with L-dopa is prolonged for several minutes, a contraction of the HC receptive field takes place (Fig. 11). Time is needed for the metabolic convertion of L-dopa into dopamine (see pages 281–305), and the receptive field contraction will be apparent only after dopaminergic cells contain excess dopamine that "leaks" out of them. Another observation provides further support for the hypothesis of dopamine mediation and is in agreement with histofluorescence observations. Repeated applications of either carbachol or substance P lead to a reduced effect, and finally no effect is observed. This could be due to some kind of desensitization but, after dopamine reapplication (and loading), a potent effect reappears [59]. Thus, it is reasonable to postulate that repeated applications of depolarizing agents lead to a depletion of dopamine from dopaminergic cells. It is of interest that in freshly isolated retinas, which show little fluorescence, carbachol and substance P produce discrete, if any, contraction of the HC receptive field and after a second or third application an effect can no longer be observed [59].

The idea of a final dopaminergic step in the HC receptive field contraction by different pharmacological agents, well supported in the fish retina, faces a major obstacle in the case of the turtle retina. In the latter, receptive field contraction can be obtained with 10^{-5} M dopamine or with several millimols of carbachol (Fig. 9). But dopaminergic cells, which in the fish are true interplexiform cells and form a rich terminal plexus at the level of HCs [62], are restricted in the turtle to the inner plexiform layer. Their cell bodies are located at the innermost part of the inner nuclear layer, separated by tens of microns from HCs. For dopamine to diffuse through such a large distance in order to exert an action is unlikely, as it would be metabolized and, if effective, very unspecific.

The contraction of the receptive field of the HC, which results in larger responses to local light stimuli and smaller responses from distant illuminated areas, could be explained if the coupling resistance between HCs did increase. This would lead to an increased total membrane resistance and a larger local response induced by equal synaptic currents, but less current flowing from neighboring cells, which for any given layer are electrically coupled [37]. In order to find what resistances, if any, vary in relation with changes in the receptive field of HCs, experiments were performed with triple microelectrodes in the isolated and perfused eugerres retina [63, 64]. The neighborhood, or separation, between two impaled cells was verified by injection of a different procyon dye into each of them. Voltage drops produced in two neighboring cells by current injection into one of them permits the evaluation of the apparent coupling resistance between them. But the problem remains as to the magnitudes of the changes in the total membrane resistance of a cell and those of the coupling resistance between neighbors. Since HCs form a mosaic in which each cell is surrounded by six cells, resistances were evaluated with a simplified linear network model for an hexagonal array of identical elements. Two values were obtained: a) the membrane resistance of the cell, inclusive of synaptic and nonsynaptic resistance between the HC interior and the bath, and excluding the six parallel coupling resistances between the cell and its neighbors; and b) the coupling resistance between the two impaled cells. The contraction of the receptive field produced by dopamine occurs in association with changes in both resistances. The apparent intercellular coupling, defined as the ratio between the measured voltage drops in the two cells due to the current injected into one of them, always inversely follows the changes in coupling resistance. The increase observed in the response to a local small stimulus is associated with an increase, variable and of up to three times, in the membrane resistance. But the reduction in the response to distant illumination does not follow the temporal course of the increase of either resistance. It depends upon the relative changes of the two of them. Obviously, the conditions of intracellular current injection and of regional illumination are not equivalent. Alternative computations, with the assumption that one of the two resistances remains invariable while only the other one is affected, led to unreasonable results.

The dopamine-induced changes responsible for the modulation of the extent of the HC receptive field should manifest themselves as changes in the gap junctions between the cells. These, in turn, should be observable as changes in the electrical coupling between the cells, as described above, and also as changes in the passage of small molecules across the junctions and as ultrastructural changes. In eugerres, injection of Lucifer yellow into an HC under normal conditions always results in pronounced fluorescence of the HCs surrounding the injected cell, and sometimes in weak fluorescence of more distant cells. Under perfusion with dopamine only the injected cell is strongly fluorescent, providing direct evidence of the increase in the effectiveness of coupling between HCs (Fig. 12).

CONCLUSIONS

The numerous studies published by Svaetichin and his co-workers throughout almost three decades have stemmed from his discovery of the electrical activity of retinal horizontal cells (HC) and were aimed at the understanding of vision and nervous functions from both an electrophysiological and a biochemical viewpoint. Though wrong on occasions, Svaetichin elaborated important and frontier-opening concepts on the metabolic control of nervous excitability and on the role and mechanism of nervous feedback control.

The manipulation of the ionic composition of the extracellular environment in the retina has permitted a better understanding of transmitter release from photoreceptors and of the ionic mechanisms responsible for the electrical behavior of horizontal cells. The roles of Na^+ and K^+ permeabilities in the modulation by light of horizontal cell responses is now better understood, although the share of different parts of the cell membrane and the mechanisms involved require further study.

The characterization of a depolarizing photoreceptor neurotransmitter remains obscure despite abundant research. Neither depolarizing amino acids nor cholinergic agents appear to have the expected specificity. Their effects are usually observed at exorbitant doses and the antagonists tested have not afforded consistent data. At least GABA is a good candidate for the horizontal cell feedback

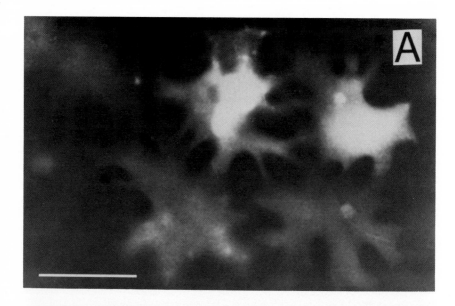

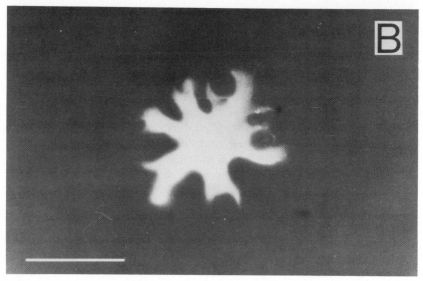

Fig. 12. Fluorescence photomicrographs of horizontal cells injected with Lucifer yellow in the perfused isolated Eugerres retina. Approximately equal injection current and time were used under normal conditions (A) and during perfusion with 200 μM dopamine (B), which produced a marked contraction of the receptive field of the cell. Calibration: 40 μm.

mediator in teleosts. Dopamine has emerged as a good candidate for the final mediator in the modulation of the receptive field extent in horizontal cells, which in turn determines the spatial and chromatic characteristics of bipolar and ganglion cells.

Horizontal cells, particularly in the retinas of lower vertebrates, which can be perfused with experimental solutions while in good functional conditions, have been and continue to be a good experimental model for the study of nonspiking interneurons participating in local circuits of the central nervous system.

ACKNOWLEDGMENTS

The author wishes to express his gratitude to Rina Lamarca, Rigoberto Guerrero, and Rafael Salas who performed many of the experiments on the eugerres retina reported in this work, and to Hersh Gerschenfeld, Marco Piccolino, and the Neurobiology Laboratory, École Normale Supérieure of Paris, where the experiments on carp and turtle retina were performed. This work was supported by grant S1-0747 from CONICIT (Consejo Venezolano de Investigaciones Científicas y Tecnológicas).

REFERENCES

1. Svaetichin G: The cone action potential. Acta Physiol Scand 29(suppl 106):565, 1953.
2. MacNichol EF Jr, MacPherson L, Svaetichin G: Studies on spectral response curves from the fish retina. Symposium on Visual Problems of Colour, National Physical Laboratory, Teddington, England, 1957, pp 531.
3. Mitarai G: The origin of the so-called cone potential. Proc Jpn Acad 34:299, 1958.
4. Tomita T, Murakami M, Sato Y, Hashimoto Y: Further study on the origin of the so-called cone action potential. Jpn J Physiol 9:63, 1959.
5. Gouras P: Graded potentials of bream retina. J Physiol 152:487, 1960.
6. Motokawa, K: Physiology of Color and Pattern Vision. Tokyo: Igaku Shoin, 1970, p 8.
7. Kaneko A: Physiological and morphological identification of horizontal, bipolar and amacrine cells in goldfish retina. J Physiol 207:623, 1970.
8. Svaetichin G, Laufer M, Mitarai G, Fatehchand R, Vallecalle E, Villegas G: Glial control of neuronal networks and receptors. In Jung R, Kornhuber H (eds): The Visual System: Neurophysiology and Psychophysics. Berlin: Springer, 1961, p 445.
9. Laufer M, Svaetichin G, Mitarai G, Fatehchand R, Vallecalle E, Villegas G: The effect of temperature, carbon dioxide and ammonia on the neuron-glia unit. Ibid., p 457.
10. Mitarai G, Svaetichin G, Vallecalle E, Fatehchand R, Villegas G, Laufer M: Glia-neuron interactions and adaptational mechanisms of the retina. Ibid., p 463.
11. Vallecalle E, Svaetichin G: The retina as model for the functional organization of the nervous system. Ibid., p 489.
12. Svaetichin G, Negishi K, Fatehchand R, Drujan B, Selvin de Testa A: Nervous function based on interactions between neuronal and non-neuronal elements. Prog Brain Res 15:243, 1965.
13. Negishi K, Svaetichin G: Effects of anoxia, CO_2 and NH_3 on S-potential producing cells and on neurons. Pflügers Arch 292:177, 1966.
14. Negishi K, Svaetichin G: Effects of temperature on S-potential producing cells and on neurons. Pflügers Arch 292:206, 1966.

15. Fatehchand R, Svaetichin G, Negishi K, Drujan B: Effects of anoxia and metabolic inhibitors on the S-potential of isolated fish retinas. Vision Res 6:271, 1966.
16. Fatehchand R, Laufer M, Svaetichin G: Retinal receptor potentials and their linear relationship to light intensity. Science 137:666, 1962.
17. Sillman AJ, Ito H, Tomita T: Studies on the mass receptor potential of the isolated frog retina-I. General properties of the response. Vision Res 9:1435, 1969.
18. Negishi K, Sugawara K: Evidence for the anoxia sensitivity of the synaptic region at the outer plexiform layer in the fish retina. Vision Res 13:983, 1973.
19. Drujan BD, Svaetichin G, Negishi K: Retinal aerobic metabolism as reflected in the S-potential behavior. Vision Res 11(suppl 3):151, 1971.
20. Drujan BD, Svaetichin G: Characterization of different classes of isolated retinal cells. Vision Res 12:1777, 1972.
21. Svaetichin G, Negishi K, Fatehchand R: Cellular mechanisms of a Young-Hering visual system. In Wolstenholme GEW, Knight J (eds): Ciba Foundation Symposium on Physiology and Experimental Psychology of Colour Vision. London: Churchill, 1965, p 178.
22. Svaetichin G: Células horizontales y amacrinas de la retina: Propiedades y mecanismos de control sobre las bipolares y ganglionares. Act Cien Venez 18 (suppl 3):254, 1967.
23. Fuortes MGF, Simon EJ: Interactions leading to horizontal cell responses in the turtle retina. J Physiol 240:177, 1974.
24. Trifonov YA: Study of synaptic transmission between the photoreceptor and the horizontal cell using electrical stimulation of the retina. Biofizika 13:809, 1968.
25. Cervetto L, Piccolino M: Synaptic transmission between photoreceptors and horizontal cells in the turtle retina. Science 183:417, 1974.
26. Dacheux RF, Miller RF: Photoreceptor-bipolar cell transmission in the perfused retina eyecup of the mudpuppy. Science 191:963, 1976.
27. Dowling JE, Ripps H: Effect of magnesium on horizontal cell activity in the skate retina. Nature 242:101, 1973.
28. Kaneko A, Shimazaki H: Effects of external ions on the synaptic transmission from photoreceptors to horizontal cells in the carp retina. J Physiol 252:509, 1975.
29. Laufer M, Negishi K: Enhancement of hyperpolarizing S-potentials by surround illumination in a teleost retina. Vision Res 18:1005, 1978.
30. Brown JE, Pinto LH: Ionic mechanisms for the photoreceptor potential of the retina of Bufo marinus. J Physiol 236:575, 1974.
31. Guerrero R: Dependencia iónica de los potenciales de células horizontales en la retina de Eugerres plumieri. Tesis IVIC, 1977, pp 1–142.
32. Laufer M, Guerrero R: In preparation.
33. Waloga G, Pak WL: Ionic mechanism for the generation of horizontal cell potentials in isolated axolotl retina. J Gen Physiol 71:69, 1978.
34. Trifonov YA, Byzov AL, Chailahian LM: Electrical properties of synaptic and nonsynaptic membranes of horizontal cells in fish retina. Vision Res 14:229, 1974.
35. Miller RF, Dacheux RF: Synaptic organization and ionic basis of on and off channels in mudpuppy retina. I. Intracellular analysis of chloride-sensitive electrogenic properties of receptors horizontal cells, bipolar cells and amacrine cells. J Gen Physiol 67:639, 1976.
36. Byzov AL, Trifonov YuA: Membrane mechanisms of the activity of horizontal cells. In Drujan B, Laufer M (eds): The S-Potential. New York: Alan R. Liss, Inc., 1982, pp. 105–122.
37. Kaneko A: Electrical connexions between horizontal cells in the dogfish retina. J Physiol 213:95, 1971.
38. Gerschenfeld HM, Piccolino M: Pharmacology of the connections of cones and L-horizontal cells in the vertebrate retina. In The Neurosciences. Fourth Study Program. Cambridge: MIT Press, 1979, p 213.

39. Graham LT: Comparative aspects of neurotransmitters in the retina. In Davson H, Graham LT (eds): The Eye. Vol 6. New York: Academic Press, 1974, p 283.
40. Bounting SL (ed): Transmitters in the Visual Process. Oxford: Pergamon Press, 1976.
41. Cervetto L, MacNichol EF Jr.: Inactivation of horizontal cells in turtle retina by glutamate and aspartate. Science 178:767, 1972.
42. Sugawara K, Negishi K: Effects of some aminoacids on the horizontal cell membrane potential in the isolated carp retina. Vision Res 13:977, 1973.
43. Murakami M, Othsu K, Ohtsuka T: Effects of chemicals on receptors and horizontal cells in the retina. J Physiol 227:899, 1972.
44. Wu SM, Dowling JE: L-aspartate, a possible neurotransmitter from carp cones. Proc Natl Acad Sci USA 75:5205, 1978.
45. Ishida AT, Fain GL: D-aspartate potentiates the effects of L-glutamato on horizontal cells in goldfish retina. Proc Natl Acad Sci USA 78:5890, 1981.
46. Lamarca R: Estudio de L-aspartato y L-glutanato como posibles neurotransmisores de los conos retinianos. Tesis IVIC, 1982, p 1–72.
47. Laufer M, Lamarca R: In preparation.
48. Lam DMK, Su YYT, Swain L, Max RE, Brandon C, Wu YU: Immunocytochemical localization of L-glutamic acid decarboxylase in the goldfish retina. Nature. 278:565, 1979.
49. Marc RE, Stell WK, Bok D, Lam DMK: GABA-ergic pathways in the goldfish retina. J Comp Neurol 182:221, 1978.
50. Murakami M, Shimoda Y, Nakatani K: Effects of GABA on neuronal activities in the distal retina of the carp. Sens Processes 2:334, 1978.
51. Djamgoz MBA, Ruddock KH: Effects of picrotoxin and strychnine of fish retinal S-potential: Evidence for inhibitory control of depolarizing responses. Neurosci Lett 12:329, 1979.
52. Lam DMK: Biosynthesis of acetylcholine in turtle photoreceptors. Proc Natl Acad Sci USA 69:1987, 1972.
53. Yazulla S, Schmidt J: Radioautographic localization of ^{125}I-α-bungarotoxin binding sites in the retinas of goldfish and turtle. Vision Res 16:1878, 1976.
54. Vogel Z, Niremberg M: Localization of acetylcholine receptors during synaptogenesis in retina. Proc Natl Acad Sci USA 73:1806, 1976.
55. Kaneko A, Shimasaki H: Synaptic transmission from photoreceptors to bipolar and horizontal cells in the carp retina. Cold Spring Harbor Symp Quant Biol 40:537, 1976.
56. Gerschenfeld HN, Piccolino M: Muscarinic antagonists block cone to horizontal cell transmission in turtle retina. Nature 268:257, 1977.
57. Marshall LM, Weblin F: Synaptic transmission to the horizontal cells in the retina of the tiger salamander. J Physiol 279:321, 1978.
58. Negishi K, Drujan BD: Similarities in effects of acetylcholine and dopamine on horizontal cells in the fish retina. J Neurosci Res 4:335, 1979.
59. Laufer M, Negishi K, Drujan BD: Pharmacological manipulation of spatial properties of S-potentials. Vision Res 21:1657, 1981.
60. Negishi K, Laufer M, Drujan BD: Drug-induced changes in catecholaminergic cells of the fish retina. J Neurosci Res 5:599, 1980.
61. Negishi K, Drujan DB: Effects of catecholamines and related compounds on horizontal cells in the fish retina. J Neurosci Res 4:311, 1979.
62. Negishi K, Drujan BD, Laufer M: Spatial distribution of catecholaminergic cells in the fish retina. J Neurosci Res 5:621, 1980.
63. Laufer M, Salas R: Intercellular coupling and retinal horizontal cell receptive field. Neurosci Lett [Suppl] 7:339, 1981.
64. Laufer M, Salas R: In preparation.

The S-Potential, pages 281–305
© 1982 Alan R. Liss, Inc., 150 Fifth Avenue, New York, NY 10011

Biochemical Correlates of the S-Potential

Boris D. Drujan

INTRODUCTION

Historical Note

The discovery of the S-potential, approximately 3 decades ago, signaled a new era in the study of retinal function. It was Svaetichin [1] who for the first time observed a unique electrical response when an isolated retina was stimulated by light. Svaetichin, believing he was recording intracellularly from a single cone, named the response the "cone action potential."

Soon thereafter, other investigators observed the same phenomenon [2–4] but were doubtful that the response originated from the cones. They suspected that the recording was obtained from a retinal level proximal to the receptor cell layer. Furthermore, the characteristics of the response were very different from those which had been described for a neuronal membrane potential, because this light-evoked, sustained hyperpolarizing response was not accompanied by an action potential. For this reason it was thought doubtful that this potential resulted from an intracellular recording. Only later, when it became possible to mark cells intracellularly by injecting various dyes, was unequivocal evidence obtained that the S-potentials in the vertebrate retina originated from horizontal cells [5–8]. In the end, Motokawa proposed that the "cone action potential" should be called the "S-potential", S being the initial of Svaetichin.

The Electrophysiological Characteristics of the S-Potential

S-potentials are classified into two main types: The L-type (luminosity) response and the C-type (chromatic) response. The L-type potentials are hyper-

Since this book is meant to honor the important contribution Gunnar Svaetichin has brought to our knowledge of the retina, this article represents a brief summary of work carried out mainly with his collaboration or which was stimulated directly or indirectly by his ideas. The article is not intended to represent a complete review of the vast number of studies accomplished by many investigators in this specific field of retinal function.

polarizing in response to all wavelengths of the visible light spectrum, while the C-type can be either depolarizing or hyperpolarizing, depending on the wavelength of the light stimulus used. Moreover, in the fish retina, the photopic L-type potential can be further subdivided into three different subclasses, based on three different response maxima (λ max) of the spectral response curve; the three λ max are at 470, 530, and 610 nm [9,10]. In addition to the three photopic responses, a fourth, scotopic L-type response (λ max = 505 nm) can also be registered.

Similarly, two classes of the C-type potential can be distinguished, depending on whether the response is biphasic or triphasic [9]. The S-potentials most commonly obtained from the fish retina are (1) the photopic L-type with a maximum at 610 nm, (2) a C-type with two maxima (R/G λ max = 620 and 479 nm), and (3) the scotopic L-type (max = 505 nm).

Each of these responses was assumed to be generated in a different class of horizontal cells [9,11]. It is now generally accepted that the cells which generate the photopic and scotopic L-type reponses receive input signals respectively from either the red cones or rods, while the cells which generate the C-type responses receive two inputs: One of these is direct from a specific class of cones, while the other one may be mediated via a postulated "feedback loop" between cones and horizontal cells [12].

Functional Aspects of the Horizontal Cells

The horizontal cells in the retina were considered by Cajal [13,14] as "short axon cells" or "Golgi II cells," and, accordingly, he considered them analogous to similar cells found in abundance in the gray substance of the higher cerebral centers. Following Cajal very little further attention was paid to the morphology or the functional role of the horizontal cell in the retina. It was only after the discovery of the S-potential that these cells received renewed attention. However, because the horizontal cells do not possess the characteristic properties of a classical neuron, the early literature still referred to them by a variety of designations, such as "nonneuronal elements," "glia cells," etc. Nowadays, largely as a result of extensive electron microscope (EM) studies [12], the horizontal cell is classified as a retinal second-order neuron.

Based on studies of the S-potential, Vallecalle and Svaetichin [15] proposed the existence of an "automatic control system" in the retina, implicating the horizontal cell. Not long thereafter Svaetichin [9] proposed that "the nonlinearity responses obtained from structures subsequent to the receptors (Weber-Fechner behavior) is due to a feedback control system, possibly consisting of (1) a linear receptor input, (2) a neuronal forward conductor line, and (3) the horizontal cells as feedback elements." In this context and on the basis of physiological criteria, the horizontal cells were named "controller cells." Lipetz [16] and Byzov [17] presented further evidence in support of the idea that horizontal cells modulate the excitability of the retina. In their studies on adaptation mechanisms in man, Naka and Rushton [18–20] suggested the existence of an automatic gain control system in the retina, which would have a logarithmic transfer function. Accordingly, the horizontal cells were proposed to be involved in the negative feedback loop of the receptor-bipolar line [21], as well as to play a role in the spread of lateral inhibition along the outer plexiform layers [22,23].

The Lateral Propagation of the S-Potential

The size of the area in the retina stimulated by a constant light intensity influences the amplitude of the S-potential [7,24,25]. However, the horizontal cells do not simply duplicate the behavior of the photoreceptors. The area effect of the S-potential depends on the fact that the electrical response of the horizontal cells, evoked by the illumination of a restricted area, propagates to the neighboring nonilluminated areas [26,27]. Moreover, certain characteristics of the S-potential spread, such as its velocity (0.3 m/sec), as well as its high temperature dependence ($Q_{10} = 3$–4), suggests that electrical coupling between such cells [20,28] cannot alone explain the phenomenon [29–31].

These considerations, therefore, stimulated a number of studies directed toward elucidating the biochemical processes which might be implicated in the generation and spread of the S-potential.

AEROBIC METABOLISM

The S-potential has been shown to be highly sensitive to anoxia, or agents which interfere with aerobic metabolism, such as cyanide, azide, or carbon monoxide [32–34].

The dependence of the S-potential on aerobic metabolism is further underlined by studies comparing the effects of compounds abolishing anaerobic metabolism, as apposed to those interfering with aerobic metabolism. The former can be inhibited by glyceraldehyde which, however, has no effect on the potential. On the other hand, sodium malonate inhibits oxydative metabolism and, in the presence of this agent, both the L- and C-type responses are abolished [35] (Fig 1).

A similar effect can be obtained by exposing retinas to a gas mixture of 85% carbon monoxide and 15% oxygen. In this case the effect can be partially reversed by light [33]. The photochemical action spectrum and the wavelength maxima at which carbon monoxide inhibition can be reversed closely resemble the absorption coefficient curve for the carbon monoxide-respiratory enzyme complex [34,36].

Despite the fact that the generation of the S-potential in the horizontal cells is oxygen-dependent, evidence now indicates that these cells are little affected by conditions inhibiting oxidative metabolism in the retina. This has become evident from studies in which the respiration of the intact retina was compared

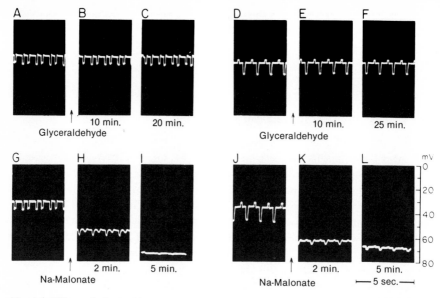

Fig. 1. Effects of glyceraldehyde and sodium malonate, anaerobic and oxydative metabolism inhibitors, respectively, on S-potentials from L-type horizontal cells (A–C and G–I) and C-type horizontal cells (D–F and J–L). Isolated fish retina. Drugs in 1 M solutions were sprayed on the retinal surface. Flashes of red and blue lights were alternated to elicit S-potentials [from 35].

with that of a retina where the receptor cell layer had been removed. The results indicated that at least 40% of the total retinal respiration can be attributed to the photoreceptors [35]. This was confirmed by measuring the oxygen consumption of single cells isolated from the retina (Table I). In such cells the receptors exhibited the highest respiratory rate, as opposed to isolated horizontal cells, which had the lowest rates of all cell types studies [31].

These observations also coincide with the morphological studies, which have revealed that the horizontal cells contain very few mitochondria, whereas the receptor ellipsoids are exceptionally rich in mitochondria. Finally, although no difference in oxygen uptake was observed between retinas during either scotopic or photopic conditions [35], intermittent light stimulation of their receptors, on the other hand, causes a sharp increase in retinal respiration [33,37]. All these findings thus indicate that the sensitivity of the S-potential to lack of oxygen is primarily a consequence of receptor properties which must initiate its generation. That was also demonstrated further by the fact that, once generated in an aerobic section of the retina, the potential can spread through an anoxic part of the retina. The propagation of the S-potential, which occurs via a definite horizontal cell layer, thus seems to be little influenced by inhibition of oxydative metabolism

TABLE I. Oxygen Consumption of the Different Types of Isolated Retinal Cells, Measured in a Magnetic Microdiver [see 31] (Receptor Cells Show Highest Respiration Rate and Horizontal Cells the Lowest; Addition of Azide to the Incubation Media Reduced the Oxygen Uptake to About 75%)

Cell	μl O_2/hr/Cell (Average of 3 Determinations)
Receptor	9.2×10^{-4}
Horizontal[1]	1.0×10^{-5}
Amacrine	1.5×10^{-4}
Bipolar[1]	9.0×10^{-5}
Ganglion	1.1×10^{-4}

[1]This value was on the border of the sensitivity of the method used and a pool of a large number of cells was used for each determination.

[34]. On the other hand, as the subsequent sections will reveal, the spread of the S-potential can be influenced in an important manner by other biochemical processes, notably those in which neurotransmitters are implicated.

CHEMICAL NEUROTRANSMITTERS IN THE OUTER RETINA

Since the retina is ontogenetically derived from the forebrain, it is not surprising that the same chemical messengers are present in this organ as are found in other divisions of the CNS. Substances like the catecholamines (CA), acetylcholine (ACh), serotonin (5-HT), substance P, and certain amino acids with possible transmitter characteristics have now been demonstrated in the retina. In the last decade or so, a vast number of studies have dealt with the localization, metabolism, and degradation of these putative neurotransmitters and their possible physiological role in retinal function.

The Cholinergic System

A possible neurotransmitter function for *acetylcholine* (ACh) is based on the following evidence: The enzymes responsible for its synthesis and degradation are present in this tissue [38]. Light [39,40] or chemical [41,42] stimulation releases ACh from the retina and a high-affinity transport system for choline is also present [40,43,44]. It was also reported that photoreceptor cells of the turtle retina are able to synthesize ACh [45]. A specific class of ACh-synthesizing amacrine cells and their distribution has been described based on labelled choline incorporation [46]. The *choline acetyltransferase* (ChAT) activity in the retina varies from species to species, being the highest in the chicken [47], and lowest in the cat [48]. The localization of ChAT also shows species variation [38]. In

TABLE II. Cholinesterase Activity in Three Different Types of Retinal Cell (Highest Activity of Enzyme Was Localized in the Ganglion And Amacrine Cells Whereas Horizontal Cells Did not Demonstrate Any Detectable Activity of Cholinesterase [From 31])

Cell Type	ChE Activity (1×10^{-3} CO_2/hr/Cell)	Diameter (μm)
Amacrine	1.3	
	2.0	40–60
	3.1	
	0.9	
Horizontal	0.005	70–110
(10 Cells)	4.8	
Ganglion	4.0	
	0.6	15–30
	2.9	
	2.1	

pigeon, rat, and frog, the retinal ChAT activity is mainly localized in the inner synaptic layer. In the outer retina very low activity of ChAT was found in the pigeon and the rat, and none in the frog. Turtle retinas possess a detectable activity of this enzyme in the receptors [45]. The *acetylcholine esterase* (AchE) shows quite similar activity in retinas of all species studied [38]. The only exceptions are the retinas from squid and octopus, where the AChE activity is ten and 20 times higher, respectively [49,50]. As to the cellular localization of AChE, it is mainly present in the inner plexiform layer with a distribution similar to that of ChAT [12,41,51–54]. Microgasometric measurements on isolated cells from the teleost Eugerres plumieri [31] show that only some amacrine, ganglion, and bipolar cells have a detectable AChE activity (see Table II).

However, EM-histochemistry has demonstrated the presence of AChE also in the outer retina, at the sites where horizontal cell processes contact photo-receptor endings, between the lateral contacts of horizontal cells in a given layer, and between their ascending processes [30,52,54] (see Fig. 6). Despite this information it is, to date, still not possible to identify the sites in the retina where ACh acts as a neurotransmitter. One likely possibility is the synapse between certain amacrine cells and ganglion cells in the inner plexiform layer and per-haps, based on the distribution of AChE, at the level of the contacts between re-ceptors and horizontal cell extensions, and at the junction between the horizontal cell bodies.

Dopamine in the Retina

Close to 2 decades ago it was demonsterated [55–57] that the retinas of vertebrates contain catecholamines (CA) and that dopamine (DA) as well as other

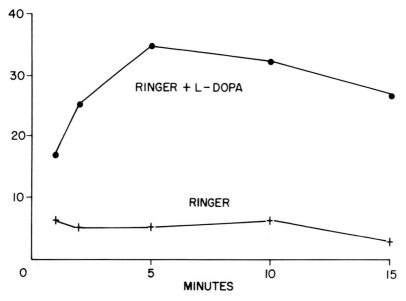

Fig. 2.   Time-course of dopamine formation in the retina of the teleost Eugerres plumieri expressed in ng/mg protein. Incubation media contained 100 μM L-DOPA. Averages of six retinas.

CA contents can be modified when the retina is exposed to different light conditions [55–58]. There also exists an active uptake and release system for DA [59]. The retina is able to synthesize DA from exogenous tyrosine [60], and from exogenous DOPA (Fig. 2). Today it is generally accepted that DA in the retina meets most of the criteria required for a substance to be considered as a neurotransmitter.

A number of studies [54,61–68] demonstrated that the DA-neurons in the retina are a separate class of cells located in the amacrine cell layer, which send their processes toward the outer plexiform layer as well as to the inner plexiform layer. Gallego [69] named these cells the "interplexiform cells." The DA-interplexiform cell (DA-IPC) shows a defined distribution pattern in the teleost retina. Their density (cells/mm^2) is highest in the peripheral region and the size of the cell bodies is larger in areas where the density of those cells is lowest. They are arranged in rows, along radial lines which appear to fan out from the optic disc. Large cells are found in the center and intermediate regions and extend three to five primary processes in various directions, while the small DA-cells in the peripheral region have two main processes arising from the opposite poles (Fig. 3). They emerge usually perpendicular to the direction of rows of cells, and parallel to the reginal margin [70].

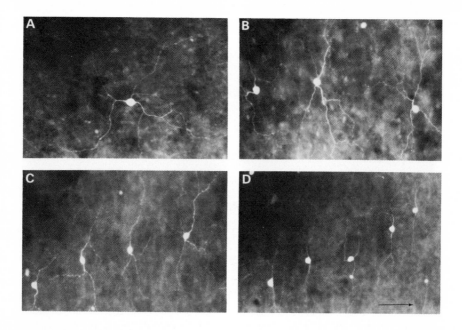

Fig. 3. Fluorescence photomicrographs from the retina of Eugerres plumieri showing DA-IPC bodies and processes. Fields were selected at retinal regions from the center (A) to the periphery (D). Modified Faglu method. Scale: 100 μm.

The ratio of the DA-IPC to other cells in the amacrine cell layer is approximately 1:200 [71]. In the teleost fish and New World monkey the interplexiform DA cells send fine processes outwards through the inner nuclear layer and their terminals from a dense network around the horizontal cells [54,70,72] (Fig. 4).

The varicosities of the extensions make contact with the somata of the horizontal cells (Fig. 5).

Amino Acids as Possible Neurotransmitters in the Retina

A number of workers have suggested that γ-aminobutyric acid (GABA), glycine, aspartate, glutamate, and taurine may act as chemical messengers in the retina [73].

The presence of GABA has been demonstrated in certain amacrine cells, as well as in the external horizontal cells in the outer retina. Those cells possess a high-affinity uptake mechanism for GABA [74–76]. In addition, the enzymatic mechanisms for synthesis and degradation of GABA is present in the retina. Succinic semialdehyde dehydrogenase is present at the site where receptor, bi-

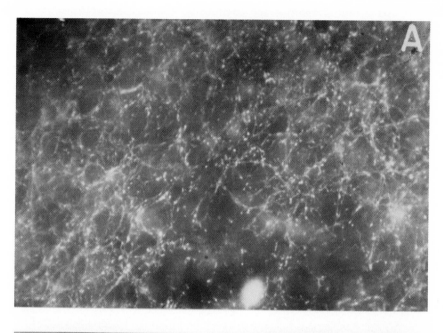

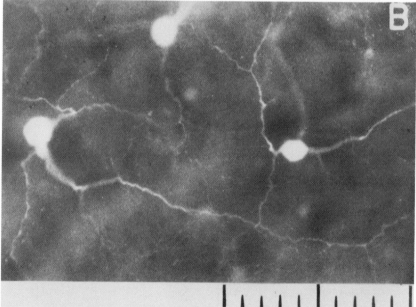

Fig. 4. Fluorescence photomicrographs from the retina of C carpio, incubated with noradrenaline. A. Fiber network at the level of the inner nuclear layer. B. Somata and processes in the inner plexiform layer. scale: 100 μm [from 70].

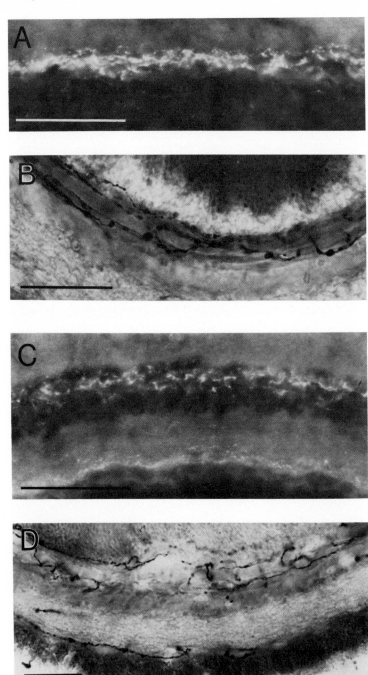

polar, and horizontal cells contact each other [77]. The activities of GAD and GABA-T appear modified, according to different light conditions [60,75,78]. The endogenous levels of GABA can be changed by light or K^+ [75,76,79,80]. It has been suggested that the feedback synapses from cone horizontal cells to cones may use GABA as a neurotransmitter [81].

Some amacrine cells and a type of interplexiform cell are reported to accumulate exogenous glycine [76]. Moreover, high- and low-affinity uptake mechanisms for glycine, as well as its K^+-evoked release, have been demonstrated. Although a relatively small and somewhat inconsistent release of glycine from the retina following light stimulation was reported [82], the endogenous changes of glycine under special light conditions are rather large. This may imply that changes of glycine may be more related to a changed metabolism rather than reflecting alterations in its release.

There is also evidence to support the postulate that aspartic acid [83] and glutamic acid [84] act as excitatory neurotransmitters on the photoreceptor cell terminals. Relatively high levels of these amino acids are found to be present in the retina [93]. The photoreceptors exhibit a substantial glutamic-aspartic transaminase activity [73], which assures a constant level of aspartate. It was also reported that light flicker (3 Hz) reduces the release of aspartate by close to 50% but does not affect the efflux of glutamate [85]. Furthermore, L-aspartate depolarizes the horizontal cells in the dark-adapted retina, and the effect of the exogenously applied aspartate, as well as that of the endogenous photoreceptor transmitter, could be blocked by DL-α-aminoadipate, a strong aspartate antagonist [83]. Nevertheless, it is possible that the type of transmitter in the photoreceptors could be species dependent and it also remains to be established if there is one or more chemical messengers in receptor cells of one and the same retina.

EFFECTS OF SOME PUTATIVE NEUROTRANSMITTERS ON THE HORIZONTAL CELL BEHAVIOR

Because the S-potential is generated in the horizontal cells of the outer plexiform layer, putative transmitters localized in this region of the retina may be of special importance when it comes to influencing this type of potential. Figure 6 summarizes the current suggested localization of the transmitters in the outer plexiform layer. The scheme is based on evidence cited in the previous section.

Fig. 5. Photomicrographs of fluorescence and Golgi preparations of the E plumieri retina. A, B. Fluorescent processes at the level of the inner nuclear layer and corresponding silver-impregnated processes. C, D. As above, but processes are seen in both the outer nuclear and the inner plexiform layers. Calibration bars: 50 μm.

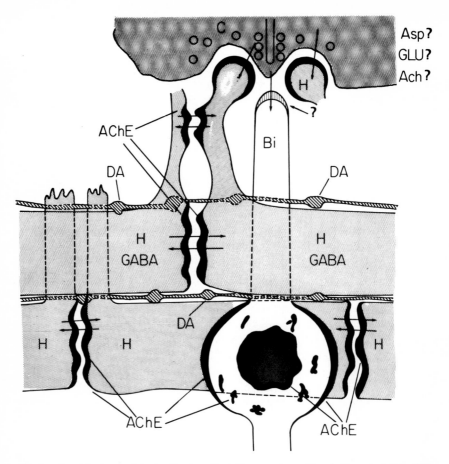

Fig. 6. General scheme of the localization of putative neurotransmitters in the outer retina. ACh, acetylcholine; AChE, acetylcholinesterase; Bi, bipolar cell; DA, dopamine; Glu, glutamic acid; H, horizontal cells [modified from 54].

Over the past years our working group has been particularly interested in the effects of several of these neurotransmitters in both the control of the resting membrane potential of the horizontal cells (dark potential), as well as on the lateral propagation of the S-potential. Most of this work was performed by observing the modifications of the S-potential when isolated retinas were perfused with solutions containing the different transmitters and/or their analogues.

Effects of Catecholamines

When the isolated retina from the teleost E plumieri is perfused with Ringer containing 100 μM dopamine (DA), the center hyperpolarizing response to spot

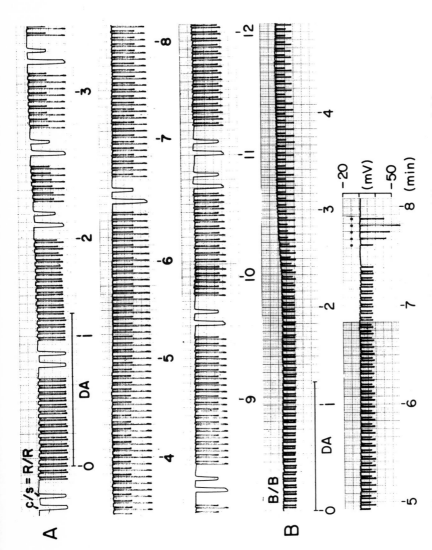

Fig. 7. Effects of 100 μM dopamine (DA) on center (c) and surround (s) responses recorded from an L-type horizontal cell of the Eugerres plumieri isolated and perfused retina. Peak of spectral response curve at 605 nm (at end of B). Alternate c and s stimuli were applied, and are shown at higher speed in A. Both stimuli were red in A and blue in B [from 86].

illumination increases and the surrounding response evoked by distant light stimulus is diminshed by 40%. The reciprocal changes in the S-potentials are reversible when DA is removed from the perfusate [86] (see Fig. 7).

The effect of DA on the dark potential of the horizontal cell, if any, is slight ($\approx$ 2 mV), which indicates that this substance does not directly affect synaptic transmission from photoreceptor to horizontal cell, but only affects the lateral propagation of the S-potential [86,87]. The action of the other catecholamines, adrenaline (AD) and noradrenaline (NA), is similar to that of DA, but not as pronounced (Fig. 8).

The precursor of DA, L-dihydroxyphenylalanine (DOPA), does not appear to have any direct action on the horizontal cell (Fig. 8D). Nevertheless, repeated and prolonged application of L-DOPA (3–6 minutes) does produce a DA-like effect (see chapter by Laufer). The late appearance of the DOPA-effect is probably related to the time required to synthesize DA from the exogenous DOPA. This is illustrated in Figure 2, which demonstrates that the time course for DA synthesis coincides with the onset of the physiological effects of the precursor.

Effects of Acetylcholine (ACh) and Carbachol

ACh has the same action as DA, but only at high concentrations, and even then, the effect seems smaller and shorter lasting. On the other hand, carbachol, the nondestructible analog of ACh, does not appear to have an action of its own, but will influence the S-potential in the same manner as DA only after the retina has been perfused previously with DA [88] (Fig. 9).

A prolonged pretreatment of the retina with the α-adrenergic blocking agent phentolamine abolishes the inhibition of the lateral spread of the S-potential produced by DA [23,89], as well as the ACh effect [54,90] (Fig. 10). However, when hexamethonium is applied, the ACh effect is abolished, but not that of DA [90]. For this reason we have suggested [54,88] that the effect of ACh is a result of the liberation of DA from the dopaminergic interplexiform cell terminals in the outer plexiform layer.

Effects of Amino Acids

The excitatory transmitters *L-aspartate* and *L-glutamate* depolarize the horizontal cells and reduce light-evoked responses [83,91]. Both amino acids do not affect markedly the spatial properties of the horizontal cells (Fig. 11). The effect of aspartate in dark-adapted state was shown to be more potent than that of glutamate.

Taurine, which was reported to be the most abundant amino acid in the vertebrate retina [92–94], did not show any significant effect on the horizontal cells, either in the rabbit [95] or fish retina [91] (Fig. 12B). The biochemical demonstration of the interrelated changes of taurine and glutamate in the retina [94] could not be registered electrophysiologically since taurine did not enhance

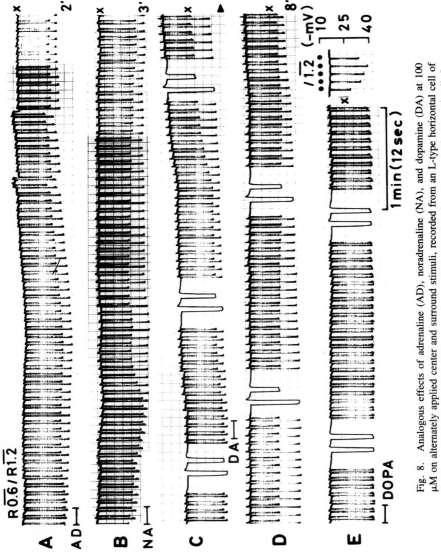

Fig. 8. Analogous effects of adrenaline (AD), noradrenaline (NA), and dopamine (DA) at 100 μM on alternately applied center and surround stimuli, recorded from an L-type horizontal cell of the Eugerres plumieri retina. Higher-speed records show pairs of responses to the two stimuli. L-DOPA did not cause significant change in the potential (E) [from 89].

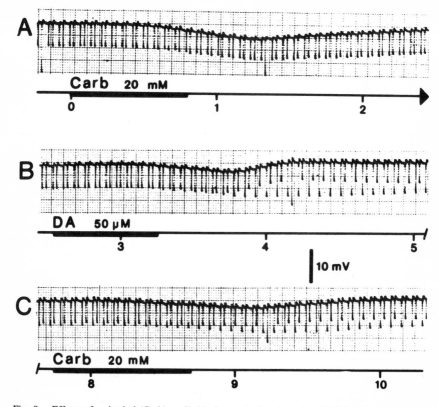

Fig. 9. Effects of carbachol (Carb) applied before and after dopamine (DA) in pairs of responses elicited by center and surround stimuli in an L-type horizontal cell of the Eugerres plumieri retina. Time in minutes [from 88].

the glutamate-induced depolarization, perhaps because the application period of the drug in this type of experiment is too short to observe a relatively long-term biochemical process [91].

GABA, which is considered to be a potent inhibitory transmitter, hyperpolarizes the cone horizontal cell (Figs. 12, 13) but has no effect on the rod-connected cells. It has been observed that only red-sensitive cells located in the horizontal cell layer are able to take up ^{3}H-GABA [76]. GABA is considered a transmitter for cone horizontal cells [81] and its effect on horizontal cells is thought to be mediated by a postulated feedback loop consisting of external (red-sensitive) horizontal cells-cones-horizontal cells [96]. Due to this and, furthermore, since the GABA-induced changes observed by us [91] are partly due to an action on cones and not on rods, it might be assumed that there is no GABA-

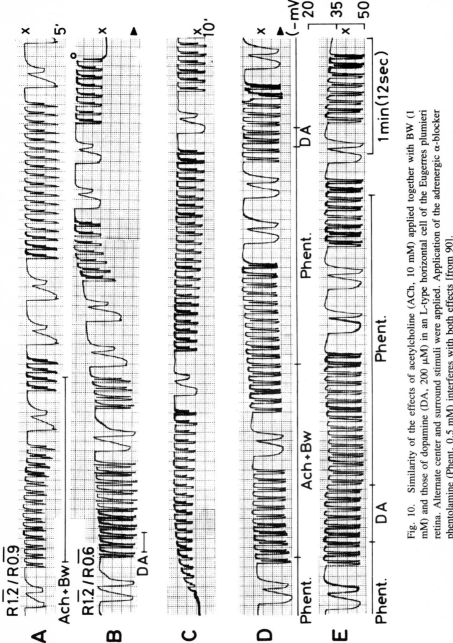

Fig. 10. Similarity of the effects of acetylcholine (ACh, 10 mM) applied together with BW (1 mM) and those of dopamine (DA, 200 μM) in an L-type horizontal cell of the Eugerres plumieri retina. Alternate center and surround stimuli were applied. Application of the adrenergic α-blocker phentolamine (Phent, 0.5 mM) interferes with both effects [from 90].

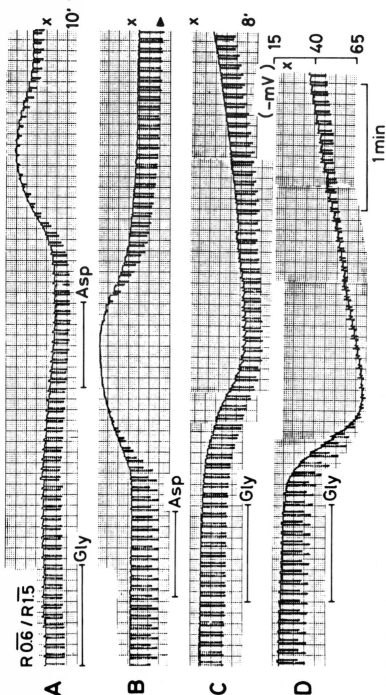

Fig. 11. Changes in the effect of Gly on a cone-connected L-type cell. All records (A–B) were obtained from a long-lasting recording. Gly (10 mM), applied first at the beginning of record A, caused an initial depolarization (2 mV) and a subsequent hyperpolarization (5 mV). Then Asp (5 mM) depolarized the cell by 20 mV (A). During interruption in the record between A and B, DA (0.1 mM) was applied (not illustrated), causing a center response slightly larger than the surround response, as seen at the beginning of record B. Asp again was applied, which caused depolarization by 18 mV, abolishing the light-evoked responses (B). Gly, successively applied, produced hyperpolarization here by 23 mV (C). Between records C and D, DA was applied (not illustrated). The third application by Gly hyperpolarized the cell by 45 mV, abolishing the light-induced responses (D). The dose of Gly applied each time (10 mM × 47 seconds) should be the same. After record D, two cone-connected cells recorded from this preparation were found to respond to Gly with a large hyperpolarization, as seen in records C and D [from 91].

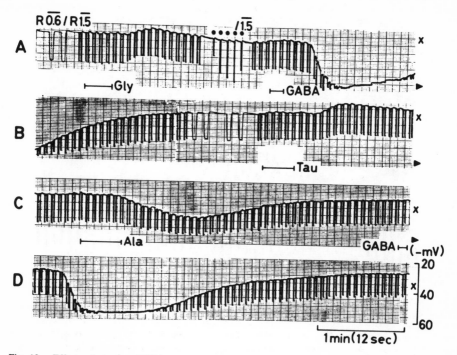

Fig. 12. Effects of glycine, GABA, taurine, and alanine (10 mM each) on an L-type horizontal cell of the Eugerres plumieri retina. Alternate center and surround red flashes were applied. Higher-speed records in A and B [modified from 91].

mediated feedback from rod-horizontal cells to rods. It was reported [97] that GABA is also affecting the lateral propagation of information in the outer retina. We have observed only in a few cases a very small and short-lasting inhibition of the surround response during perfusion of the retina with GABA [91]. Nevertheless, since GABA plays a role in the regulation of DA levels in the CNS, as well as in the retina [98], the observed effect could rather be due to an increase in the endogenous DA levels in the retina when this tissue is being perfused with relatively high concentrations (10 mM) of GABA.

Contradictory information as to the effect of *glycine* on the horizontal cells is found in the literature. It was reported [99,100] that glycine hyperpolarizes the horizontal cells, whereas others [83] demonstrated that glycine has no effect on those cells. We have observed [91] (Fig. 11A) a very small, short-lasting, and inconsistent, first depolarizing (2 mV) and then hyperpolarizing (5 mV) effect of this amino acid on the horizontal cells. Nevertheless, with preloading of the retina with DA (100 μM) prior to the perfusion with glycine, a rather large

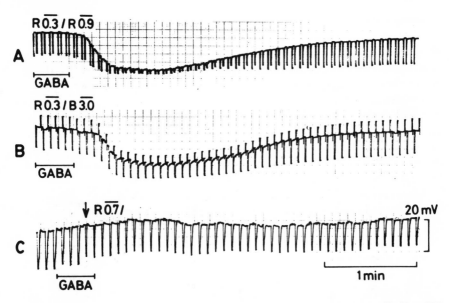

Fig. 13. Different effects of GABA (10 mM) on cone-connected L- and C-type cells (A and B) and on a rod-connected L-type cell (C). In record A red spot and annulus (R/R) stimuli, and in record B red spot and blue annulus (R/B) stimuli were used. In record C, only red spot stimulus (R/) was used and the intensity was fixed at 0.7 log unit a response 7 from the beginning (↓) [from 91].

hyperpolarizing (45 mV) effect on the horizontal cell was observed [91] (see Fig. 11) which suggests that the glycine effect is DA dependent.

Therefore, we assume that the discrepancy in the results obtained by different authors might be due to the levels of endogenous DA present in the retina during the conducting of the experiments.

THE EFFECTS OF SUBSTANCE P

Several reports on the presence of substance P in the retina are available [101–104]. This substance was localized in a specific type of amacrine cell [105]. It was proposed that substance P is a neurotransmitter released by amacrine cells and affects receptors located on ganglion cells [106]. No action of substance P on the horizontal cells was detected. Nevertheless, after preloading the retina with DA, a pronounced effect of this peptide on the spatial properties of the horizontal cell was observed [88] (See chapter by Laufer).

CONCLUSIONS

Most of the information at hand to date suggests the following biochemical characteristics of the S-potential: While the generation of the S-potential itself depends on the state of aerobic metabolism of the receptor cell, its lateral propagation is not oxygen dependent. The relatively slow propagation of this potential (0.3 m/sec) and the temperature changes that are able to modify its propagation velocity with such a high Q_{10} (Q_{10} = 3–4), suggest that other mechanisms than purely electrotonic conduction must also play a role in this process.

The neural activity of the inner plexiform layer could influence the behavior of the horizontal cells through the dopaminergic interplexiform cell, which closes a feedback loop between the external and inner plexiform layers. Transmitters like ACh and its analogue carbachol, as well as substance P, may also influence the propagation of the S-potential, but indirectly, probably by interacting with DA. Therefore, DA plays a particular key role in the outer retina.

Amino acids with neurotransmitter characteristics like aspartate, glutamate, GABA, and glycine are able mainly to modify the dark potential of the horizontal cells but show little or no direct action on the spatial properties of the S-potential. These amino acids, as far as the outer retina is concerned, evidently play an important role in the function of the receptor-horizontal-bipolar-cells' synaptic circuitry.

Still, the mechanism of the observed neurotransmitter interaction is not yet known and represents an interesting and challenging task.

ACKNOWLEDGMENTS

The author wishes to express his gratitude to Dr. Nico van Gelder for his help in the preparation of the manuscript, and to Valentin Parthe, Yvonne Drujan, and Mary Urbina for their collaboration.

REFERENCES

1. Svaetichin G: The cone action potential. Acta Physiol Scand 29 (Suppl 106):1953.
2. Mitara G, Yagasaki Y: Resting and action potential of single cone. Ann Rev Res Inst Environment Med Nagoya Univ 2:54, 1955.
3. Motokawa K, Oikawa T, Tasaki K: Receptor potential of vertebrate retina. J Neurophysiol 20:186, 1957.
4. Tomita T, Murakami M, Sato Y, Hashimoto Y: Further study on the origin of the so-called cone action potential. Jpn J Physiol 9:63, 1959.
5. MacNichol EF Jr, Svaetichin G: Electric response from the isolated retina of fishes. Am J Ophthalmol 46:26, 1958.
6. Mitarai G: The origin of the so-called cone potential. Proc Jpn Acad 34:299, 1958.
7. Werblin FS, Dowling JE: Organization of the retina of the mudpuppy *Nectourus maculosus*. II. Intracellular recordings. J Neurophysiol 32:339, 1969.
8. Kaneko A: Physiological and morphological identification of horizontal, bipolar and amacrine cells in goldfish retina. Proc Natl Acad Sci USA, 78:5890, 1970.
9. Svaetichin G, Negishi K, Fatehchand R: Cellular mechanisms of young-herring visual system. In Dereuck AVS, Knight J, eds: Ciba Symposium on Color Vision: Physiology and Experimental Psychology. London: Churchill, 1965, pp 178.
10. Laufer M, Millan E: Spectral analysis of L-type S-potentials and their relation to photopigment absorption in fish *Eugerres plumieri* retina. Vision Res, 10:237, 1970.

11. Svaetichin G, Negishi K, Parthe V, Drujan G: Estudios electrofisiológicos en las células horizontales de la retina. Acta Cient Venez 21(Suppl 1):16, 1970.
12. Stell WK: The morphological organization of the vertebrate retina. In Fourtes MGF, ed: Handbook of Sensory Physiology, Vol VII/2. Berlin: Springer Verlag, 1972, pp 111.
13. Cajal SR: Textura del Sistema Nervioso del Hombre y de los Vertebrados, Tomo I. Madrid: N. Moya, 1899.
14. Cajal SR: Textura del Sistema Nervioso del Hombre y de los Vertebrados, Tomo II. Madrid: N. Moya, 1904.
15. Vallecalle E, Svaetichin G: The retina as a model for the functional organization of the nervous system. In Jung R, Kornhuber H, eds: The Visual System: Neurophysiology and Psychophysics. Berlin: Springer Verlag, 1961, pp 489.
16. Liptetz LE: Glial control of neuronal activity. IEEE Trans Mil Electr 7:144, 1963.
17. Byzov AL: Horizontal cells of the retina as regulators of synaptic transmission. Fiziol Zh SSSR 53:1115, 1967 (from Neurosci Transl 3:268, 1967–1968).
18. Rushton WAH: Visual adaptation. Proc R Soc Lond [Biol] 162:20, 1965.
19. Rushton WAH: Bleached rhodopsin and visual adaptation. J Physiol (Lond) 181:645, 1965.
20. Naka KI, Rushton WAH: The generation and spread of S-potential in fish (Cyprinidae). J Physiol (Lond) 192:437, 1967.
21. Svaetichin G, Laufer M, Negishi K, Muriel C: Retinal automatic control mechanisms responsible for Weber's and Steven's laws. Proc Intern Union Physiol Sci 7:1267, 1968.
22. Svaetichin G, Muriel C: Función retiniana y control automático. Rev Oftalmol Venezolana 24:41, 1970.
23. Hedden WL, Dowling JE: The interplexiform cell system. II. Effects of dopamine on goldfish retinal neurons. Proc R Soc Lond [Biol] 201: 1978.
24. Svaetichin G, Krattenmacher W, Laufer M: Photostimulation of single cones. J Gen Physiol 43 II:101, 1960.
25. Tomita T: Electrophysiological study of the mechanisms subserving color coding in the fish retina. Cold Spring Harbor Symp Quant Biol 30:559, 1965.
26. Mitarai G, Svaetichin G, Vallecalle E, Fatehchand R, Villegas J, Laufer M: Glia-neuron interactions and adaptational mechanisms of the retina. In Jung R, Kornhuber H, eds: The Visual System: Neurophysiology and Psychophysics. Berlin: Springer Verlag, 1961, pp 463.
27. Negishi K, Sutija V: Lateral spread of light-induced potential along different cell layers in the teleost retina. Vision Res 9:881, 1969.
28. Kaneko A: Electrical connections between horizontal cells in the dogfish retina. J Physiol (Lond) 213:95, 1971.
29. Svaetichin G: Células horizontales y amacrinas de la retina: Propiedades y mecanismos de control sobre las bipolares y ganglionares. Acta Cient Venez (Suppl 3):254, 1967.
30. Drujan, DB, Svaetichin G, Negishi K, Brzin M: Biochemical and electroctrophysiological studies on the functional controls of the horizontal cells. In Broda E, Locter A, eds Proc 1st Europ Biophys Congress. Bader: Springer, 1971, 89.
31. Drujan BD, Svaetichin G: Characterization of different classes of isolated retinal cells. Vision Res 12:1777, 1972.
32. Fatehchand R, Svaetichin G, Negishi K, Drujan B: Effects of anoxia and metabolic inhibitors on the S-potential of isolated fish retinae. Vision Res 6:271, 1966.
33. Negishi K, Svaetichin G, Laufer M, Drujan BD: Polarographic and electrophysiological studies on retinal respiration. Vision Res 15:527, 1975.
34. Drujan BD, Svaetichin G, Negishi K: Retinal aerobic metabolism as reflected in the S-potential behavior. Vision Res Suppl 3:151, 1971.
35. Santamaria L, Drujan BD, Svaetichin G, Negishi K: Respiration, glycolysis and S-potentials in teleost retina: a comparative study. Vision Res 11:877, 1971.

36. Warburg O: Das Sauerstoffubertragende Fermet der Atmung. Angew Chem [Engl] 45:1, 1932.
37. Sickel W: Retinal metabolism in dark and light. In Fuortes MGF, ed: Handbook of Sensory Physiology, Vol VII/2 Physiology of Photoreceptor Organs. Berlin: Springer, 1972, pp 667.
38. Graham LT: Comparative aspects of neurotransmitters in the retina. In Davson H, Graham LT, eds: The Eye, Vol VI. New York: Academic Press, 1974, pp 283.
39. Masland RH, Livingstone CJ: Effect of stimulation with light on synthesis and release of acetylcholine by an isolated mammalian retina. J Neurochem 39:1210, 1976.
40. Vivas IM, Drujan BD: Certain aspects of acetylcholine metabolism in the teleost retina. Neurochem Res 5:817, 1980.
41. Neal MJ: Acetylcholine as a transmitter substance. In Bonting SL, ed: Transmitters in the Visual Process. Pergamon Press, 1976, pp 127.
42. Massey SC, Neal MJ: The light-evoked release of acetylcholine from the rabbit retina in vivo and its inhibition by -aminobutyric acid. J Neurochem 32:1327, 1979.
43. Atterwill CK, Mahoney A, Neal MJ: The uptake and subcellular distribution of ^{3}H-choline by the retina. Br J Pharmacol 53:447, 1965.
44. Neal MJ, Gilroy J: High-affinity choline transport in isolated retina. Brain Res 93:548, 1975.
45. Lam DMK: Biosynthesis of acetylcholine in turtle photoreceptors. Proc Natl Acad Sci USA 69:1987, 1972.
46. Masland RH: Acetylcholine in the retina. Neurochem Int 1:501, 1980.
47. Hebb CO: Cholineacetylase in mammalian and avian sensory systems. Q J Exp Physiol 40:176, 1955.
48. Hebb CO: The problem of identifying cholinergic neurons in the retina. Acta Physiol Pharmacol Neerl 6:621, 1957.
49. Minami M: The location of cholinesterase in the retina. Acad Soc Ophthalmol Jpn 56:604, 1952.
50. Leo PR, Florey E: The distribution of acetylcholine and cholinesterase in the nervous system and in innerfated organs of Octopus dofleini. Comp Biochem Physiol 17:509, 1966.
51. Nichols CW, Koelle GB: Comparison of the localization of acetylcholinesterase and non-specific cholinesterase activities in mammalian and avian retinas. J Comp Neurol 133:1, 1968.
52. Brzin M, Drujan BD: Activity of histochemical and cytochemical localization of cholinesterases in fish retina. Proc Sec Int Meeting Neurochem 110, 1969.
53. Drujan BD, Díaz Borges JM, Brzin M: Histochemical and cytochemical localization of ace-tylcholinesterase in retina and optic tectum of teleost fish. Can J Biochem 57:43, 1979.
54. Drujan BD, Negishi K, Laufer M: Studies on putative neurotransmitters in the distal retina. Neurochem Internat 1:143, 1980.
55. Drujan BD, Díaz Borges JM, Alvarez N: Relationship between the contents of adrenaline, nor-adrenaline and dopamine in the retina and its adaptional state. Life Sci 4:472, 1965.
56. Häggendal J, Malmfors T: Identification and cellular localization in the retina and the chorioid of the rabbit. Acta Physiol Scand 64:58, 1965.
57. Nichols S, Jacobowitz D, Hottenstein M: The influence of light and dark on the catecholamine content of the retina and choroid. Invest Ophthalmol 6:642, 1967.
58. Drujan BD, Díaz Borges JM: Adrenaline depletion induced by light in the dark-adapted retina. Experientia 24:676, 1968.
59. Sarthy PJ, Lam DMK: The uptake and release of (^{3}H)dopamine in the goldfish retina. J Neurochem 32:1269, 1979.
60. Lam DMK: Synaptic chemistry of identified cells in the vertebrate retina. Cold Spring Harbor Symp Quant Biol 40:571, 1975.
61. Dowson and Pérez: Unusual retinal cells in the dolphin eye. Science 181:747, 1973.
62. Dowling JE, Ehinger B: Synaptic organization of the amine-containing interplexiform cells of the goldfish and cebus monkey retinas. Science 188:173, 1975.

63. Dowling JE, Ehinger B: The interplexiform cell system. I Synapses of the dopaminergic neurons of the goldfish retina. Proc R Soc Lond [Biol] 201:7, 1978.

64. Boycott BB, Dowling JE, Fisher SK: Interplexiforms cells of the mammalian retina and their comparison with catecholamine-containing cells. Proc R Soc Lond [Biol] 191:353, 1975.

65. Kolb H, West RW: Synaptic connections of the interplexiform cell in the retina of the cat. J Neurocytol 6:155, 1977.

66. Negishi K, Hayashi T, Nakamura T, Drujan BD: Histochemical studies on catecholaminergic cells in the carp retina. Neurochem Res 4:473, 1979.

67. Negishi K, Laufer M, Drujan BD: Drug-induced changes in catecholaminergic cells of the fish retina. J Neurosci Res 5:599, 1980.

68. Dowling JE, Ehinger B, Hedden WL: The interplexiform cell: A new type of retinal neuron. Invest Ophthalmol 15:916, 1976.

69. Gallego A: Horizontal and amacrine cells in the mammallian retina. In Shipley T, Dowling JE, eds: International Symposium on Visual Processes in Vertebrates, Santiago de Chile. Vision Res 2:33, 1971.

70. Negishi K, Drujan BD, Laufer M: Spatial distribution of catecholaminergic cells in the fish retina. J Neurosci Res 5:621, 1980.

71. Negishi K, Drujan BD, Laufer M: Counterstaining of fluorescent retinal preparations: Cell densities in different layers. Neurosci 6:2047, 1981.

72. Ehinger B: Biogenic monamines as transmitters in the retina. In Bonting SL, ed: Transmitters in the Visual Process. London: Pergamon Press, 1976, pp 147–163.

73. Neal MJ: Amino acid transmitter substances in the vertebrate retina. Gen Pharmacol 7:321, 1976.

74. Ehinger B: Cellular location of the uptake of some amino acids into the rabbit retina. Brain Res 46:297, 1972.

75. Lam DMK, Steinman L: The uptake of gamma-^{3}H-aminobutyric acid in goldfish retina. Proc Natl Acad Sci USA 68:2777, 1971.

76. Marc RE, Stell WR, Bok D, Lam DMK: GABA-ergic pathways in the goldfish retina. J Comp Neurol 182:221, 1978.

77. Moore CL, Gruberg ER: The distribution of succinic semialdehyde dehydrogenase in the brain and retina of the tiger salamander *(Ainbystoma tigrinum)*. Brain Res 67:467, 1974.

78. Kuriyama K, Sisken B, Haber B, Roberts E: The -aminobutyric acid system in rabbit retina. Brain Res 9:165, 1968.

79. Graham LT, Baxter CF, Lolley RN: In vivo influence of light or darkness on the GABA system in the retina of the frog *(Rana pipiens)*. Brain Res 20:379, 1970.

80. Drujan BD, Ciarletta E: The effect of light and darkness on the metabolism of adrenaline, -aminobutyrate, glutamate and aspartate in the visual system of the teleost *Eugerres plumieri*. Proc ISN Tokyo p 318, 1973.

81. Lam DMK, Lasater EM, Naka KI: -Aminobutyric acid: A neurotransmitter candidate of cone horizontal cells of the catfish retina. Proc Natl Acad Sci USA 75:6310, 1978.

82. Ehinger G, Lindberg-Bauer B: Light evoked release of glycine from cat and rabbit retina. Brain Res. 113:535, 1976.

83. Wu SM, Dowling JE: L-Aspartate: Evidence for a role in cone photoreceptor. Synaptic transmission in the carp retina. Proc Natl Acad Sci USA 75:5205, 1978.

84. Ishida AT, Fain GL: D-Aspartate potentiates the effects of L-glutamate on horizontal cells in goldfish retina. Proc Natl Acad Sci USA 78:5890, 1981.

85. Neal MJ, Massey SC: The release of acetylcholine and amino acids from the rabbit retina in vivo. Neurochem Int 1:191, 1980.

86. Negishi K, Drujan BD: Reciprocal changes in center and surrounding S-potentials of fish retina in response to dopamine. Neurochem Res 4:313, 1979.

87. Negishi K, Drujan BD: Effects of catecholamines on the horizontal cell membrane potential in the fish retina. Sen Processes 2:388, 1978.
88. Laufer M, Negishi K, Drujan BD: Pharmacological manipulation of spatial properties of S-potentials. Vision Res 21:1657, 1981.
89. Negishi K, Drujan BD: Effects of catecholamines and related compounds on horizontal cells in the fish retina. J Neurosci Res 4:311, 1979.
90. Negishi K, Drujan BD: Similarities in effects of acetylcholine and dopamine on horizontal cells in the fish retina. J Neurosci Res 4:335, 1979.
91. Negishi K, Drujan BD: Effects of some amino acids on horizontal cells in the fish retina. J Neurosci Res 4:351, 1979.
92. Orr HT, Cohen AI, Lowry OH: The distribution of taurine in the vertebrate retina. J Neurochem 26:609, 1962.
93. Pasantes Morales H, Klethi J, Leding M, Mandel P: Free amino acids of chicken and rat retina. Brain Res 41:494, 1972.
94. Van Gelder NM, Drujan BD: Interrelated changes of amino acids in the retina and optic tectum of a marine fish with alterations of illuminating conditions. Brain Res 189:137, 1978.
95. Cunningham R, Miller RF: Taurine: Its selective action on neuronal pathways in the rabbit retina. Brain Res 117:341, 1976.
96. Murakami M, Shimoda Y, Nakatani K: Effects of GABA on neuronal activities in the distal retina of the carp. Sens Processes 2:334, 1979.
97. Mooney RD: GABA and the lateral spread of tonic activity in frog retina. Vision Res 19:501, 1978.
98. Marshburn PB, Yuvone PM: The role of GABA in the regulation of the Dopamine/Tyrosine hydroxylase-containing neurons on the rat retina. Brain Res 214:355, 1981.
99. Murakami M, Ohtsu K, Ohtsuka T: Effects of chemical on receptors and horizontal cells in the retina. J Physiol (Lond) 227:899, 1972.
100. Sugawara K, Negishi K: Effects of some amino acids on the horizontal cell membrane potential in the isolated carp retina. Vision Res 13:977, 1973.
101. Duner H, von Euler US, Pernow B: Catecholamines and substance P in the mammalian eye. Acta Physiol Scand 31:113, 1954.
102. Winder AF, Patsalos PN: Substance P and retinal neurotransmission. Biochem Soc Trans 2:1260, 1974.
103. Kanasawa I, Jessel T: Post mortem changes and regional distribution of substance P in the rat and mouse nervous system. Brain Res 117:362, 1976.
104. Reubi JC, Jessel TM: Distribution of substance P in the pigeon. J Neurochem 31:359, 1978.
105. Karten HJ, Brecha N: Localization of substance P immunoreactivity in amacrine cells of the retina. Nature 283:87, 1980.
106. Glickman RD, Adolph AR, Dowling JE: Inner plexiform circuits in the carp carp retina: Effects of cholinergic agonists, GABA and substance P on the ganglion cells. Brain Res 234:81, 1982.

The S-Potential, pages 307–310

Gunnar Svaetichin: Man of Vision

Dorothea Jameson and Leo M. Hurvich

Gunnar Svaetichin showed us graded DC potentials that reversed in polarity with a change from shortwave to longwave light stimulation as he recorded them from a cell in the fish retina in his laboratory at IVIC in the summer of 1959. The occasion was charged with suspense and elicited considerable collegial admiration, because this was not an ordinary laboratory visit by a couple of fellow scientists, but rather a spontaneously arranged demonstration for a group of participants in a Symposium on Visual Mechanisms being held by IVIC at their beautiful mountain site high above Caracas. In addition to ourselves, as we now remember it, those "looking over Gunnar's shoulder as he worked," so to speak, included Tomita, Wagner, De Valois, MacNichol, Verzeano, Mitarai, Wolbarsht, De Robertis, and probably others. Gunnar was indeed gratified. The electrode was perfect, the isolated retina preparation was in good physiological condition, and the spectral stimulating apparatus was functioning just as it should. The cell went on responding so that Gunnar was able to demonstrate the sustained response to a steady light, its monotonic relation to light intensity once the polarity was determined by a chosen wavelength, and the transitory, plus/minus response at the transition region of the spectrum between the regions that elicited hyperpolarizing potentials on the one side and depolarizing ones on the other. For some of us, at least, the demonstration had a seeing-is-*really*-believing flavor.

Svaetichin's original publications [1] had aroused much attention, but also some understandable resistance and skepticism. His findings were novel, unorthodox, and in direct conflict with conventional expectations of electrophysiologists. Grundfest [2] summarized the situation by his statement that if Svaetichin's findings were to be accommodated, electrophysiological theory of that time had to be modified. Early on, Hartline had required MacNichol's assurance from on-the-spot collaborative experiments with Svaetichin in his Caracas laboratory [3] that the unexpected findings did indeed constitute an important discovery about visual physiology and not some strange electronic quirk in his amplifier circuitry.

We empathized with Gunnar's wish to demonstrate his phenomenon to fellow visual scientists at that Symposium, and we understood his euphoric delight that this occasion broke the law that under such circumstances, anything that can go wrong, will.

Our own feelings about Gunnar's demonstration were related to the fact that if, at that time, wavelength-dependent opposite responses were disturbing to electrophysiologists, they were anathema to most visual psychophysicists. Our research in human color vision had gotten under way in Ralph Evans' Color Control Department at Eastman Kodak Company in 1947 with a study that confirmed the stability of metameric color matches (unpublished), followed by psychophysical studies on the binocular fusion of yellow, a series concerned with the determination of perceived white and its implications for color adaptation, and another series concerned with the spectral sensitivity of the fovea. What we were trying to do was to develop a framework that would encompass both the quantitative data of visual psychophysics and the qualitative phenomena of color perception. What we kept running into was the need to modify the conventional framework that placed the whole physiological burden of color vision on three cone mechanisms. The kinds of modifications needed could best be summarized as interactions, pairings, and mutual oppositions, and, not surprisingly, we expanded our attention to include not only the receptor mechanisms but also the hypothetical neural processes of Hering's [4] opponent color theory. In our 1951 Science paper [5] that re-examined, repeated, and revised Hecht's [6] landmark demonstration of what was claimed to be the synthesis of a yellow hue by binocular fusion, we found that the binocular mixture of lights that are seen separately as unique red (neither yellowish nor bluish) and unique green (neither yellowish nor bluish) yielded a white or gray sensation; red and green did not generate yellow at some visual center in the brain but rather cancelled each other. Yellow remained only if the red and green stimuli were both yellowish when seen separately by each of the two eyes. In our papers on perceived whiteness [7] and on spectral sensitivity [8], we were forced to consider the possibility of a separate brightness or whiteness process, in addition to those associated with hue coding.

Our serious consideration of Hering's theoretical proposals was looked upon as somewhat bizarre by many visual scientists. Perhaps, they wondered, we failed to understand the three-variable nature of color vision—a pseudo-issue, but one that caused a British colleague to make a stop in Rochester en route to Indiana to "straighten us out" on color arithmetic. That pseudo-issue was easily resolved, but we were not prepared to provide any physiological evidence for wavelength-dependent opposite neural processes in the retina. It was in 1934 that Hecht had remarked that "Hering's ideas of assimilation and dissimilation mean nothing in the modern physiology of sense organs and of nerves," and Hecht's estimate was still generally endorsed by researchers in color vision in the late 1940s and early 1950s.

The Journal of the Optical Society papers reporting our psychophysical cancellation measures of opponent hue responses and development of a quantified opponent-process model of color vision appeared in 1955 [9] and 1956 [10], and we moved our laboratories to New York University in 1957. It was in our laboratory there that Gunnar Svaetichin appeared one day, unannounced but welcome. Our friendship took root over lunch, and the long afternoon conversation back at our nearby apartment was only the first of many that we remember with warmth and pleasure. Whether it was at a meeting in Paris, Oxford, Freiburg, Munich, New York, Los Angeles, Philadelphia, or during our protracted stay in 1965 as guests of IVIC at the Caracas laboratories, our discussions with Gunnar were always stimulating, often informative, sometimes exasperating when the poet side of his complex intellect tried to outreach too far the analytical, scientific side.

We must, in turn, have exasperated Gunnar at times during our collaborative work with him in his laboratory. We were interested, as was he, in the receptive field properties of the horizontal cells, and we worked out experimental protocols much as we would for a psychophysical experiment. Gunnar, who might have spent much of the night alone in the lab making and testing microelectrodes and checking out electronic equipment for our joint experiment, would occasionally locate a cell that responded in just the way needed to check out an idea he had about the effect of some particular drug on the retinal tissue. But, while he called for the chemical solution, we would insist on his waiting until we had finished the series of light intensities, or annulus diameters, in our stimulus program before he changed the state of the retinal preparation.

We believe, however, that it was just this spontaneous, insightful personality characteristic, combined with the skill with which he used his hands, the depth and breadth of his anatomical and physiological knowledge, and his willingness to entertain novel or unorthodox ideas and accept unanticipated phenomena that made his contribution to visual science one of discovery rather than incremental data gathering.

REFERENCES

1. Svaetichin G: Spectral response curves from single cones. Acta Physiol Scand 39, Suppl 134: 17–46, 1956.
2. Grundfest H: An electrophysiological basis for cone vision in fish. Arch Ital Biol 96:135–144, 1958.
3. Svaetichin G and MacNichol EF Jr: Retinal mechanics for chromatic and achromatic vision. Ann NY Acad Sci 74:385–404, 1958.
4. Hering E: Grundzüge der Lehre vom Lichtsinn [Outlines of a Theory of the Light Sense]. Berlin: Springer, 1920. (Trans. by Hurvich LM and Jameson D) Cambridge: Harvard University Press, 1964.
5. Hurvich LM and Jameson D: The binocular fusion of yellow in relation to color theories. Science 114:199–202 1951.
6. Hecht S: On the binocular fusion of colors and its relation to theories of color vision. Proc Nat Acad Sci USA 14:237–241, 1928.

7. Hurvich LM and Jameson D: A psychophysical study of white. I. Neutral adaptation. J Opt Soc Am 41:521–527, 1951.
8. Hurvich LM and Jameson D: Spectral sensitivity of the fovea. I. Neutral adaptation. J Opt Soc Am 43:485–494, 1953.
9. Jameson D and Hurvich LM: Some quantitative aspects of an opponent-colors theory. I. Chromatic responses and spectral saturation. J Opt Soc Am 45:546–552, 1955.
10. Jameson D and Hurvich LM: Theoretical analysis of anomalous trichromatic color vision. J Opt Soc Am 46:1047–1089, 1956.

Index

PROGRESS IN CLINICAL AND BIOLOGICAL RESEARCH

Series Editors

Nathan Back
George J. Brewer
Vincent P. Eijsvoogel
Robert Grover

Kurt Hirschhorn
Seymour S. Kety
Sidney Udenfriend
Jonathan W. Uhr